Foundations of
COGNITIVE
PROCESS
in Remedial and Special Education

Lester Mann
Hunter College of the City University
of New York

David A. Sabatino
University of Wisconsin–Stout
Menomonie, Wisconsin

CARL A. RUDISILL LIBRARY
LENOIR RHYNE COLLEGE

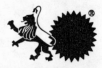

AN ASPEN PUBLICATION®
Aspen Systems Corporation
Rockville, Maryland
Royal Tunbridge Wells
1985

Library of Congress Cataloging in Publication Data

Mann, Lester.
Foundations of cognitive process in remedial and special education.

"An Aspen publication."
Bibliography: p.
Includes index.
1. Remedial teaching. 2. Cognition in children. 3. Exceptional children—Education. I. Sabatino, David A. II. Title.
LB1029.R4M35   1985   371.9   85-7557
ISBN: 0-87189-115-8

371.9
M31f
137017
may 1986

Editorial Services: Ruth Bloom

Library of Congress Catalog Card Number: 85-7557
ISBN: 0-87189-115-8

Printed in the United States of America

1 2 3 4 5

Table of Contents

Preface

This book is intended to provide remedial and special educators with a broad perspective on and understanding of cognition. It will be helpful both as an introduction to the topic of cognition and as a review for those who already are familiar with it. It is an appropriate text for graduate students.

We limited our range of topics and simplified our discussions in order to make the scope of cognition more manageable and meaningful to these readers. As a consequence, we have dealt minimally with certain cognitive areas while neglecting others entirely. We do not feel apologetic for our actions. Let us take a leaf from cognitive education itself to make our point. The reader will encounter the term *schemata* in Chapter 6. The term is used generally in cognitive psychology education to represent general knowledge structures that guide the human learner (Resnick, 1981). By studying our book, readers will develop cognitive schemata-knowledge structures that will enable them to learn and understand cognition more readily in greater detail later. An excess of coverage would have been detrimental to the development of such schemata.

While we frequently refer to cognitive training and remediation, this book is not meant to serve as a guide for either. It is intended rather to provide our readers with a variety of perspectives so that they can better understand the theories and research that guide modern cognitive remediation and training. But it cannot be used as a cookbook for cognitive assessment and training.

Acknowledgments are in order, first, to Rosalie Villanova, Debbie Garzone, and Jane Stevens for having assisted in typing chores. Second, a note of gratitude is due to students who evaluated earlier versions of this text.

Chapter 1

Introduction to Cognition

The topic of cognition often intimidates people so that they become confused when they encounter it in a textbook. Like so many other mysteries, however, those surrounding cognition reveal themselves, on closer examination, as being a matter of appearances. The basic issues involved in the study of cognition can be understood with a small amount of time and effort. This chapter introduces the reader to cognition and attempts to justify its place in special and remedial education.

DEFINITION OF COGNITION

We explain cognition in this chapter from a number of different standpoints in the belief that this will help the reader understand the topic.

The *Random House Dictionary of the English Language* defines *cognition* as follows: "1. The act or process of knowing; perception. 2. The product of such a process; thing thus known, perceived, etc. 3. knowledge" (1971 ed., s.v. "cognition").

Webster's Third New International Dictionary gives an expanded definition of the word. *Cognition*, it states, is (a) "the act or process of knowing in the broadest sense; . . . [specifically] an intellectual process by which knowledge is gained about perceptions or ideas—distinguished from *affection* and *conation* (b): a product of this act, process, faculty or capacity" (1971 ed., s.v. "cognition").

Cognition As Knowing and Knowledge

These definitions, although they differ from most current textbook ones, provide us with an excellent starting point. The definitions make it clear, first of all, that cognition, both as a term and as an area of study, concerns itself with knowing and knowledge, that is, in the sense of our knowing what goes on, both about and within us, and the implications of our knowledge for behavior.

If some readers find the definition of *cognition* in terms of *knowing* and *knowledge* a little confusing, it is because most of us have come to use the latter words in certain everyday ways that limit their meaning. Most people would interpret the term *know* as meaning that we are sure about something or, as the *Random House Dictionary* puts it, are able to "perceive or understand (it) as fact of truth" (1966 ed., s.v. "know"). Thus, we *know* the lesson we studied yesterday, we *know* how to repair an automobile, we *know* a person whom we met at a party last year. Similarly we usually think of *knowledge* as being 1. "an acquaintance with facts, truths, principles, as from study or investigational general erudition . . . 2. familiarity with a particular subject . . . 3. acquaintance or familiarity gained by sight, experience or report" (1966 ed., s.v. "knowledge").

Cognitive experts, too, are sometimes hesitant to equate cognition with *knowing* and *knowledge* because the latter words seem too imprecise and even blurred in meaning; they have been spoiled, as it were, by everyday, casual usage. Nevertheless, the equation is a fundamental one. The terms *knowing* and *knowledge* broadly encompass how, why, and what we as functioning organisms receive, interpret, and manage in the way of information; information reaching us through our sense organs, as a result of our movements (also sensed), or in the form of what we call perceptions, images, memories, ideas, thoughts, and the like. And it is these implications of knowing and knowledge that are the essentials of cognition, as the latter is scientifically studied today. Thus, Bower (1975) states, "Cognitive psychology is concerned with how organisms cognize or gain knowledge about their world, and how they use that knowledge to guide decisions and perform effective actions" (p. 25). Neisser (1976) begins a recent book on cognition with the observation that "cognition is the activity of knowing: the acquisition, organization, and use of knowledge" (p. 1).

Cognition As Process, Product, and Capacity

Our dictionary definitions of cognition further help us understand what is meant by cognition by calling attention to the different ways in which we can study cognition. Thus, the *Random House Dictionary* describes *cognition* as an act or process whereas *Webster's Dictionary* tells us that we are also able to interpret cognition in terms of special capacities, i.e., aptitudes, abilities, skills, or (as cognition was talked about years ago) faculties.

Our dictionary definitions suggest that we can study cognition from three standpoints. First, we can study it in terms of the cognitive processes that we engage in when dealing with information, e.g., the processes through which we go in perceiving an object, making a judgment about it, deciding how to use it, and then creating the behaviors to use it. Second, we can study cognition in terms of the cognitive capacities, structures, aptitudes, abilities, skills, etc., that create or otherwise make cognitive processes possible. Third, we can study cognition through the products that are the result of the first two standpoints. These may be entirely cognitive in nature, e.g., perceptions, images, concepts, decisions; they may also be expressed behaviorally, e.g., in oral language, written composition, or drawing.

These three ways of studying cognition are clearly interdependent. Let us use an example to illustrate this point. Students are assigned a homework topic. This engages them in a variety of cognitive processes, i.e., ones that go on during reading, others that are used to conceptualize the topic, still others that direct preparation of the homework assignment. The students must possess the cognitive abilities that make these processes possible. And the cognitive processes result in a number of cognitive products, e.g., thoughts about the topic, decisions how to prepare a paper on the topic, the paper written to complete the assignment. The cognitive processes, structures, and products are also expressed behaviorally, e.g., when the students physically turn in the homework to the teacher and give a speech about it to the class.

What the dictionaries do not state, and what is most important to keep in mind always, is that cognition is always inferred and it is inferred from behavior. We never directly observe cognition.

Inclusiveness of Cognition

Our dictionary definitions of *cognition* raise the question as to what the topic should include. It was often restricted to so-called higher thought processes, e.g., comprehension, judgment, problem solving, decision making. Currently, however, the meaning of cognition has been broadened considerably to include sensory, perceptual, memory, and even motor phenomena. Both the Random House and Webster definitions are responsive to these broader implications of cognition.

Webster's Dictionary excludes cognition from motivation (conation) and emotions (affection). This distinction was first clearly made by the Greek philosopher Plato (427–347 BC). It was popularized during the eighteenth century by the philosopher Immanuel Kant (1724–1804). It is still a popular distinction. Now, however, cognitive scientists clearly recognize that it is an arbitrary one and that it is incorrect to consider emotion and motivation as separate and distinct from cognition. How and what we perceive, remember, or think, clearly affect our motives and feelings—indeed are part of them. And it is equally clear that our motives and feelings affect what and how we perceive, remember, and think, etc. We do not carry out cognitive activities in a motivationless, nonattitudinal, and emotion-free vacuum (Bolles, 1975).

Webster's separation of *cognition* from *affection* and *conation* is thus clearly artificial—it does not and cannot hold up in real life. Many of the cognitive theories reviewed in this book deal with cognition as separate and distinct from feelings, attitudes, and the like. They usually do this, however, as a matter of convenience and efficiency. Increasingly, cognitive scientists are attending to cognition in its broader, e.g., emotional and motivational aspects (Scott & Osgood, 1979).

These two dictionary definitions have surely helped us to understand better what is meant by cognition. Proceeding from them, we have decided that cognition can be defined in terms of knowledge and knowing, insofar as the latter words imply the utilization and management of the information that organisms receive through their senses and through their cognitive activities, i.e., images, memories, ideas. We have also determined that cognition can be studied from a number of standpoints—in particular those of processes; "inner" capacities, abilities, powers, skills, etc.; and products. We have further decided that it is inferred from behavior and that the topic of cognition can be a broad one. We agreed that although distinctions can be made between cognition and feelings (affections, emotions) and motivation, these distinctions are arbitrary and artificial and can be justified only as a matter of convenience.

COGNITION AND THE MIND

Cognitive Equated with Mental

Many readers by this time have decided that *cognition* is another name for the *mind* and that *cognition* means *mental*. If so, they are correct. Many, if not all, of the phenomena that we call *cognitive* were in previous years considered as properties or acts or qualities of the mind, for example, perception, memory, problem solving, thinking, dreams, and consciousness. A number of cognitive theorists still insist on equating cognition and mental activities. Thus, we find statements of two recent defenders of cognition: "The subject matter of cognitive psychology would be broadly defined as 'how the mind works'" (Lachman, Lachman, & Butterfield, 1979, p. 6); "Cognitive psychology is concerned with the general principles of how the mind works" (Wickelgren, 1977, p. ix).

But if these defenders are correct, why don't all the experts talk and write about the mind and mental activities, rather than about cognition and cognitive processes? What is wrong with talking about the mind?

Let us provide a few answers to these questions. New times require new terms. New terms can cast new light on topics. For example, the term *energy*, as applied to coal, oil, the sun, nuclear fusion, etc., is quite recent; previously we talked about coal, oil, etc., as fuels or sources of power. However, considering them now in terms of *energy* creates a clearer understanding of their interrelatedness and commonalities and of the fundamental uses to which we put them. It is the same in psychology and education. The use of new terminology often helps us to understand matters better.

There are other reasons why cognitive theorists and practitioners usually prefer the term *cognitive* over the term *mental*. To understand this, we need a bit of history.

Early Cognitive Psychology

Mental phenomena—the study of the mind and its content—were psychology's major concern well into the twentieth century. The study of the mind—the conscious mind—was carried out under laboratory conditions by psychological introspectionists, who sought to determine the basic mental elements of their subjects' conscious experiences (Boring, 1950). These subjects would give reports on what was going on in their minds while under controlled experimental conditions. The introspectionists, however, could not agree among themselves, either about the data that these reports provided or on their interpretations. Some of them insisted on having their own theories confirmed at all costs.

The introspectionists also failed to recognize that the data produced depend on the particular methods of research. This failure is not at all uncommon in cognitive psychology (Neisser, 1976). The introspectionists were also overly dependent on their subjects' verbal reports; reports are frequently low in reliability.

BEHAVIORISM'S DISCREDITATION OF COGNITIVE PSYCHOLOGY

John Broadus Watson, in a stunning article "Psychology As Behaviorists View It" (1913), dismissed the introspectionist's work as being untrustworthy and called for the study of behavior rather than the mind. Watson said in effect that science can deal only with physical realities and that all references to the consciousness should be eliminated from psychology. He and his behaviorist followers insisted that the mind and all mental activities should be reduced to and explained in terms of behavior. For example, Watson explained thinking to be "covert" acts of speech, thought to be nothing more than "talking to ourselves." He attempted to prove this point by demonstrating that subject's throat and jaw muscles were activated (though not visibly to the human eye) when the subject thought about something.

Early Watsonian behaviorism was built on foundations created by Thorndike (1931). Thorndike explained that learning results from the "stamping in" and "stamping out" of sensory-motor neural connections or bonds in the nervous system. This process, he said, is governed in large part by the law of effect, according to the satisfying or unsatisfying consequences of associations made between stimuli and the responses to them. There are "satisfiers" (what we call *reinforcements*) and "annoyers" (*aversive stimulations*). The process of learning, he said, is also governed by the law of exercise, which affects the frequency, duration, and vigor of the bonds that are formed.

Later scientific justification was also claimed by Watson and his behaviorist followers on the basis of Pavlov's discovery of the conditioned response. Pavlov showed ways in which a response could be attached or conditioned to a stimulus and how this process could be explained in purely physical, i.e., physiological, terms. His work (1927) also shows how behavior could be clearly, carefully, and precisely observed and reported. The way seemed clear for behaviorism to make psychology as objective and scientific as biology and the physical sciences (Schultz, 1969).

Watsonian behaviorism came to be known as *stimulus-response (S-R) behaviorism*. It became the dominant force in scientific psychology in America. Psychological scientists began more and more to talk about mind and mental processes as figures of speech or metaphors rather than as meaningful subjects for scientific study. In fact, those who still believed that mental phenomena were worthy of investigation were often considered naïve and unsophisticated. Behaviorists believed that the same principles of learning, governing associations among stimuli and responses, could explain any type of human activity, from the maze learning of a laboratory rat to the solving of mathematical problems by humans. The fundamental mechanisms and processes were presumed the same for the latter as those for the former—only more complexly developed and expressed. Much of the behaviorists' research was with animals (since Watson had proclaimed that there was no real dividing line between human and infrahuman behavior). Studies of human learning were, by and large, reduced to narrow types of research that sought to determine the ways that associations are formed between stimuli and responses during learning.

Later behaviorists, sometimes called *neobehaviorists*, were not satisfied with simply studying responses to stimuli on an overt basis since these did not suffice to explain how organisms performed in more complex learning situations. They explained their results in terms of implicit, i.e., nonvisible "mediating," behaviors (responses) going on within the organism, these in turn creating implicit stimuli (Hull, 1952; Kendler & Kendler, 1975; Spence, 1950).

Both early "primitive" (Watsonian) behaviorism and the later, more sophisticated neobehaviorist research and theories created a great deal of intellectual ferment in psychology and education. They also stimulated a considerable amount of educational research directed to the improvement of school learning, e.g., Gagné's learning hierarchies (1965). However, S-R behaviorism proved of limited use when applied to instruction (Lachman et al., 1979).

Skinner's Radical Behaviorism

Fortunately for education, behaviorism spawned a particular variant that did prove exceedingly helpful in a practical sense. In 1938 B.F. Skinner wrote *The Behavior of Organisms*. In this book he recommended that psychologists divert their attention away from the make-up of stimuli and the reinforcements and focus their attention directly on the organism's responses, i.e., the behaviors. The study of behavior, he claimed, would permit the development of a scientific psychology, one that would effectively lend itself to practical results in education and training. Like Watson, Skinner (1977) would not deign to bother with cognitive processes as such: "We can define terms like 'information,' 'knowledge' and 'verbal ability' by reference to the behavior . . . [from] their presence. We may then teach the behavior directly" (pp. 49–50).

Skinnerian behavioral theories and research were originally designated as operant conditioning because they focused on operant or behavioral responses rather than on the relationship between these responses (r) and the stimuli that invoked them. Later his work came to be called *operant behaviorism*. More recently it has been called *radical behaviorism*—partly because it resists influences from other fields of psychology—and has taken a strong antitheoretical stand.

Whatever it is called, Skinnerian behaviorism has proven of great value to educators, generating as it does some truly effective ways of helping pupils. It led to the development of programmed learning and stimulated the development of behavioral objectives. The techniques of behavioral modification, which have been found so effective with handicapped pupils, emerged from Skinnerian behavioral psychology. Thanks to behavior modification techniques teachers are better able to control unruly pupils, help individuals to learn word lists more effectively, overcome reversals in reading, and correct defective speech. In special education, in particular, it is difficult to conceive of being able to help severely handicapped pupils without Skinnerian techniques.

THE REVITALIZATION OF COGNITIVE PSYCHOLOGY

It would be surprising if any one particular approach or set of technologies—no matter how effective—could satisfy the interests and needs of enterprises as vast as psychology and education—or even of the more limited objectives of the audiences for which this book is intended: remedial and special educators. Even during behaviorism's years of its greatest achievements and popularity, counterforces began to challenge it. Some of these eventually brought cognition to the fore once again in the interests of psychologists and educators.

These counterforces developed from a number of different sources. New discoveries and theories in neurological science (reviewed in Chapter 3) made it clear that an understanding of cognitive processes vis-à-vis brain function would eventually be necessary to comprehend and explain human behavior fully. Jean Piaget's (1952) explanation of children's development cast serious doubts on explanations of behavior that didn't include cognitive components. Psycholinguists like Noam Chomsky (1957, 1968) and E.H. Lenneberg (1967) successfully challenged Skinner's behavioral explanations of language. Educational psychologists like J.S. Bruner (1966) and David Ausubel (1968) set out to prove that school learning could be enhanced by cognitive theories. Benjamin Bloom and others (1956) offered a cognitive taxonomy to aid in the classification of educational objectives. Even behaviorists and learning theorists (of a non-Skinnerian persuasion) developed cognitive concepts of a sort (Kendler & D'Amato, 1955; Miller, Galanter & Pribam, 1960; Osgood, 1957).

These were but a few of the many cognitive counterforces that came to the fore to challenge purely behavioral approaches to psychology and education. However, major credit for the resurgence of cognitive psychology may be due to the growing popularity of the computer.

A major problem that has always confronted cognitive psychologists is obtaining scientific consensus that cognition is real. But if we cannot directly observe cognition, how can we assume that anything cognitive is going on? We respond to this problem in some detail later in this chapter. For the moment we wish to observe simply that the computer strikes many researchers as operating like a mind. Like people's minds, computers are information processors. Like minds, computers receive information, transform (code) it in special ways, store coded information in memory banks, and later "remember" and recall the information so that it can be used to answer questions, solve problems, and even direct goal-oriented actions (robots).

Can a computer "think" like a human being? Some computer programs truly try to make it think (Simon, 1976). Does human cognition work in computer fashion? We respond to this question later in this book. What is important here is that the computer has provided a sense of reality to cognitive processes. And by so doing it has served to overcome many researchers' hesitancies in turning to the study of cognition. The computer and its operation are real. Since the mind, i.e., cognition, operates in ways similar to that of a computer (Newell & Simon, 1972), it too may have reality. In addition, the computer field has provided cognitive psychology with special ideas and terminology that give it additional scientific respectability (see Chapter 7).

There are other reasons why cognition again became popular in psychology and education. The newer cognitive scientists tend to be more precise and modest in their claims than their predecessors. They no longer claim to study the whole conscious mind but rather concern themselves with specific aspects of how the mind (cognition) works. They have reduced their reliance on verbal reports (which had been severely criticized as unreliable) and have made their methods of study more behavioral and objective. They also use methods of scientific logic and mathematics in formulating their theories; Shannon and Weaver's (1949) mathematical theory of communication was a trail breaker in this respect. Thus did the mind, now described as *cognition,* come back into scientific favor.

Let us once again consider the current preference for the terms *cognition* and *cognitive* over those of *mind* and *mental.* Among the reasons for this preference is that many cognitive scholars now believe that the old conceptions of the mind are too controversial and confused or too limited in meaning to readopt for modern purposes. Still others (though not all) feel that the terms *mind* and *mental* have too many popular associations and that these limit their value in scientific study. The public, for example, often talks of the mind as a disembodied spiritual substance. The cognitive psychologist usually prefers to talk about information processing, cognitive structures, cognitive channels, schemata, and the like—all of which can be precisely delineated theoretically and experimentally anchored in observable behaviors and measurements.

Nevertheless, readers may feel more comfortable about cognition if they remember that it represents a modern version of one of the oldest and most fervent topics of interest to humanity: the mind.

THE NATURE OF COGNITION

Why should it be so hard to agree on the nature of cognition and the processes that constitute it? Every day of our lives, all of us go through experiences in which we perceive things, think about things, use our imaginations, solve problems, dream, etc. Our cognitive activities characteristics seem real enough to us. Why should there be any problem in agreeing as to what they are?

There are a number of reasons for this. The most critical one is that cognition, e.g., cognitive structures, cognitive processes, etc., does not have directly observable physical characteristics. Cognition's structures, mechanisms, and processes cannot ever be observed or studied directly. No one, for example, ever saw a thought or thinking going on. Cognition is always a matter of inference.

Because cognition in all its aspects does not exist as something real, it must be considered as a hypothetical construct. That is, it physically represents assumptions that we cannot directly prove are true. Perception, imagination, memory, intelligence, etc., are all hypothetical constructs.

Let us assume that a man runs away when he sees a criminal point a gun at him. Did he think that the criminal was a source of danger? This appears to be a reasonable assumption. However, we do not know what actually transpired within this person's cognitive structures. Nor could we directly assess his perceptions, thoughts, decisions, i.e., the cognitive processes, that directed his running away. We were able to assess directly his pulse rate, perspiration, the rate at which he accelerated before, after, and during his running. We could also have questioned him later about his motives in running away; his answers constitute behaviors or (when written) behavioral products. These types of behavioral information are directly observable, as is the act of running away. And it is from such observables that we are able to draw our inferences about his unobservable cognitive processes and to make educated guesses about them. The fact that cognitive processes can be studied only indirectly, i.e., on the basis of certain behaviors and behavioral products, is perhaps the major reason why staunch behaviorists still try to avoid involvement with cognition.

Turning to the classroom, we observe a pupil marking answers on a test paper. The answers are correct by our standards. On the basis of the pupil's (test) behavior and its products (the test answers) we may assume that the pupil was *able to read* the questions, *understood* them, possessed enough *knowledge* to formulate the answers, and had the *ability* to write the answers (or if it were a multiple-choice test to *decide* whether to mark the test choices as correct). However, the italicized words by which we have described the pupil are cognitive inferences on our part. They took place (if they took place at all) internally, i.e., within the pupil. We could not and cannot directly observe them. We assume their existence, i.e., their reality, on the basis that they plausibly explain the pupil's behaviors and behavior products, which were directly observed.

What were these behaviors and behavior products? The pupil looked at the test paper, sat still awhile, squinted, then began to write (or mark multiple-choice items). The child also made a number of erasures and corrections and finally turned the paper in and left the room. We have no way of directly knowing whether the pupil actually read the questions, thought about them, formulated answers, made decisions. For all we know, the student may have answered the test purely on the basis of rote memory or by cheating—without the slightest understanding of the questions' meaning and without any attempt to think them through. Even if we asked the student to explain how he or she arrived at the answers, we would obtain incomplete and partly inaccurate information, because people have great difficulty in precisely and accurately explaining what they do and why.

COGNITION AS A HYPOTHETICAL CONSTRUCT

Let us once again emphasize that cognition is a hypothetical construct. We cannot ever directly observe cognition. No one ever heard, touched, felt, or saw a person's cognitive processes. Cognitive processes do not exist in the physical sense. They can be assessed and measured only indirectly.

Some Problems with Hypothetical Cognitive Processes

Cognitive processes are hypothesized because they are helpful in understanding and predicting behavior. Their relationships to behavior are, however, far from certain. For example, the cognitive processes that we identify as intelligence are supposed to predict how well a pupil does in school. Yet pupils with high intelligence test scores often fail in their school work while others with mediocre IQs do well. Similarly a pupil may score high on a test of musical ability or on one of motor aptitude. But that does not necessarily ensure being a good composer or a good athlete. While we may make assumptions about the cognitive processes that are associated with particular behaviors, we are never fully sure that we are right.

This is one of the major reasons for the popularity of behavioral objectives. Let us assume that we see a student hit another pupil. If all of us were watching, we could reach a 100 percent agreement as to what actually happened in the event. On the other hand we might greatly disagree as to the cognitive processes that might lie behind the incident. Did Pupil A make a decision to strike Pupil B, or was he trying to touch his shoulder and hit him accidentally instead? If we assume he intended to hit the pupil, did he do so to bully him, was he angry, was he afraid, did he plan it? If it were an accident, was it because he thought of pointing to something or was he reaching for something clumsily? Or did he wish to hit another pupil and hit the wrong one? If we ask Pupil A for his reasons, we have no guarantee he will tell the truth or is even fully aware of why he did what he did. At the very best, we will never be quite sure about the cognitive activities behind his behaviors even though we might be in 100 percent agreement about the behaviors themselves, which can be directly observed and measured.

A thorough behaviorist might well ask why we should concern ourselves at all with cognitive inferences about behaviors. Would we be better off, after all, in limiting ourselves to directly observing, charting, and controlling the pupil's behaviors, rather than in engaging in inferences that are—at best—a matter of belief or faith? There was, and is, much to be said for this point of view as being both more scientific and useful.

This type of behaviorist viewpoint receives additional support from the fact that the terms we use to describe cognitive processes are of an abstract nature. Abstract terms usually have a multiplicity of meanings and tend to be vague and uncertain. The same (presumably) cognitive processes may be labeled differently by one theorist than by another. For example, a child may stare at an object and be described by one investigator as having unusually strong powers of concentration (a cognitive term). Another investigator may see the same child and describe the fixed looking as due to a lack of *flexible attention* (another cognitive term).

Investigators can use the same cognitive terms to refer to entirely different events. Lachman and his colleagues (1979) tell an amusing story along these lines. One chapter of a book on attention written by Donald Broadbent, a most distinguished cognitive scientist, was titled "Stimulus Set and Response Set: Two Types of Selective Attention." It had 34 bibliographic references to attention. In the same book another chapter was written by the well-known cognitive scientist, Werper Honig. It was titled "Attention and the Modulations of Stimulus Control." It had 38 references to attention. There were thus a total of 72 references in the bibliographies of both articles. Yet not one of these appeared in both bibliographies. Both authors were writing about attention. But were Broadbent's ideas of attention the same as Honig's? It does not appear likely. Which chapter should teachers use to understand attention and problems in attention? It is probable they would come away with entirely different slants on these topics, depending on which chapter they read.

Similar language problems exist in other areas of cognitive study. Such seemingly clear terms as *memory, perception, reasoning, judgment,* and *intelligence* receive quite different interpretations by different writers.

Many authors who write books on cognition must devote an entire chapter or more to the definition of their cognitive terms, in seeking to define them for their specific purposes. Otherwise one might read a book about a particular cognitive topic with an entirely wrong idea as to what a particular author means and is writing about.

Thus, uncertainty and inaccuracy of cognitive terms are still another argument given by behaviorists like Skinner (1978) for not getting involved with cognitive theory. It is a strong argument with which many people agree.

Is it possible, then, in the face of all these problems, to justify our interest in cognition and to make particular efforts to apply its tenets in remedial and special education? We believe that the answer to this question is yes.

A Defense of Cognition's Hypothetical Construct

As we have observed throughout much of this chapter, no matter how we choose to deal with cognition, we often must rely on inferences and assumptions rather than direct observations. No one ever directly saw perception, memory, or problem solving going on (or heard or touched them either). We assume that such cognitive states exist because they help us to explain various behaviors or products that we do directly observe, e.g., the explanations that a pupil makes when we question that person or the answers given on one of our tests. Cognition, in all its aspects, represents a group of hypothetical constructs, i.e., theoretical ideas that we use to explain things and events, for example, to help understand why a particular pupil, after repeated instruction, using ordinarily effective reinforcers, persists in making the same carrying errors in addition.

Cognition is in good company when it uses hypothetical constructs to explain cognition. The physical sciences also use hypothetical constructs to generate their laws and theories and to understand, predict, and control the events of the "real," i.e., physical, world.

Indeed it is hard to imagine physical scientists working without hypothetical constructs. Concepts like time and gravity are hypothetical constructs. The inner structures of an atom are hypothetical constructs. No one ever directly saw a proton or a neutron. Light, scientifically speaking, consists of a number of hypothetical constructs. Indeed, distinctly different, and incompatible, constructs are used to explain light; each of them is useful for different practical purposes.

The physical sciences have long recognized that their ideas are provisional, i.e., not true in any final or ultimate sense. Physical scientists justify their ideas (constructs) on the basis of their heuristic value. That is, they justify them because they help make sense of things and because they are useful in stimulating and guiding thought, research, and practical applications.

Physical scientists use their constructs as theoretical scaffolding within which they can organize their facts. When these constructs cease to explain things effectively or to be otherwise useful, they are revised or discarded. The atom is a case in point. Scientific conceptions (constructs) of the atom have been repeatedly revised. Early ones were useful for a while but then found to be incomplete or inaccurate in various particulars; for example, certain observations were made that they couldn't explain properly. Newer conceptions were then developed to overcome their limitations or errors. We still do not have a final version of the atom. We may never have it. Yet the atom's theoretical constructs have proven their scientific and practical values time and time again.

Do hypothetical constructs ever prove to be real in some physical sense? Sometimes they do receive physical verification, often because of advances in technology. There was a time when genes were hypothetical. They now can be seen by microscope. Indeed advances in microscopic technology also make it possible to distinguish one atom from another actually (physically). Similarly many phenomena in astronomy were hypothetical until sophisticated telescopes and photography "proved" that they physically existed. Other hypothetical constructs like gravity and time can never be observed. They are real, nonetheless, in the sense that they represent, describe, and explain physical phenomena that can be precisely measured.

Will the hypothetical constructs used in cognition ever achieve the precision, the power, or the reality of the constructs used by physical science? Some scholars believe that this may be possible if we explain cognition in terms of the nervous system and its functions (Gerschwind, 1980). But even if it is, its achievement is far away. We must continue living with the fact that cognition's hypothetical constructs do not have the precision or the rigor of those used by the physical sciences.

Beyond such considerations, cognitive constructs are real in a personal way. We think of ourselves as organisms that perceive, think, and solve problems, rather than in terms of being stimulus-response mechanisms. Even behaviorists do not actually deny that something that might be called *cognition* goes on inside us, i.e., images, memories, thoughts (Skinner, 1978). Some behaviorists indeed have tried to interpret cognition as a form of behavior (Wolpe, 1978). We, as well as most cognitive scientists, e.g., Newell and Simon (1972), Lachman et al. (1979), do not think that this is necessary. The study and uses of cognition can stand on their own (more about this in Chapter 2).

Cognitive constructs, at the least, are a productive source of ideas for use with pupils, while in some cases suggesting actual ways to help improve the student's behavior and academic performances. On the other hand one should reject attempts by anyone to promote their particular cognitive ideas or practices as being proven. At best, cognitive constructs can only be considered as approximations to the inner events they represent. Assumptions to the contrary are naive. When cognitive constructs are used to promote extensive programs of cognitive training—like those of perceptual training—at the cost of teaching pupils educational basics, they can be dangerous.

SOME CRITICISMS OF BEHAVIORISM FROM A COGNITIVE STANDPOINT

Remedial reading teachers are frequently guided by cognitive constructs such as encoding and comprehension skills. Special education teachers are more likely to be guided by behavioral principles. Both benefit from a better understanding of the differences and distinctions between behavioral and cognitive ideas. It is helpful to review some criticisms that cognitive educators and psychologists have offered regarding an exclusively behavioral approach to education.

Carroll, a distinguished educational psychologist, has stated that behaviorism is unable to deal with effectively, explain, or help teachers to manage many of the important things that go on in education. Behaviorists, he says, have failed to recognize that "reinforcers" affect a student's cognitive states rather than the student's "responses." He also points out that behaviorism cannot satisfactorily deal with the kinds of "knowledge" that education is usually engaged with. It cannot, for example, explain language acquisition in a satisfactory way. Furthermore, cognition, in contrast to behaviorism, is concerned with the learner, as well as with what is learned. Thus, it recognizes that students respond (behave) differently to instruction when they have different personal (cognitive) characteristics, that learning proceeds in different ways at different ages, and that the nature of what has been learned significantly affects what is being learned. Cognition also emphasizes attention and motivation as learning factors and takes education's purposes and guiding principles into consideration during instruction. And, in contrast to behaviorism, cognition explains rather than merely describes behaviors (Carroll, 1976a,b).

Competence versus Performance

Apropos of Carroll's remarks, it can be said that behaviorism is primarily interested in behaviors and their successful control, while cognition is concerned with why these behaviors occur and what they mean. Or, putting it another way, behaviorism is essentially interested in performance, while cognition is also interested in the competencies that make performance possible.

An interesting example of the distinction between performance and competence is given by Elkind in his discussion of Piaget's cognitive approach to education (1979). Elkind uses the telling of time to compare competence and performance.

Let us say that teachers of a mentally retarded or learning disabled pupil wish to teach that child to tell time. This can be done in a number of ways. The pupil can be taught to read the hands on a dial watch or to read time from the numerals that flash on the face of a digital one. Similar performances, i.e., behaviors, can be obtained from one child reading time from the digital watch and the other from the dial watch. These behaviors, however, are vastly dissimilar in their implications. A mental age of about four years is required for a child to read hours, minutes, and seconds from the face of a digital watch, but it usually takes a mental age of six to seven for a child to identify the same time features from a dial watch. In our teaching of time, therefore, it will clearly help us if we understand the cognitive competencies behind the telling of time. Thus, we might want to use digital watches with four-year-old children and dial watches with seven-year-old ones.

Let us go further. Time is a hypothetical construct that implies much more than the mere telling of time from the face of a digital or dial watch. We usually want our students to know more about time than what time it is. If possible, we want them to understand the broader perspectives of time such as the interrelationship of its various units—seconds, minutes, and hours. We might further want them to understand the relationship of these units to those of AM, PM, days, weeks, months, years, decades, etc. We might desire some of them to understand the importance of time variables in the scientific world, e.g., how considerations of time can affect measurements in space. Perhaps we might want to help them to appreciate time in a psychological or philosophical sense. Time is indeed a complex construct or set of constructs. Telling time deals with but a little part of time. And behaviorism cannot do time.

Nor does it appear that behavioral principles by themselves can do full justice to either basic or advanced learning processes. As Carroll observed, they cannot adequately explain language acquisition. Nor can they entirely explain learning reading, writing, and arithmetic. They are most certainly insufficient for a full understanding of advanced skills and advanced knowledge areas. Algebra, calculus, and trigonometry require more than a simple production of answers for their mastery. An understanding of the implications of the War of Independence requires more than the writing of the dates of particular battles. An appreciation of Marxism requires that a student do more than point to an item on a test illustrating Communist activities.

Our interest in cognition, therefore, as remedial and special educators, is justified on the basis of our needs for deeper insights and broader perspectives into the educational needs of our pupils.

A Reconciliation of Cognition and Behaviorism

A final point should be made before we move on to the next section of this chapter. This is to make it clear that remedial and special educators can feel free to adapt both behaviorism and cognition to their instructional purposes. It is important to distinguish between behaviorism as a theory and behaviorism as a set of techniques, i.e., methodological behaviorism. One does not have to be a behaviorist, or to agree with their philosophies, in order to use their methods. It is quite possible for a teacher wishing to teach certain ideas of a cognitive nature to utilize behavioral approaches to get across cognitive objectives as well as behavioral ones and to teach both according to specific behavioral criteria of performance.

In fact, a teacher can take a purely behavioristic approach in one area of instruction, e.g., teaching dressing skills, and a purely cognitive one in another area of instruction, e.g., teaching a pupil to understand justice. Both behaviorism and cognition are best regarded as paradigms for instructional purposes rather than either/or ways in education (Lachman et al., 1979). We do not have to give up one to accept the other as having a place in education under particular circumstances. And remedial and special education teachers should become conversant with the principles and methods of both so that they are able to apply them, as needed, in instruction. Readers of this book should be able to both deal more intelligently with the cognitive aspects of education and to relate them more effectively to those of behaviorism.

EXPERT DEFINITIONS OF COGNITION

We are ready to review some definitions of cognition that have been suggested by experts. These will help guide us in subsequent discussions.

A broad definition of cognition is offered by Kagan and Kogan (1970):

> *Cognition stands for those hypothetical psychological processes invoked to explain* overt verbal and motor behavior as well as certain physiological reactions. Cognitive process is a subordinate term subsuming the more familiar titles of imagery, perception, free association, thought, mediation, proliferation of hypotheses, reasoning, reflection and problem solving. . . . All verbal behavior must be a product of cognitive processes as are dreams and intelligence test performances. (p. 125)

Hayes (1978) makes a case for the reinterpretation of mental processes in terms of cognitive ones: "Cognitive psychology is a modern approach to the study of the processes by which people come to understand the word, such processes as memory, learning, comprehending language, problem solving and creativity" (p. 3). Bower (1975) interprets cognition in terms of knowledge: "Cognitive psychology is concerned with how organisms cognize or gain knowledge about their world and how they use that knowledge to guide decisions and perform effective actions" (p. 25).

Scott and Osgood (1979) take a particularly broad perspective of the topic: "Cognition is the representation of reality that the person experiences as reality itself" (p. 7).

Neisser (1967) provides a definition in terms of information processing: "Cognition is all the processes by which the sensory input is transformed, reduced, elaborated, stored, recovered, and used" (p. 8). Lerner (1981) addresses cognition from the standpoint of a learning disabilities expert: "The term *cognitive skills* refers to a collection of mental skills that enable one to know, to be aware, to think, to conceptualize, to use abstractions, to reason, to criticize, to be creative" (p. 159).

These are but a few of the many definitions offered by cognitive experts in the field. Not all of them are in agreement. Their differences stem from the particular perspectives that various theorists and researchers take. They all generally agree, however, in indicating that cognition refers to inner states, i.e., activities, processes, and that the individual possesses particular structures or traits that underlie, accompany, or determine the ways in which they act.

Almost all would agree that cognitive constructs are inferential in nature. Most experts readily admit that their conceptions of cognition are imperfect and inevitably will change with time (Neisser, 1976). They nevertheless believe, as we do, that to study human behavior while ignoring cognition limits our understanding of that behavior and our ability to predict or manage it. They further tend to agree that behaviorist approaches to behavior are not by themselves sufficient to develop a comprehensive appreciation of any human learner, from a competent scientist to a mentally retarded pupil.

COGNITIVE TERMS USED IN THIS BOOK

As pointed out in this chapter, there is a great deal of imprecision and uncertainty in definitions and explanations of cognition. This is in part because of the indirect nature of the observations that we make in cognition. It is further due to the imprecision of the language that we use to describe and explain cognition. It is still further due to the fact that various cognitive scientists and practitioners interpret their terms in ways that are quite different from those chosen by their colleagues.

Beyond all of this, there is a general tendency for cognitivists to write on two different levels. The first level is that of ordinary communication, i.e., what they would use in ordinary conversation; they do not bother as a rule to be too concerned about precision when writing at this level. The second level of writing is that of a cognitive scientist. Here they make every effort to define and explain their terms precisely so as to be explicit about the issues they are discussing.

By and large, we are not overly concerned in this book about precision. Most certainly, whenever precise cognitive descriptions and explanations are required, we make every effort to be as exact as possible so that our readers and ourselves (as well as the theorists and researchers we are writing about) can be in agreement about our topics. But the readers should usually respond in a commonsense, everyday way to such terms as *memory, perception, dreaming, thinking,* and *language.* Nevertheless, we should put our readers on notice regarding some of the more important terms in this book.

Abilities usually refer to a persistent type of inner potential to perform various types of behaviors. *Traits* are sometimes a preferred way of talking about abilities. *Capacities* and *aptitudes* are other variations. *Skills* usually refer to limited types of abilities, e.g., as required for specific acts of motor skill, math, decoding. The term *structure* "refers to the form or forms that mental abilities take and how they are organized" (Sternberg, 1979, p. 214). The term *process* usually refers to the way an ability or structure functions or operates. *Cognitive content* "refers to the identity" of particular cognitive processes, e.g., whether the latter are perceptual, memorial (Sternberg, 1979, p. 214).

These are some of the terms that the reader faces in this book. It is not always clear or certain whether the distinctions among them amount to much more than a play of words. In any case, precise distinctions are more likely to be more important to researchers than to practitioners. Readers need not be alarmed if they occasionally become confused.

THE FOCUS OF THIS BOOK

The literature on cognitive processes is vast. Most of it is, and should continue to be, areas reserved for researchers and theorists. This book deals with cognition from the standpoint of the practitioners in remedial and special education. It attempts to provide them with a general understanding of cognition and some of its implications for their work. Thus, some narrowing of the field of cognition is required.

For example, it is quite proper for cognitive theorists to study cognitive processes in animals (of which we form a particular species) (Premack, 1982; Spear & Miller, 1981). However, for us to do so in this book would take us rather far from the purposes of remedial and special education.

We could also devote a large part of this book to language. We, however, deal with it in this book only as it bears on the broader problems of cognition. This is not to slight the importance of language as a major field of cognitive investigation. It is rather done in recognition that the cognitive aspects of language cannot be done full justice in an introductory book. Those readers who wish specifically to study the cognitive aspects of language will be better prepared to do so on completion of this book.

Cognition clearly enters into schoolwork, from the simplest discriminations of letter and number forms up through the problem solving of physics. Many educational efforts attempt to approach schoolwork directly from the standpoint of cognition, often with very exciting results (Mayer, 1981). Nevertheless, we are in this book more concerned with the more basic of cognitive processes, e.g., intelligence, perception, memory, problem solving, rather than with the specific cognitive processes involved in school learning. As with language, the interested reader is better prepared to proceed with a detailed study of the latter at the close of this book.

Having discussed topics that we intend to pass, let us consider those that are dealt with in detail. Chapter 2 attempts to review some critical concepts and issues applicable to the study of cognition. Chapter 3 discusses the central nervous system and its implications for cognition. Chapter 4 reviews intelligence (and its components) as a cognitive construct. Chapter 5 covers specific abilities. Chapter 6 deals with Piaget's theories of developmental cognition. Chapter 7 is concerned with information processing—which most cognitive researchers agree to be the most important approach to cognition. Chapter 8 reviews the topic of cognition and learning styles, e.g., the persistent cognitive ways in which people differ from each other in learning and dealing with problems. Chapter 9 takes up the topic of cognitive strategies and metacognition; these are among the newest areas of investigation in cognitive psychology. Chapter 10 reviews cognitive behavioral therapy, which is a recent attempt at rapprochement between cognition and behaviorism. Chapter 11 deals with cognitive task analysis. Chapter 12 discusses the implications of cognition for remedial and special education.

The reader will not find much discussion of specific ways to assess, remediate, or correct cognitive problems in this book. Our intent, rather, is to help the reader know about cognition. We leave the doing about it to others.

Chapter 2

General Cognitive Issues

In Chapter 1 we defined cognition and discussed some aspects of its study. In this chapter we provide some additional perspectives on cognition. They should make it easier to understand the various ways in which cognition is studied.

PARADIGMS, THEORIES, AND MODELS

Cognitive research and its application are guided by and stabilized within particular paradigms, theories, and models.

Paradigms

There is no single point of view on cognition that we can point to and state as fully representing cognition. Rather, a variety of paradigms guide the study of cognition and the application of cognitive ideas to education. An understanding of the paradigmatic nature of cognitive approaches is essential if we are to understand cognitive science and cognitive education.

The *Random House Dictionary* defines the word *paradigm* in a number of ways. It is, for example, "a set of forms . . . based on a single . . . theme," or, "a model, ideal, standard" (1966 ed., s.v. "paradigm"). There has been a great deal of discussion about the paradigmatic nature of science (Lachman, Lachman, & Butterfield, 1979). The term *paradigm* is perhaps best summed up as constituting an agreed set of rules that guide the investigation of scientific phenomena: A paradigm suggests the types of problems that should be studied, the types of questions that should be asked, and the methods to be used in seeking answers.

While some general rules guide all types of scientific investigation, scientists differ in the ways they interpret and observe these rules, often because they have adapted different paradigms. Thus an astronomer investigates phenomena in different ways, e.g., uses methods and seeks answers differently, than does a biologist. Indeed, even within the same area of science, and studying the same phenomena, scientists proceed according to different types of paradigms. Some neurologists may view the brain as an integrated organ and study it as such. Other neurologists may study it from the standpoint of the individual neurons. An educational researcher studying cognitive methods of teaching can be expected to take a different paradigmatic approach than one studying behavioral modification techniques.

This book reviews a variety of cognitive paradigms. Some are quite similar, even interrelated. Others may appear to contradict each other. The readers of an introductory book such as this need not be concerned about contradictions. The proof of any paradigm lies ultimately in its value in guiding research or practice. Remedial and special educators may find different, even contradictory, cognitive paradigms useful under various conditions. In any case we offer our readers a number of different cognitive perspectives rather than present or support only one of several points of view. This does not mean, however, that we do not have our preferences or our biases.

Theories

Scientists develop theories that conform to the paradigms they have accepted to guide their work. They use assumptions and hypothetical constructs to make sense of certain types of facts. This is no less true of cognitive scientists than it is of those working in the fields of physics, chemistry, and biology. Within cognition, there are, as we noted, a number of paradigms, and for any particular paradigm we find a number of theories.

Cognitive theories, like all theories, are not to be confused with facts. They are rather to be regarded as tools that help scientists organize and explain their works. Theories have been described as temporary scaffolding that holds the known facts in an area of investigation together and guides the accumulation of new ones. Theories should be changed when they do not agree with the facts or, for that matter, altogether discarded if new theories explain and predict the same facts in better ways. Theories play important roles in day-to-day instruction and remediation even though their influences are not clearly visible. Behavioral theories, for example, have been dominant within special education in the 1970s and 80s, and much of special education instruction has proceeded in accordance with the ways that behaviorists believe pupils learn. Similarly many remedial education efforts are guided by the theoretical belief that learning is created through perceptual experiences.

It is important that remedial and special educators be aware of the theoretical influences in their work, particularly of those that may suggest they teach their pupils in special ways. Remedial and special educators should not accept any theories as true in any absolute sense; theories should be judged on the basis of their usefulness in guiding research and instruction.

Models

Similar words of caution are in order about models. A *model* is a physical way (pictorial or three-dimensional) of demonstrating a concept or theory. Scientists use models to organize their data and to clarify ideas. They can be useful. Physicists use models to represent the interior of atoms. Chemists use them to display molecular structures. Similarly, cognitive theorists often use models to show how the mind may function.

Models may stimulate research that seeks to confirm their "validity" or to discover ways the models should be changed to make them useful. Some cognitive theorists rely more on models than others. In Chapter 4 what is called the *SI theory of intelligence* is described as dependent on a model while Spearman's *g* theory doesn't require one. While Piaget has not emphasized the use of cognitive models for his theories, his followers have done so (Kirby & Briggs, 1980). Information-processing paradigm (IPP) theories (Chapter 7) are heavily dependent on models.

It is important to remember that cognitive models, like theories, are based on assumptions and hypothetical constructs. They thus do not necessarily represent anything real even though modelers sometimes talk and write about them as if they were real.

Keeping these points about paradigms, theories, and models in mind helps minimize confusion in the chapters to come.

REDUCTIONISM AND COGNITION

Science constantly seeks the simplest explanations of the phenomena it studies. Einstein's formula $E = MC^2$ is an example of this. This simple statement has greatly expanded our knowledge of the universe while it ushered us into the atomic age. Some aspects of the scientific search for simplicity are identified with what is called *scientific reductionism*.

Scientific reductionism represents attempts to explain phenomena regardless of their apparent complexity, in their simplest terms, for example, to try to analyze some chemical substance into its simplest elements or to explain some physical action on the basis of a few simple principles or laws. Scientific reductionism has a long and distinguished history and has successfully guided many scientific achievements. In atomic research, the atom at one time appeared to be the simplest unit in the universe, the ultimate reduction possible for physical matter. But then physicists went still further in their reductionist efforts and identified protons, neutrons, and ions. With each of their reductions they have achieved greater understanding, and control, of the physical world.

Chemistry can truly be described as a child of reductionism. Chemists literally develop their science by determining how complex compounds can be reduced to simple elements and by demonstrating that these simple elements can be combined or transformed to create extraordinarily complex products. The term *synthetics* stands testimony to chemistry's success in taking the same basic hydrocarbon elements and changing (synthesizing) them into an extraordinary range of diverse and complex forms.

Reductionistic efforts in biology have also been extremely productive. We can identify the molecular and chemical natures of cells and their components when once they appeared to be unsolvable mysteries. By so doing, we have increasingly come to understand how the cells carry out their functions and with this knowledge are able to carry out genetic engineering.

In medicine, reductionist efforts have been responsible for many of our modern miracles. Medical scientists have isolated the specific carriers or causes of many once-baffling diseases. In neurology we can partly explain the functioning and dysfunctioning of the nervous system in terms of the activities of specific brain cells and by the workings of specific neuroenzymes.

PSYCHOLOGICAL REDUCTIONISM

Psychology is the field of scientific study that more than any other provides remedial and special education with its scientific basis. Here too reductionist efforts have prevailed in many ways.

There are a number of different efforts at psychological reductionism. One may be called *physical reductionism*. This is an effort to explain cognition and behavior in terms of biological or physicochemical activities. Some psychologists believe that a truly scientific psychology must eventually explain all human behavior in terms of actual biological processes.

The dominant form of psychological reductionism, however, over the past 40 years, is usually identified broadly with the doctrines of associationism and specifically with the associationistic doctrines of stimulus-response learning and behaviorism.

Modern doctrines of association date to the British empiricists of the eighteenth century. These associationists attempted to explain cognition in terms of mental bonds formed through experiences. Early versions of associationism held that mental phenomena are simply collections, combinations, or syntheses of associated sensations. Later versions, after it was discovered that the nervous systems were organized along sensorimotor lines, emphasized the association of simple motor and sensory mental elements.

During the twentieth century, associationism continued to dominate psychological theory. But rather than study associations among mental elements (which they believed to be unscientific), many psychologists chose to study the associations among physical phenomena—specifically those between stimuli (Ss) and responses (Rs). Learning thus came to be interpreted as the creation or strengthening of associations between stimuli and responses, e.g., in terms of S-R, S-S, R-R, and R-S relationships.

The earliest forms of behaviorism were clearly S-R in nature. Behaviorists such as Watson (1925) believed that, through learning, behaviors become associated with particular stimuli that can later elicit them. Early behaviorists claimed that relationships among observable stimuli and responses could explain so-called cognitive phenomena such as perception, memory, reasoning, creativity, imagination, as well as behavioral ones. Their neobehaviorist post–World War II successors (see the discussion of mediation in this chapter) were more willing to entertain hypothetical constructs. These too were reductionist in nature.

Such earlier types of behaviorism were later to become identified as types of respondent behaviorism, which indicated that they were concerned with the way organisms respond to stimuli. However, the form of S-R behaviorism that present-day remedial and special educators are most likely to be familiar with is operant behaviorism. While operant behaviorism is a form of S-R associationism (Travers, 1977), it is more concerned with stimuli as reinforcement or as aversive stimuli subsequent to responses (R-S) and in the relationship of responses to each other (R-R) rather than with the specific Ss to which the subject might be responding (S-R). Thus teachers of handicapped pupils are more likely to attempt to reinforce behaviors (R-S) or to chain them (R-R) than they are in identifying the precise stimuli (S-R) to which their pupils are responding.

Both respondent and operant behaviorists have dealt with cognitive phenomena in reductionist ways. One way they do this is by saying that cognitive terms are dummy terms that simply provide labels that identify certain stimulus-response events (a respondent explanation) or behaviors (an operant explanation) (Kendler & Kendler, 1975). Thus perception can be explained as being nothing more than a label that identifies the fact that people react a certain way to particular types of stimulation. Similarly memory can be considered as a dummy term describing the fact that people may respond (behave) in ways that are the same or similar to the ways they responded on earlier occasions. Thus Watson (1925) observed that "by 'memory,' we mean nothing except the fact that when we meet a stimulus again after an absence, we do the old habitual thing . . . that we learned to do when we were in the presence of that stimulus in the first place" (p. 190). And he "reduced" thought in the same way: "The behaviorist advances the view that what the psychologists have hitherto called thought is in short nothing but talking to ourselves" (p. 191).

Another way behavioral reductionism proceeds is to study the physiological aspects associated with so-called cognitive phenomena (from an S-R point of view). From this standpoint, fear (a cognitive construct) can be studied by observing the subject's behavior in a dangerous situation, by studying the (physical) tension of the muscles, or by measuring the amount of perspiration exuded in that situation. Behavioral research into language (another cognitive construct) may study oral speech (behavioral acts) or written compositions (behavioral products). It may also study physiological behavior, e.g., the EEGs (brain waves) from a student's skull, while the student is reading a book.

Some behaviorists have begun to identify cognitive phenomena as behaviors or behavioral equivalents. They do this to eliminate distinctions between cognition and behavior or to reconcile them in some fashion. Thus Wolpe (1978) has stated, "Cognition is behavior and subject to the same lawful inevitability as other behavior . . . [it obeys] the same mechanistic laws as motor or autonomic behavior" (pp. 437–438). Further,

> Thoughts are responses [Rs] whether they are perceptions or imagining. Like other responses whether they are evoked when the relevant neural excitations occur and, in as much [as] they have stimulus characteristics, may be conditioned to other thoughts and responses in other categories. They are not part of a separate mechanism of learning that only humans possess. (p. 441)

Where do cognitive psychologists stand concerning reductionism? We find many of them, past and present, also in favor of reductionism. In fact, the early associationists, who were clearly reductionist in outlook, would be considered cognitive psychologists today. Indeed, many modern cognitive researchers attempt to "reduce" cognition to a few basic elements and governing principles.

At the same time most modern cognitive psychologists work with larger and more varied types of units than do behaviorists. Furthermore, even those who emphasize careful dissection of cognition into component structures, processes, and contents are more prone to recognize complexities than do behaviorists. And many cognitive theorists believe that efforts to explain human cognition in terms of simple elements or units are in the long run detrimental to an understanding of both cognition and behavior. Along these lines Carroll (1976) has criticized behaviorism for what he regards is its reductionist oversimplification of learning:

> The only thing that behavior theory regards as being learned is some overt response or some integrated combination of responses, which occur under appropriate circumstances or stimulus conditions. A strict form of behavior theory makes no assumptions about information, memories, knowledge or even habits. . . . (p. 14)

An instructive example of nonreductionism in cognition is provided by a particular type of cognitive reductionism. This is the construct of schema. This construct has a long history; in its modern version it can be traced to Barlett's (1932) work in memory in the 1930s. Schemata became particularly prominent in postwar years as an essential construct in Piaget's (1972) developmental theory of cognition. In the last 10 years, it has become popular in many other cognitive circles (Resnick, 1981).

What are *schemata*? *Schemata* are construed to be generalized, active, cognitive structures that allow us to make sense of information that we receive from the environment, to organize that information, and to use it to direct our thinking and behavior. But these basic cognitive units may be quite complex, and there are a variety of them. There are perceptual schemata, memory schemata, motor, etc. There are schemata that organize schoolwork, while others organize social experiences and the ways we feel about ourselves. Indeed schemata are not identical with those of Bartlett (1932) or entirely congruent with more recent usages of the construct (Resnick, 1981). And while schemata can be construed as a reductionist construct, they still have considerable complexity. They are not simple elements.

The point is that the reader will usually find modern cognitive theorists dealing with more complex and a much greater variety of constructs than do behaviorists, and less inclined, as well, to adhere to a simple policy of reductionism. In this respect, the modern study of cognition parallels some current trends in physical and biological sciences. For while physical and biological scientists have made many of their great strides forward through reductionism, they are increasingly inclined to recognize that reductionist points of view are not suitable for certain phenomena. Thus physics and biology are often studied from dynamic, interactionist, even holistic points of view, as well as through reductionist perspectives.

The Reduction of Cognition to Behavior

Efforts to explain cognition in behavioral terms have been helpful in supporting the fact that cognition is a physical phenomenon, and no more supernatural than a TV picture or the computations a computer performs. Behaviorism's principles and constructs may also help us to understand some aspects of cognitive phenomena and help to support cognitive types of instruction. Beyond this, however, we believe that cognition and behavior are distinctly different ways of studying and helping people. It is not necessarily useful to reduce cognition to behavior through S-R explanations or renaming cognitive activities as behaviors.

Such attempts may beg the question as to what cognition is. They do not truly explain cognition any more than a chemical analysis of food explains the delight of a fine meal, the examination of one's pulse rate explains love, or conditioning experiences explain our belief in justice. Cognition has qualities and aspects that are beyond, i.e., not reducible to, behavioral explanations. These qualities and aspects should be studied on their own terms.

MEDIATION

In the previous sections of this chapter we have discussed the implications of associationism, behaviorism, and reductionism for cognition. These topics are an essential introduction to the concept of mediation. And the concept of mediation is an essential one for cognition, since it helps us understand how cognition affects behavior.

To understand how the concept of mediation first developed, we must return to reconsider the S-R behaviorism. One of its advantages was that it forced people to think of human behavior in clear concrete terms. As Kendler and Spence (1971) observed, attempts made by S-R behaviorists were admirable in that "S-R language [clarified] the experimental and theoretical task of the psychologist by focusing attention on the empirical relationships to investigate and explain" (p. 32).

Classical S-R behaviorism had problems, however, in comprehensively explaining behavior in that it could not easily explain what goes on inside the organism (animal or human) in order to make an S result in an R. Indeed, in a simple S-R model the input side of behavior is "directly linked, in a figurative sense, to the output component, the response. . . . [and the model simply] predicts the . . . responses of subjects from the physical characteristics and the number of pairings they had with reinforced and non-reinforced responses" (Kendler & Kendler, 1975, p. 203). Simple S-R models do not explain why an organism responds the way it does. They have been identified with what has been called *empty-box* conceptualizations of behavior; i.e., they don't concern themselves with what goes on inside the organism.

Since empty-box explanations of behavior made it difficult for S-R psychology to account for complex behaviors, a latter-day group of behaviorists known as *neo-behaviorists,* e.g., Hull (1943) and Spence (1950), attempted to bridge the gap (fill the empty box) between external stimuli and external responses by proposing that physical mediational mechanisms are at work within organisms that affect the relationships between external Ss and external Rs. Because they studied rats, they first conceptualized these mediational activities in terms of the learning behaviors of these animals. For example, rats learn to run through mazes in order to reach goals at which there is food. While running, they show anticipatory goal responses, i.e., behaviors showing that they are anticipating food at the end of their runs. Specifically they have been found to engage in the partial (fractional) responses of chewing and salivating while running, as if they anticipated the food they would find at the goal.

Hull, Spence, and their followers hypothesized that such fractional responses create internal, unobservable stimuli within rats that help to guide their searching and running behaviors. They speculated that rats respond to the external stimuli (S) in a maze with anticipatory response (r_m). These intervene or remediate between the external stimuli and the terminal responses of running and produce mediating stimuli (s_m) that guide the execution of the terminal response (the running behaviors). In effect, the neobehaviorists conceptualized hypothetical inner chains of inner responses (r_m) and stimuli (s_m) that mediate between stimuli in the mazes (S) and the response (R) of rats to them. They were thus better able to explain how rats' responses to external stimuli develop into the organized behaviors that eventually guide them to their goals (see Figure 2–1).

Figure 2–1 Simple S-R Mediation

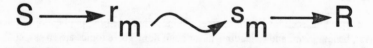

The initial, external stimulus situation (S) arouses (⟶) a mediating response (r_m) that produces a mediating stimulus (s_m). This arouses (⤳) a terminal response (R). The use of the lower case letters for mediating responses and stimuli is to suggest that they are not usually directly observed, but rather inferred.

Source: Adapted from *Basic Learning Processes in Childood* by Hayne W. Reese, © 1976 by Holt, Rinehart and Winston. Adapted by permission of Holt, Rinehart and Winston, CBS College Publishing.

Through such simple S-R mediational conceptualizations it became possible for neo-behaviorist learning theorists to predict more accurately how laboratory rats and other lower organisms act and learn. Some of them proposed that similar mediation sequences might go on in humans and explain what others called *cognitive activities*.

An example of how this may be done is explaining the processes of children in picking up blocks. The model (Figure 2–1) that explains rats' maze-running behavior can also be used to explain how children pick up blocks (Reese, 1976).

Suppose that the first stimulus (S) in the sequence is a block. If the subjects say to themselves the word *block* on seeing it, they will get feedback from the muscles used in saying the word. Using the model shown in Figure 2–1, the children's saying of the word produces an (r_m) (a mediating response), which creates a mediating stimulus (s_m); actually there are chains of mediating responses and stimuli through all this. It is the (s_m) rather than the S that triggers the terminal response (R) of picking up the block. Let us review this application of our simple mediational model once again. The block (S) causes the subjects to produce a mediating response (r_m) (saying the word *block* to oneself) in anticipation of moving the block. This r_m produces a mediating stimulus (s_m) that arouses the terminal response (R) of picking up the block.

Sequences of mediation may sometimes be examined almost directly. We might thus see the children actually saying the word *block,* prompting themselves to pick it up. However, these sequences are more likely to go on invisibly within the children. They may produce mediating responses and stimuli simply through muscular anticipations of picking the block up or saying the word *block* silently.

The implications of this mediational model have proven most important to behaviorism and to cognition. The initial (mediating) responses that we make to stimuli may be different from the terminal responses we make to them. Furthermore, the terminal responses we eventually produce are not responses to the original stimuli but are rather made to the mediating stimuli generated by mediating responses.

Using such mediational models, behaviorists were much better able to deal with what we would consider *cognitive concepts*. For example, they could explain how concepts develop. In behavioral terms, if different stimuli (S) produce the same terminal responses (R), a concept may be said to have formed. Such a concept is created by mediating responses and stimuli. That is, different stimuli can produce the same terminal responses because these stimuli, even though they are different, activate the same mediating responses that make them (the original stimuli) identical as far as the organism's terminal responses are concerned because they create the same mediating stimuli. That is, the organisms respond to mediators created by external stimuli rather than directly to the external stimuli themselves.

The construct of mediation similarly explains why the same external stimuli may produce different terminal responses. They do so even though they have for one reason or another triggered different chains of mediating responses and stimuli, which in turn trigger different types of external responses.

Let us use a table as an example to explain the type of S-R mediation we have been discussing. As to the type of concept we have discussed, a person produces the same mediating language response of table to the great variety of stimuli created when seeing different tables. This table r_m produces an s_m (we are simplifying things) that conceptually makes those different tables into equivalents. Thus the person does not necessarily respond to a particular table as a unique object but rather as a representative of the concept table. That is, the person will act in response to that table in terms of the mediating properties associated with the table stimulus. Seeing any table, the individual can be expected to make the same types of terminal responses to it as to other (different) tables, e.g., sitting down by it, putting things on it. In short, the person responds to any and all tables with the same similar mediating responses and mediating stimuli and responds (behaves) according to these rather than responding directly to the external stimuli provided by the physical tables.

Let us look at an example of the same stimuli resulting in different responses at different times. Again let us use responses to a table to illustrate how this is done through mediation, which changes the relationship between stimuli and terminal responses. The person may thus look at the table on one occasion and produce mediating responses and stimuli to it that identify it as a table. On another occasion, in a fit of rage, the person may respond with mediation responses and stimuli that identify the table as something to throw. On the first occasion the table is responded to terminally as a place to put a plate. On the other occasion it is responded to terminally as a weapon.

This sort of simple mediation S-R model has proven a useful one, but it is too simple to explain complex types of stimulus and behavioral generalizations or to explain cognition in all its complexities. Consequently a broader mediational S-R model was proposed by H.H. Kendler and his associates (Kendler & D'Amato, 1955; Kendler & Kendler, 1975). In contrast to the S-r-s-R linkages of the earlier S-R model, this mediation model "involves an additional theoretical link, a mediational mechanism that intervenes between the observable stimulus and response operating to *transform* incoming stimulation into some internal representation that guides subsequent behavior" (1975, p. 203).

As Kendler and Kendler put it, mediation in the earlier Hull-Spence S-r-s-R model behavior (R) is regarded as directly connected to specific attributes of physically defined discriminatory stimuli (Ss), i.e., the features of stimulus situation that the organism is responding to, through a simple chain of internal motor responses and the stimuli they generate. In a true mediation model, Kendler and Kendler suggest there is more going on. The organism's behavior is actually controlled by the organism's inner transformations of the discriminatory stimuli that result in new types of "inner representation." It is with this type of conceptual mediational model that mediation emerges as a truly useful, explanatory, cognitive construct, one that can be used apart from S-R explanations.

Production and Control Deficiencies

Originally developed from S-R theory, the idea of production and control mediation deficiencies is an important one in cognitive circles, where it has been applied to a variety of cognitive issues.

Using S-R terminology and conceptualization to help us understand the idea of production and control deficiencies, we find two phases of training required for the use of mediators. In the first phase the mediating response (r_m) is conditioned to the initial stimuli (S) so as to form an association between the S and r_m. In the second phase the mediating stimulus (s_m) generated by the r_m must be conditioned so as to form an association between it and the terminal response (R).

Although we train organisms (animals or humans) to establish these associations, mediation may fail to take place. One type of mediation failure results when the external stimulus does not arouse mediating responses even after training. That is, even though a child may be capable of producing the mediating response, the child for some reason does not do so. This type of failure is identified as a *production deficiency* in mediation. In the second type of mediation failure the mediating stimulus fails to arouse terminal response (R) for some reason or another. That is, while the organism produces necessary mediating responses to an external stimulus, the stimuli produced by these fail to control the terminal response. This is a mediational control deficiency. Though developing from S-R behavioral theories, the idea of mediation deficiencies has been used to explain cognitive limitations and failure with a variety of cognitive theoretical frameworks. Indeed, the current concept of mediation and mediation deficiencies owes much to ideas generated by Soviet psychologists such as Pavlov (1927), Vigotsky (1962), and Luria (1961), who viewed inner speech as a major mediating system that controls human behavior (see Chapter 10).

The concepts of production and control deficiencies can be useful ones in remedial and special education. Thus, when a pupil is having difficulties in school, we might want to ask ourselves whether the child is suffering from production or control difficulties. The student may not have effectively developed the cognitive mediators that make school performance possible, so that the child lacks the concepts, ideas, plans, etc., necessary to succeed in school; the pupil is suffering from production deficiencies. On the other hand the pupil may have learned the correct mediators but is unable to use them properly, so that the child cannot use concepts, ideas, plans, etc., to behave properly; the student is suffering from control deficiencies. Much of what we discuss in this book derives from or uses mediational constructs.

CHARACTERISTICS OF COGNITIVE PARADIGMS

There are some generally recurring themes in cognitive paradigms and theories. This is particularly true of those that became popular during the past 30 years. We try to illustrate them through contrasts with behaviorism.

Competencies

Cognitive theorists typically make the distinction between performance and competencies (capacities) (Chomsky, 1957, 1968; Fodor, 1975; Lenneberg, 1967). Cognitive theories are usually concerned with both of these aspects of human behavior: (1) with what the pupil can do and the conditions under which the child can do them, and (2) with the type of learner characteristics, abilities, competencies, properties, traits, etc., that make performance possible. Behavioral theories on the other hand usually focus on performance, on what the learner can do, and does, rather than why they can be done.

Activity

A second type of theme found in much of cognitive research is an emphasis on the learner's active role in learning. Behaviorism typically casts learners into a passive role. Their behavior is interpreted as created by repetitive association of responses and stimuli, the consequences of reinforcements, etc. (see Carroll's statement earlier in this chapter). In contrast, cognitivists, particularly those in the 1970s, conceptualize the learners as actively engaging with and transforming information (Lachman et al., 1979). Even the traditional construct of intelligence, which has often been accused of being a static construct, was originally conceived of as an active force used by organisms to master environmental challenges.

Nature As Well As Nurture

Behaviorists are inclined to deal with learners as products of their learning histories. The latter are considered to be an accumulation of past stimulus-response associations and behaviors. While behaviorists most certainly acknowledge that genetic and developmental factors play significant roles in behavior, their knowledge of such factors does not usually affect their theories or methods significantly. As a rule they are by sympathy, if not with full conviction, environmentalists, believing in the power of nurture rather than of nature.

Cognitive theorists usually support nature as well as nurture. They often insist that we are preprogrammed genetically to perceive, think, and act in certain ways, that, for example, language consists of "emergent functions that appear at certain times of life in certain ways" (Fodor, 1975). Even those cognitivists who favor the nurture side of the nature-nurture debate acknowledge the importance of inherited abilities (capacities), e.g., the fact that cognitive functioning is determined by internal cognitive structures, abilities, traits, or the like.

Despite its emphasis on the observable, behaviorism is a complex system of constructs and principles. It is fair to say, however, that cognitive theories are much more varied and more complex.

Chapter 3

Cognition and the Nervous System

Throughout history, efforts have been made to interpret cognitive functioning in terms of the nervous system (Mann, 1979). Concepts like brain damage, cerebral dysfunction, minimal cerebral palsy, and chronic brain syndrome were used to explain language disorders, learning disorders, learning disabilities, dyslexia, hyperactivity, and mental retardation. Remedial and special education strategies and techniques were based on neurological theories (Bannatyne, 1971; Gillingham & Stillman, 1966; Luria, 1961; Myklebust, 1973).

During the late 1960s and 1970s protests were raised against remedial and special education's dependence on neurological conceptions. Their point was that knowledge of the nervous system, and of neurological disorders, was of little help in the training of handicapped pupils or in the remediation of school disabilities. Some experts advised that teachers should study rather their pupils' cognitive strengths and weaknesses through tests (Bateman, 1964; Kirk & Kirk, 1971; Minskoff, Wiseman, & Minskoff, 1972). Others, behaviorist in orientation, recommended that educators devote their efforts to applied behavior analysis and behavioral objectives. As a consequence, many remedial and special educators turned their interest away from neurological functioning.

Remedial and special educators are showing renewed interest in neurology. There are good reasons for this. Knowledge about the nervous system is expanding at a rapid rate. So many different professions are contributing to this knowledge, like chemists, computer scientists, and engineers (as well as physicians, psychologists, and educators), that we speak about the study of the nervous system as the *neurosciences*.

It is still true that most of this knowledge does not yet have much direct application to the classroom. Nevertheless, we may not be far from the time when it will have practical application. An increasing number of books are addressing themselves to this possibility, e.g., Chall and Mirsky (1978), Wittrock (1977), and Hynd and Obrzut (1981). In 1976 the U.S. President's Committee on Mental Retardation published a review of neurological factors in mental retardation, while at the Seventeenth International Conference of the Association for Children with Learning Disabilities, a number of presentations were made concerning the implications of such factors for learning disabilities (Cruickshank & Silver, 1981).

In any case, knowledge of the nervous system is important to remedial and special educators interested in cognitive processes simply from the standpoint of understanding those processes. It is hard to ignore the nervous system if we want to understand what it is about or in our pupils that contributes to their behavior, whether it be the writing of a fine essay, the accomplishment of some athletic feat, or the failure to decode and comprehend reading.

We would like to complete this introduction with several cautionary notes. The first is that our account of the nervous system is a simplified one, intended only as an introduction to the topic. Second, we have written about the nervous system in terms of its implications for cognition. This has meant an emphasis on some of its aspects, while others are discussed only minimally.

Third, it is incorrect to think that the nervous system, either as a whole or in its parts, creates or causes cognition—even though we may sometimes speak as if it does. Our whole body participates in cognition. We cannot think without our heart pumping blood any more than we can do so without a brain. And cognitive activities are greatly dependent on the interrelationships of our sense organs, musculature, and glands (McGuignon, 1978).

Finally, a great deal about the nervous system still remains a mystery. Many of the ideas that we present in this chapter are still speculative. They may later prove either incomplete or incorrect. The knowledge explosion in the neurosciences is producing new insights every day, some of which make yesterday's ones obsolete.

THE NEURON: BUILDING BLOCK OF COGNITION

Educators' interest in the nervous system usually focuses on the brain. However, the brain, despite its singular importance to cognition, is, like all other bodily organs, composed of cells. To understand cognition, we must understand these cells.

The most important of them is the neuron, or nerve cell. Each of them (5 to 100 microns in diameter) is a miniature biochemical-electrical information-processing system. Figure 3–1 shows some typical neurons.

We do not know exactly how many neurons there are in the nervous system. Estimates of those in the brain alone (which has approximately 90 percent of the neurons in the entire nervous system) are on the order of 100 billion. All of the neurons we will ever have are present at birth; indeed they diminish in numbers from that time on. There is a normal loss of neurons as we mature. This may be partly responsible for the development of more precise cognitive functions as we mature—a sloughing off of superfluous nerve cells that might get in the way of the ones that are essential to specific cognitive activities. On the other hand, severe neuronal losses, such as might result from disease or injury, can cause severe and irreparable cognitive impairments. Unlike other bodily cells, neurons once lost cannot be replaced.

Though the neuron is highly specialized, it shares a number of structural and functional characteristics with other bodily cells. Like other cells, it has a continuous cell membrane that encloses cytoplasm and a nucleus. Like other cells, too, a neuron engages in various biological processes that sustain its life and enable it to carry out its specialized functions.

Supporting and nourishing the billions of neuronal cells in our nervous systems are vast networks of vessels. A variety of accessory cells support and protect the neurons. Among the most important of these are the glial (Greek for *glue*) cells, which outnumber neurons 10 to 1. Glial cells act as a sort of packing material; they help neurons remain in place and separate them from each other. Glial cells also control neurons' interactions with the vascular system (blood vessels) and carry away their waste products.

Neurons come in a variety of shapes and sizes, which specialize them for different purposes within the nervous system (see Figure 3–1). There are more than 60 different

Figure 3–1 The Neuron

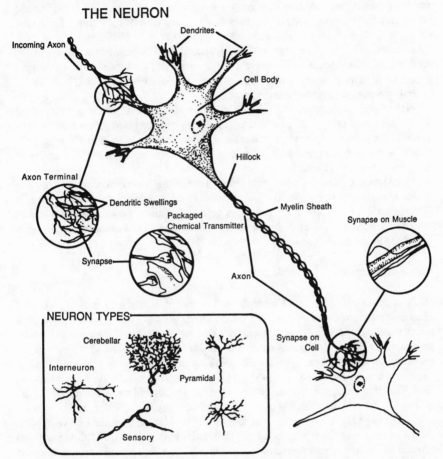

THE NEURON

Source: Reprinted from *The Human Brain* by M.C. Wittrock et al., p. 18, with permission of Prentice-Hall, Inc., © 1977.

types, based on appearance alone. We can generally distinguish between small neurons that send local messages and large ones that transmit information to relatively distant locations. The degree of neuronal specialization is, however, much more than that.

Despite their great numbers, neurons would not be sufficient by themselves to support the complexities of human cognition if they operated independently. They in fact operate in complex networks. Yet each individual neuron is a marvelous cognitive structure in its own right—functionally polarized to receive, integrate, and transmit electrical signals—out of whose composites cognition emerges.

Neurons receive information, i.e., are stimulated by nerve impulses transmitted from other neurons, through specialized receptor sites that they have on their cell bodies and dendrites. Dendrites are afferent (receiving) processes that branch from the neurons' cell bodies in elaborate forms. A single dendrite may have thousands of receptor sites on it.

Neurons also send information. Each neuron has a single axon, an efferent (sending) fiber extending from its body. A neuron, when effectively stimulated, generates a nerve impulse that travels down its axon. Nerve impulses may be the physical equivalents of cognitive information. Some axons branch extensively (see Figure 3–1), but they do so at their terminations, unlike dendrites, which always branch close to the neuron's cell body. Just as dendrites, with their receptor sites, make it possible for a single neuron to receive messages from other neurons, so do an axon's branching terminals make it possible for a single neuron to send information to many other neurons.

Some of the nervous system's glial cells form a special covering for neurons called *myelin*. Myelin is a waxy white substance. A neuron's cell body is never covered by it, its dendrites sometimes are, its axons always are—hence the term *gray matter* for the brain cortex, which is rich in neuronal cell bodies and the term *white matter* for bundles of myelinated axons and dendrites.

Myelin wraps itself around a neuron's axon in a sheath that leaves naked spaces known as the *nodes of Ranvier* (see Figure 3–1). As a nerve impulse travels down an axon, it jumps from one node of Ranvier to another over its myelinated sections. Because myelin acts as an insulator, the nerve impulses that travel down heavily myelinated axons tend to be faster than those in less myelinated ones.

Neuronal Information Transmission

The neuron is able to transmit information, i.e., neural impulses, because of its unique electrochemical properties (Figure 3–2). Its membrane has many tiny pores or "gates" that permit small molecules and charged atoms (ions) to pass through it. The neuron's electrical state, at any given time, depends on its sodium (Na^+) and potassium (K^+) balance. In periods when it is electrically inactive, it maintains an electrical resting potential, and its membrane acts as a *pump*, expelling sodium ions from its interior and pumping in potassium ions. This produces a negative membrane potential, i.e., one in which the interior of the neuron is -60 to -70 millivolts more negative than its exterior (Teyler, 1977).

In order to "trigger" a neuron so as to make it "fire," i.e., transmit a nerve impulse down its axon, it must be stimulated to move the resting potential toward a "threshold" and produce an electrical state called an *action potential*. The action potential travels down the length of the axon, opening the miniature gates in its membrane. When this happens, sodium ions rush into the axon's interior while potassium ions rush out. As a result the interior of the axon becomes less negative in relation to its exterior; that is, the transmembrane potential drops to approximately -10 to -20 millivolts. This generates an electrical impulse in the axons that travels from its hillock (see Figure 3–1) down to its terminals.

After a neuron fires, its Na^+/K^+ "pump" is activated to restore it to a state of resting potential by reestablishing its original negative transmembrane balance. The importance of sodium and potassium to cognition is apparent. Deficiencies or excesses of either, as a consequence of our diets or of other conditions, can seriously interfere with neural transmission and impair cognitive functioning.

An important characteristic of the neuron's electrical impulse is its uniform strength. There is no such thing as a strong or weak neural impulse. A neuron either transmits an electrical impulse or does not. This is called its *all-or-none response*. This response, however, is enhanced by factors of number and rate that greatly increase the neuron's information-transmitting capacities. Thus a neuron may generate different numbers of electrical impulses when stimulated, and these can follow each other at different rates of speed. A telegrapher can use combinations of dots and dashes to send messages. The computer manages a great variety of information through its manipulations of a simple binary code consisting of 1s and 0s. So, too, can a single neuron create a complicated information pattern from its simple yes-no system of electrical impulse.

The Synapse: The Juncture of Cognition

The neuron's ability to transmit information is greatly diversified by its synapses. The transmission of information from one neuron to another (or to a muscle) takes place at the synapse. It is here where the axonal terminals of one neuron make contact with the specialized receptor sites of another. Synapses greatly increase the communication capability of individual neurons, providing each of them with thousands of points of contacts with other neurons. There are perhaps 100 trillion in our nervous system.

In higher animals, including man, the synapse is usually a region of communication between neurons rather than a physical connection. Typically a space called the *synaptic gap* (1.5 billionth or so of a millimeter) separates the terminal of a sending neuron and the receptor site of a receiving one.

This gap is bridged by chemical means. That is, an electrical impulse traveling down a neuron's axon does not directly stimulate another neuron. Rather it causes the release of small amounts of specialized chemical substances called *neurotransmitters* from tiny boutons (buttons) to stimulate the receptor sites of receiving neurons. The released neurotransmitters are then destroyed by other chemical processes in the nervous system or are reabsorbed by the neuron that created them (Figure 3–2).

Neurotransmitters

Neurotransmitters are either excitatory or inhibitory in nature. Excitatory neurotransmitters increase the chances of a neuron generating an electrical impulse. Inhibitory neurotransmitters make the neuron more resistive to firing. At any given time a single neuron is receiving perhaps thousands of conflicting excitatory and inhibitory influences. In fact, it may be stimulated by an excitatory neurotransmitter on one of its receptor sites while being simultaneously stimulated by an inhibitory one on a neighboring site. How it resolves all of this information is one of the most fascinating aspects of its operations.

We still do not know how many different types of neurotransmitters there are in our nervous system. Over 60 have been identified to date, but many more will undoubtedly be discovered. The various neurotransmitters are located in different parts of the nervous system and appear to have specific effects beyond their excitatory and inhibitory actions. Acetylcholine, an excitatory substance, is found in parts of the brain associated with memory and is also found at nerve-muscle junctures. Dopamine, an inhibitory neurotransmitter, seems to play a role in controlling the motor directions issued by our brains; it is found in part of the brain whose degeneration is linked to Parkinson's disease. Norepinephrine is an inhibitory neurotransmitter that has been linked with alertness (Teyler, 1977).

Many of the effects that nutrition and drugs have on cognition appear due to their influence on neurotransmitters (Barbeau, Growden, & Wurtman, 1979). Also the powerful effects that such drugs like amphetamines and LSD have on our mental states seem to be due

Figure 3–2 The Neuron and Its Electrochemical Properties

THE SYNAPSE

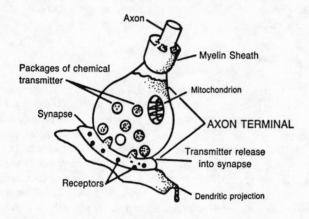

RESTING NEURON

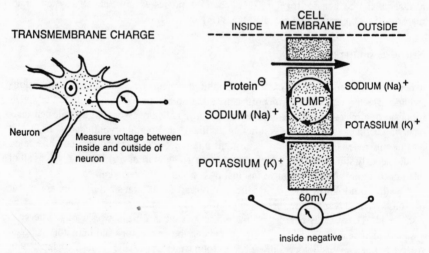

Source: Reprinted from *The Human Brain* by M.C. Wittrock et al., p. 19, with permission of Prentice-Hall, Inc., © 1977.

to their mimicking of the effects of specific neurotransmitters in exaggerated ways. Some neuroscientists believe that we shall someday be able to influence learning, memory, and other cognitive processes significantly by placing specific dosages of neurotransmitters (or their chemical equivalents) at specific locations within the brain.

Neural Factors Influencing Information Transmission

The transmission of information through the nervous system is dependent on a number of the neural phenomena. Two of the more important of these are summation and facilitation (Gomez, 1978).

A single nerve impulse passing down an axon may not release enough neurotransmitter material to stimulate another neuron. However, should that impulse, before it entirely dies away, be succeeded by additional impulses, they together may release enough neurotransmitter to do so. This is *temporal summation*—the combining of nerve impulses over time to achieve neural transmission of information.

In *spatial summation* there is the combination of the effects of a number of different neurons, any one of which by itself does not release sufficient neurotransmitter substances to cause another neuron to fire but which, when simultaneously working together, are effective.

Facilitation is a process in which the influence of one neuron on another has a sub-threshold effect. That is, its transmission of a neural impulse may not be sufficient to cause a state of excitation or inhibition in another neuron, but it can make that neuron more prone to excitation or inhibition by other neurons that later act on it. Facilitation helps us understand the effects of stimulant drugs and so-called painkillers. The first may make neurons more readily excitable. The second makes them less ready to respond to pain.

Neuronal Decision Making

It is obvious that what neurology textbooks describe as the neuron's "stereotyped and obligatory" all-or-none response to stimulation is a complex affair. Our appreciation of its complexity is increased when we observe how the neuron comes to grips with the different types of stimulation (information) that it receives from other neurons—how it, in fact, "decides" whether to release an action potential on its own and to fire a neural impulse, whether, from a cognitive reference point, it "decides" to pass information on to other neurons or to halt the transmission of this information.

The neuron makes its decision on the basis of a statistical analysis. That is, every neuron at every moment averages all of the excitatory and inhibitory inputs (stimulations) that it receives from other neurons. If the average of these inputs is on the excitatory side, the neuron will discharge an electrical impulse of its own. If on the other hand the average of inputs is on the inhibitory side, the neuron will not fire. Indeed it may become less receptive to later excitatory stimulation (Gomez, 1978).

Convergence and Divergence

Two additional neuronal phenomena remain to be considered before we consider higher units of neurological functioning. They are critically important to our understanding of the higher units and of the ways in which the nervous system can sustain cognition. Single neurons are able to organize themselves into complex communication networks and systems through convergence and divergence.

Convergence takes place when the axonal terminals of several neurons converge in a synapse with the receptor sites of another (see Figure 3–2). Divergence takes place when the branches of a single neuron's axon terminate in synaptic relationships with the receptor sites of several other neurons (see Figure 3–3).

Figure 3–3 Neuronal Convergence and Divergence

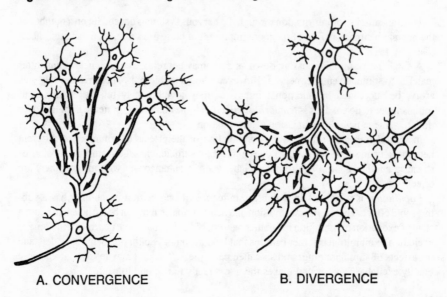

A. CONVERGENCE   B. DIVERGENCE

Source: Reprinted from *Common Neurologic and Language Disorders* by A.J. Gomez with permission of Center for Disorders of Communication, Medical Center Hospital of Vermont, © 1978.

Because of convergence a number of neurons can receive information from many other neurons; the phenomenon of spatial summation is an example of this. Because of divergence a single neuron can pass its information on to many others, thus expanding its range of information transmission. Many of the nervous system's functions are dependent on these phenomena.

Cognition in the Neuron

Before we consider broader units within the nervous system, let us ask whether we can conceive of cognition in simple neuronal terms. It is obvious that nervous functioning must in the final analysis be considered in terms of the nervous system functioning as a system. And yet the basic unit of this system is the neuron. And the more we learn about the neuron, the more impressed we become about its role in cognition. Some scientists have suggested that some of the highest of mental activities can be explained in terms of the composition and activities of single neurons (Kandel, 1979; Stevens, 1979).

We have already reviewed the importance of neurotransmitters—created by individual neurons—and suggested that they be critical to much of what we call *cognition*. Indeed, learning experiences have been found to increase neurotransmitter concentrations in certain parts of the brain, while conditions of environmental deprivation result in their depletion.

Much of cognition, e.g., learning and memory, may in the final analysis be explained on the basis of alterations of neuronal processes. The brains of rats that have been actively trained are considerably heavier than those of other rats. This increase is due to the growth in numbers of axons and dendrites. On the other hand lack of adequate stimulation results in neuronal atrophy and destruction. For example, the cells in the part of the brain that connect with the eyes shrivel (atrophy) in blind people. As we come to understand the neuron better, we can expect to understand cognition better.

NEURONS IN THE AGGREGATE

In the previous section we studied cognition from the standpoint of single neurons. It is true that we often had to consider the single neuron in relationship to other neurons. This was illustrative of the fact that even the simplest of units in the nervous system are, and function as, interrelated components of larger totalities. However, we are ready to examine directly the broader units of the nervous system, for it is in terms of these large units that cognition's relationships to the nervous system begin to emerge.

Neuronal Nuclei and Ganglia

Neurons tend to group together physically when they carry out specific types of functions together. Within the central nervous system (CNS), i.e., brain and spinal cord, a group or cluster of neurons is called a *nucleus* (not to be confused with the structure in the neuron's cell body). A group or cluster of neurons outside the CNS is called a *ganglion*. The brain has many nuclei. The retinas of our eyes are partly controlled by ganglia.

Although some neuronal cell processes, i.e., dendrites and axons, are located in the nervous system's nuclei and ganglia, others extend beyond these neural centers. They do in the form of fibers that extend into all corners of the body. These fibers usually are clustered together and held together by connective tissue in bundles that are called *nerve tracts* if in the CNS or *nerves* if outside the CNS. Those that are myelenated appear white on inspection by the naked eye.

Damage to the nervous system's nuclei and ganglia is likely to have devastating effects on specific cognitive functions, e.g., visual, auditory, and memory ones. Destroy the retinal ganglia, and perception is disrupted. Destroy the nuclei of the amygdala (which is on the lower side of the brain), and an individual may be unable to recall any recent information.

Damage to the nerve tracts can also cause major cognitive impairments because these tracts serve as the highways of communication within the nervous system. As indicated earlier, myelin insulates as well as protects, and it improves the speed of neural transmission in those nerve fibers covered with it. Disturbances of the myelenization process cause neurological dysfunctioning and in many instances cognitive impairments as well. It has been suggested that delays in myelenization can cause learning disabilities. Severe disruptions cause muscular dystrophy.

STUDY OF COGNITION BY NEUROSCIENCES

We are ready to study the larger structural units of the nervous system, particularly that part most responsible for cognition: the brain. Before we proceed to this study, it is essential that we review some of the ways that the neurosciences study the nervous system because our conceptions about the latter's role in cognition are dependent on the information provided by these techniques.

Anatomical and Physiological Studies

From ancient times the study of the nervous system has fascinated medical and psychological researchers. It was once illegal to dissect the human body. Ancient Greek and Roman physicians dissected apes, pigs, and cattle and then guessed how the nervous system was constructed in humans. Once dissection of humans was allowed, knowledge of neural anatomy began to grow slowly and then with the development of advanced instruments and methods moved rapidly ahead.

Such study was greatly assisted by the development of the microscope in the seventeenth century, which permitted a closer study of the tissues that constitute the various organs of the nervous system. The usefulness of this instrument was greatly enhanced by the development of stains that made the neurons easier to study under microscopic inspection (Hubel, 1979).

A major breakthrough in staining techniques—one that greatly accelerated the study of the brain—was accomplished by Italian anatomist Camillo Golgi in 1895. Before his time, the stains used to distinguish neurons from each other often caused blurring and confused pictures. For one, there are so many neurons in any particular slice of brain tissue that they are ordinarily difficult to distinguish from each other. Golgi's method stained only a small number of the neurons in any particular tissue and did this seemingly at random. These stained neurons stood out clearly from the rest and could be studied individually in their entirety. By using many samples of tissues, it became possible to understand the cellular make-up of the brain structures. Thus Golgi's contemporary Ramon Cajal was able to show that neurons joined together in networks (Hubel, 1979). A later staining method developed by Nissl stained only the neuron's cell body (and not its axon and dendrites). This provided another way of seeing how neurons are organized. The development of light microscopy also furthered neuronal study.

A recent giant step forward in understanding how the neuron operated was made in the 1950s by the Dutch scientist Walter J.H. Natau. His method capitalized on the fact that when a neuron is destroyed, its nerve fibers degenerate but before this happens, it is possible to stain them so that they leave an impression that is distinctly different from the fibers of neighboring undamaged neurons. It thus became possible to destroy certain parts of the brain in experimental animals and to observe the paths that the fibers from the destroyed regions took to other parts of the brain. In this way we have been able to find many previously unsuspected connections among brain cells and larger components that have broadened our understanding of cognitive processes. For example, where we once may have thought only a certain part of the brain is involved in a particular type of cognitive activity, we can now see that other parts are also critically engaged (Hubel, 1979).

Lately chemical advances have improved our understanding of brain processes. Transport autoradiography has been one of the most important of these. A radioactive chemical is injected into a brain structure. The latter's cell bodies transport the chemical along the axon so that it accumulates in the latter's terminals. When a photographic emulsion is later put in contact with a slice of tissue from this structure, the destination of the axons is revealed. In a reverse application, chemicals are picked up by the axon's terminals and transported back to the cell bodies. In this way the origins of particular axons can be distinguished (Hubel, 1979).

The most exciting of recent advances in neural tracing is a technique developed by Louis Solokoff of the National Institutes of Health during the 1970s. Neurons use glucose as their fuel. The more active they are, the more glucose they consume; the glucose is metabolized and disappears. When radioactive deoxyglucose is absorbed by neurons, it is metabolized like regular glucose, but unlike the latter it does not break down all the way. Instead it accumulates in the nerve cells. Thus the more active particular neurons have been, the more radioactive they become when they are "fed" radioactive glucose. And if the radioactive deoxyglucose has been stained, the level of their activity can actually be studied on dissection.

This method has made it possible to identify the brain cells that participate in specific types of cognitive processes and to determine how active they have been. For example, deoxyglucose was injected into the veins of laboratory animals that were then stimulated with certain kinds of sounds. When brains of these animals were later studied, it was possible to determine which of their parts had responded to the sounds (Hubel, 1979). Variations of this method are applicable to live humans.

Clinical Studies

Much of what we know about cognitive processes has come from our work with individuals whose nervous systems have been affected by disease and injury. Sometimes this is revealed by establishing the presence of certain cognitive deficits in these individuals through observations, tests, or their histories and then by dissecting their brains after death to determine what parts were damaged and might be associated with the deficits. There are problems with this approach. Brain damage usually is not precise or clearly localized. It is often so widespread or severe so as to damage brain structures we would prefer to leave intact in our studies. For such reasons many neurological researchers prefer to rely on experimental research in which they can more precisely deal with the nervous system even though they may have to limit their work to animals.

Experimental Studies

In experimental studies parts of animal brains may be surgically removed. The cognitive and behavioral effects of this surgery are then studied through specialized tests and observations. We have come to understand a great deal about our own cognitive functioning from such studies. Cats' brains have certain similarities to our own; those of chimpanzees, even more. For that matter, squids' nerve fibers have electrical properties that are similar to our own.

Other forms of experimental investigation utilize recordings from electrodes placed into nervous tissue. Using microelectrodes, we can even measure the activity of a single neuron. Electrodes have also been used to stimulate the brain and have helped us to determine what parts of the brain are associated with various kinds of sensation and movement. Electrical stimulation has also helped us find locations in the brain that are associated with experiences of hunger, fear, and rage. It is thus possible to stimulate a cat's brain to make the cat afraid of a mouse placed in its cage (Masserman, 1943).

Noninvasive Studies

The term *noninvasive* in medicine means exactly what it says: A patient is not "invaded" to find out what is going on. Opening up a patient's chest to study the heart is invasive. To study the heart with a stethoscope is noninvasive. In neurology a number of noninvasive methods are being used to study cognition.

Electroencephalography

In 1924 the German psychiatrist Hans Berger attempted to record the electrical activities of a patient's brain without injuring him in any way; the patient was his son. He placed a pair of electrodes on the center of the boy's head and obtained electrical "readings." From this beginning developed the modern electroencephalogram, which records the electrical impulses from the brain through electrodes placed on the skull, amplifies them so they can be recorded, and records them by a pen writing on paper or on a cathode tube (Duane, 1981).

Electroencephalographic readings (EEGs) show how the brain responds to different types of stimulation and under various conditions of neurological health, stress, disease, and injury. EEGs have been helpful in the diagnosis of neurological difficulties such as epilepsy and brain tumors. They have also been of value in studying the brain's electrical activity in various states of consciousness, work, and rest. They have, however, not been precise enough by themselves to be of great use in assessing specific cognitive processes such as memory and problem solving.

Average Evoked Responses

The average evoked response method is a recent computerized application of EEG technology that appears to hold considerable promise for the study of cognition (Duane, 1981). The method makes computer-controlled repetitive presentations of special stimuli of a visual, auditory, or tactile nature to a subject. These stimuli are repeated as few as 12 times or as many as a thousand. They evoke electrical responses from specific parts of the subject's brain, which are recorded through electrodes placed at different points of the skull. Each time the subject is stimulated, the responses evoked are transformed by the computer into a digital code and averaged. The average responses can be recorded and used to provide computer printouts or to display brain activity on a cathode tube.

The ordinary EEG can show only a gross and general picture of the brain's electrical activities. Averaged evoked responses are much more precise. They are able to indicate the parts of the brain that respond to specific types of stimulation and their levels of activity while so doing. The technique has been used to study such conditions as hyperactivity, mental retardation, and learning disabilities (Duane, 1981). Recent improvements in the evoked response method can now generate video color images of brain activities showing the ebb and flow of electrical functioning in the various points of the brain over time. The acronym *BEAM* is used to identify such approaches. It stands for *brain electrical activity mapping*.

Computerized Axial Tomography (CAT)

Computerized axial tomography (CAT) has proven a recent improvement of x-ray technology that can be said to have revolutionized our understanding of the brain (and other bodily organs). X-rays by themselves can show only the length and width of a bodily organ. The CAT scan can reveal the organ's depth as well. For example, CAT sends beams of x-rays through various parts of the brain. The information from these beams is transmitted to a computer, which can display three-dimensional slices of it on a TV screen. Thus, for the first time the brains of living subjects could actually be "seen."

The CAT has contributed enormously to our ability to diagnose brain abnormalities, e.g., tumors and other neurological conditions. Beyond this it is providing fascinating information about the brain-cognition relationship. For example, we are able to compare visually the brains of living people and to see whether differences in their brain structure are related to differences in their cognitive abilities. Thus we have found that certain parts of the brain are less well developed in some individuals with language difficulties than they are in normal individuals. "Like an electronic knife the DSR can pictorially slice open an organ and expose its interior . . . [showing it] . . . pulsing with the flow of blood and oxygen" (Fincher, 1981).

Nuclear Magnetic Resonance (NMR)

This is a technique that is just now being applied to the study of the brain. It may have certain advantages over CAT. First, it seems to be able to penetrate through bone better than the CAT and may thus be able to detect abnormalities more precisely. Unlike the CAT, which uses x-rays, NMR relies on a combination of magnetic fields and radio waves, so that it appears risk-free. Most important, it can actually make possible a mathematical analysis of actual brain tissue from outside the body. The technique is still in its infancy in medical applications.

Positron Emission Transaxial Tomography (PETT)

The PETT is another new contender for honors in the repertoire of methods for studying brain-cognitive relationships. Like BEAM methods the PETT provides color pictures of the brain's activities during cognition. But it provides a different focus on them. Subjects are injected with radioactively treated glucose, and x-rays are taken of their brains during various types of cognitive activity. As discussed, the more active a part of the brain, the greater is its consumption of glucose. This shows up through the PETT. We can thus literally "see," on a TV screen, those parts of the brain that are active when we are stimulated in different ways, e.g., when we hear music or noise.

The PETT is so precise that we can even identify the parts of a rat's brain, one by one, that respond when the rat has individual whiskers stroked. When a child moves a hand, we can see all the activation in various parts of the brain that are sequentially involved in the movement. When a schizophrenic child hallucinates voices, the specific parts of the brain that respond to the voices show up in different colors—depending on their rates of glucose use. PETT promises to increase enormously our knowledge of brain physiology and of the latter's involvement with cognition (Duane, 1981).

There are, of course, other techniques for the study of neurological, neuroanatomical, and neurophysiological aspects of the brain besides the ones discussed, for example, chemical methods used to study the concentrations and types of neurotransmitters in different parts of the nervous system. But space considerations make it necessary for us to limit ourselves to the brief sampling presented.

MAJOR STRUCTURAL COMPONENTS OF THE NERVOUS SYSTEM

The three major structural components of the nervous system are presented in Table 3–1 and Figure 3–5. Our major interest in this chapter is with the first two of these: the peripheral and central nervous system. The autonomic nervous system, involved as it is with our appetites and emotions (hunger, thirst, sexual arousal, fear, and anger), is obviously of great importance to cognitive functioning. However, it has not yet drawn much interest from cognitive psychologists.

Table 3–1 Major Structural Divisions of the Nervous System

1. Central nervous system	forebrain—prosencephalon
a. brain	midbrain—mesencephalon
b. spinal cord	hindbrain—rhombencephalon
2. Peripheral nervous system	
a. cranial nerves (12 pairs)	
b. spinal nerves (31 pairs)	
3. Autonomic nervous system	
a. parasympathetic	
b. sympathetic	

Source: Reprinted from *Common Neurologic and Language Disorders* by A.J. Gomez with permission of Center for Disorders of Communication, Medical Center Hospital of Vermont, © 1978.

The central nervous system (CNS) consists of those neurons that are enclosed in the bony coverings of the skull and spinal column. The system is protected by coverings called *meninges*, and it "floats" in a protective primitive sea of cerebral spinal fluid.

The peripheral nervous system consists of neurons and cell processes outside the CNS. It carries information from the CNS to the body's muscles and glands.

Segmental and Hierarchical Organization

It will help us to understand the relationships of both nervous systems, as well as some major characteristics of neurological functioning, if we keep in mind that they both are organized along segmental and hierarchical lines. All vertebrates, including humans, have segmental nervous systems, even though the latter are physically continuous. This is reflected in the separate vertebrae of our spinal cords. It is difficult to think of our brains being organized segmentally, but photographs of the human embryo make this aspect quite clear.

Structurally organized on a segmental basis, the nervous system is also functionally organized in a hierarchical way. That is, as we move up the length of the spinal cord and through the brain, physically higher structures may dominate, modulate, and even control the functions of lower ones. In man and higher animals the cerebral cortex, the most highly developed, and newest phylogenetic, component of the brain modulates the functioning of subcortical brain structures. Subcortical structures such as the brain stem, the physically lowest part of the brain, monitor the functions of the spinal cord. Within the spinal cord higher spinal levels affect the functions of lower ones.

What this means for cognition, in its broadest aspects, is that we can expect the higher parts of the brain to be the ones that are particularly involved with complex cognitive processes such as those of language and reasoning. It also means that when higher brain structures are impaired, the activities of lower ones take over and exercise control in respect to cognition. Thus in an individual with severe injuries affecting the higher brain centers, language might be lost though the person still may be able to perceive quite well and otherwise manage bodily functions. In coma, where there is incapacitation or even "death" of higher brain structures, lower structures, e.g., those of the brain stem, continue to function. In such cases patients are still able to breathe and carry out other vital functions but unable to remain conscious or capable of what we would ordinarily consider to be cognition.

One well-known school of education-rehabilitation thought—that of Doman-Delacato—bases techniques on restoring neurological hierarchies (Delacato, 1966a; Doman, Spitz, Zuchman, Delacato, & Doman, 1967). The system tries to restore lower functions first and later build higher ones on them as treatment continues.

THE PERIPHERAL NERVOUS SYSTEM

The peripheral nervous system consists of cranial and spinal nerves. Some cranial nerves are mixed; i.e., they have both sensory and motor fibers. Others are entirely motor or sensory. All spinal nerves are of the mixed variety.

Cranial Nerves

There are 12 pairs of cranial nerves (see Table 3–2). Five of these are purely motor nerves, 3 purely sensory nerves, while 4 are mixed (sensory and motor nerves). Most of them originate (motor fibers) or terminate (sensory fibers) in the brain stem. The cranial

Table 3–2 The Cranial Nerves

Number	Name	Modality	Function
I	Olfactory	Sensory	Transmits smell.
II	Optic	Sensory	Transmits vision.
III	Oculomotor	Motor	Moves the eye.
IV	Trochlear	Motor	Moves the eye.
V	Trigeminal	Mixed	Sensory fibers—transmits sensation from face area. Motor fibers supply the muscles of mastication.
VI	Abducens	Motor	Moves the eye.
VII	Facial	Mixed	Motor fibers supply the muscles of the face. Motor fibers also supply the mandibular, sublingual, and lactimal glands. Sensory fibers are taste fibers from the anterior two-thirds of the tongue.
VIII	Acoustic	Sensory	Acoustic or cochlear fibers carry impulses for hearing. Vestibular fibers transmit impulses for equilibrium maintenance.
IX	Glosso-pharyngeal	Mixed	Sensory fibers carry taste from the posterior one-third of the tongue as well as sensation from upper pharynx. Motor fibers supply the upper pharyngeal muscles and the parotid glands.
X	Vagus	Mixed	Supplies motor fibers to the pharynx, larynx, thoracic and abdominal organs. Sensory fibers transmit sensation from the same areas.
XI	Spinal accessory	Motor	Supplies sternomastoid and trapezius muscles.
XII	Hypoglossal	Motor	Supplies muscles of the tongue.

Source: Reprinted from *Common Neurologic and Language Disorders* by A.J. Gomez with permission of Center for Disorders of Communication, Medical Center Hospital of Vermont, © 1978.

nerves serve organs in the body's thoracic and abdominal cavities as well as those in the head and neck regions.

Because they receive information from or send commands to key organs in the eye, ear, tongue, etc., the cranial nerves have been topics of keen interest to cognitive theorists. Remedial and special educators, whether concerned with improving tachistoscopic recognition of words, better auditory discrimination, or speech improvement, are intimately engaged with them on a daily basis.

Spinal Nerves

There are 31 pairs of spinal nerves. They enter (sensory fibers) or leave (motor fibers) the spinal cord through spaces between the spinal column's vertebrae. They terminate in cell bodies located in the gray matter of the spinal cord. In cross section, this gray matter has a butterfly shape (see Figure 3–4).

Sensory and motor fibers join together away from the spinal cord. They divide into separate bundles of nerve fibers (roots) near it (see Figure 3–4). The afferent (sensory) fibers of the dorsal (posterior) root terminate in the dorsal (top) horns of the spinal cord's central gray matter, where they make contact with the cord's sensory neurons and bring information from the body into the cord, both for local action and for transmission to higher centers. The efferent (motor) fibers of the ventral root (anterior) are actually the axons of large motor neurons located in the lower horns of the spinal cord's central gray matter. They carry information from the cord out to muscles and glands; their responses are based on reflexive actions, but they also respond to commands from the higher nerve centers.

Modern special education and remedial education are inevitably concerned with the peripheral nervous system. A vast amount of literature indicates that its impairments mean qualitative and quantitative impairments in cognition (Frailberg & Frailberg, 1979; Rosenzweig, 1981).

THE CENTRAL NERVOUS SYSTEM

The central nervous system consists of two components: the spinal cord (see Figure 3–4) and the brain. While these components are distinct systems in their own right, they also constitute a still larger unit whose function, as its name implies, is that of central information processing.

The Spinal Cord

The spinal cord is a pathway between the brain and the body's senses and muscles. Indeed the spinal cord's neuronal core of gray matter is sheathed by bundles of white myelenated nerve tracts of axons that carry (sensory) messages to and (motor) messages from the brain. The spinal cord, however, also processes information by itself at local levels. And even at these local levels a great deal of complexity of functioning can be found.

Thus, while the spinal cord consists of many sensory and motor neurons, most of its neurons are interneurons, which integrate information flow between its input (sensory) and output (motor) conduits. Even what may seem to be a simple reflex, e.g., removing a finger from a hot stove, results from the complex spinal interaction of sensory and motor impulses.

Figure 3–4 Organization of the Spinal Cord

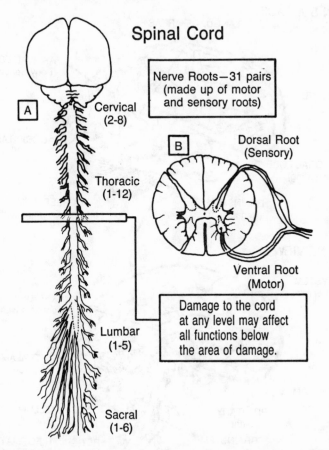

Source: Reprinted from Howell I. Runion and Sandra L. McNett-McGowan, "An Illustrated Review of Normal Brain Anatomy and Physiology," in *Bridges to Tomorrow, Volume 2, The Best of ACLD*, edited by William M. Cruickshank and Archie A. Silver (Syracuse, NY: Syracuse University Press, 1981), p. 182.

The spinal cord does not usually receive much attention from cognitive theorists. But the information it provides the brain, the motor commands it carries from the latter to our glands and muscles, and the role it plays in the integration of behavior cannot be ignored in any neurological accounts of cognition. Certainly remedial and special educators concerned with tactile and kinesthetic information processing should pay it some attention.

The Brain

The human brain is the most complex of neurological structures. It is large—three pounds or more in human beings—and it consists of billions of neurons. The surface (the cerebral cortex) of the brain is convoluted (see Figure 3–5)—folded in on itself—which permits

Figure 3–5 Views of the Brain

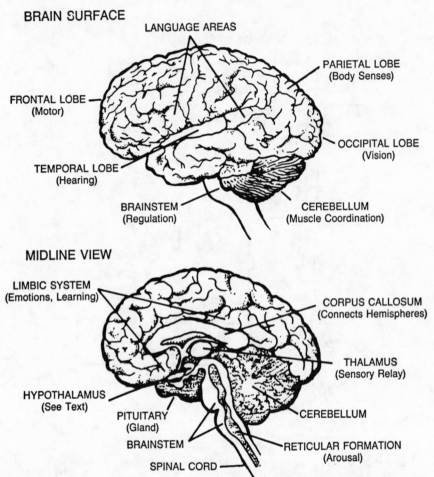

BRAIN SURFACE

LANGUAGE AREAS

PARIETAL LOBE
(Body Senses)

FRONTAL LOBE
(Motor)

OCCIPITAL LOBE
(Vision)

TEMPORAL LOBE
(Hearing)

BRAINSTEM
(Regulation)

CEREBELLUM
(Muscle Coordination)

MIDLINE VIEW

LIMBIC SYSTEM
(Emotions, Learning)

CORPUS CALLOSUM
(Connects Hemispheres)

THALAMUS
(Sensory Relay)

HYPOTHALAMUS
(See Text)

PITUITARY
(Gland)

CEREBELLUM

BRAINSTEM

RETICULAR FORMATION
(Arousal)

SPINAL CORD

Source: Reprinted from *The Human Brain* by M.C. Wittrock et al., p. 7, with permission of Prentice-Hall Inc., © 1977.

many more neurons to be fitted into the skull than would be possible if it were smooth. The more convolutions, and these convolutions increase in animal brains as we move up the evolutionary scale to man, the more neurons there are; generally speaking, they are representative of a more sophisticated cognitive process.

The most prominent structure of the brain is the cerebral cortex, an outer shell of gray matter enclosing and otherwise physically dominating other brain structures. There are also large bundles of white matter—nerves—connecting the various parts of the brain, both with other parts and with the spinal cord. Buried within these nerve tracts are a number of subcortical neurological structures such as the thalamus, hypothalamus, basal ganglia, and brain stem (see Figure 3–5), the latter connecting the brain to the spinal cord.

How shall we study the brain—this mighty organ—which according to one group of authors "pumps behavior" like the heart pumps blood (Filskov, Grimm, & Lewis, 1980, p. 39)? We choose to do so moving from its lower structures up through the cerebral cortex, since this route seems to us to allow the best appreciation of how the brain serves cognition.

The Brain Stem

The brain stem holds most of the structures below the cerebral cortex. These connect the brain, so to speak, with the spinal cord and other sources of information.

The medulla is the major connecting structure between the brain and the spinal cord. It is a conduit for nerve tracts traveling between the higher parts of the brain and the spinal cord. The brain stem is also an entrance and exit point for certain cranial nerves. Some of the nuclei of these lower brain structures hold the cell bodies of these cranial nerves. Others control the information flow within the nervous system. Still others are responsible for basic life processes like the circulation of blood and breathing and for such behaviors as blinking, coughing, and vomiting.

The roles of such lower brain structures in higher cognition were often overlooked in the past. This is changing as we make new discoveries. Thus, the now heavily researched reticular formation has its origin in the structures of the medulla oblongata. It extends from these in a network of neurons into the pons and the thalamus and then into the cerebellum and cerebral cortex. The reticular formation is of great importance in managing the flow of sensory and motor information between various levels of the nervous system. It further plays a significant role in the cognitive processes associated with the attention. Disruptions or impairments of its functions may be one of the causes of childhood autism (Rimland, 1964). Lesser problems associated with its dysfunctions may be inattentiveness or inability to concentrate.

Midbrain Structures

Moving beyond the medulla and other brain structures, we find a small structure called the *hypothalamus*, located in the diencephalon, which is a relay station between lower and higher parts of the brain. It is associated with the pituitary gland, the master gland of the body, which controls the activity of other glands. The hypothalamus has many critical regulatory functions, including those of hormone and neurotransmitter production. It also regulates bodily temperature and activity levels. As to its implications for cognition, the hypothalamus is a center for integrating the cognitive and affective aspects of behavior. It regulates our appetites, e.g., thirst, hunger, and sex, and our emotions, e.g., rage and fear, all of which affect cognitive functioning. We can electrically stimulate the hypothalamus in a docile animal to make it go into a fury or make a cat afraid of a mouse by stimulating its fear centers (Masserman, 1940, 1943). We can make a rat hungry or thirsty after it is satisfied by food or water by stimulating its hunger and thirst centers (Olds & Olds, 1965).

The Thalamus

The thalamus (including the basal ganglia) can be considered the major relay station of the brain. Sensory information ascending to the brain from our body and visual and auditory receptors first passes to centers in the thalamus and is sorted out and integrated there before passing on to the cerebral cortex. The thalamus also helps to direct the motor activities set in motion by the cerebrum.

The Cerebellum

The cerebellum is adjacent to the brain stem and communicates through it to the other parts of the brain and the spinal cord. The reticular formation plays an important role in monitoring and modulating its functions. The cerebellum affects motor control and integration of gross and fine motor activities. It plays a major role in modulating posture, balance, and antigravity control and as such is often spoken of as a center of coordination. Lesions to the cerebellum or the brain stem tracts that lead it result in a variety of handicaps. These can be severe loss of muscle control in walking (ataxias), tremors in writing, and cerebellar speech, which is characterized by excessive slowness and disjuncture in saying words (Runion & McNett-McGowan, 1981).

The Cerebrum

It is the cerebrum that most of us picture in our mind's eye when we think about the brain and about the brain's role in cognition. There are some good reasons for this. First, the cerebrum is the most visible part of the brain, covering or concealing the other structures that we have just discussed. Second, the cerebrum is the largest part of the brain. In fact, over 90 percent of the neurons in the nervous system are to be found in it. Still further, it is the most accessible part of the brain. We can much more easily study its electrical activities than those, let us say, of the hypothalamus. Finally, and most importantly, it is the most important part of the nervous system from the standpoint of cognition.

The *cerebral cortex* (another name for the cerebrum that refers to its role in covering the rest of the brain) consists of horizontal sheets of neurons generally separated by groups of perpendicular axons. In most places there are six. The fifth and sixth lowest layers have a great concentration of motor neurons; these send axons down into the spinal cord to activate the body's muscles. The fourth layer is the cortex's main receiving platform for sensory information from our receptor organs, which receive these through the perpendicular axons from the neurons in the thalamus. The first through third layers have a great concentration of association neurons, e.g., internuncial neurons, which process, coordinate, and interpret information from various regions of the cerebrum.

The cortical layers are not uniform in make-up throughout the cerebrum, being thicker or thinner and having different cell compositions in different locations. Because of this it is possible to develop precise "maps" of the cortex, i.e., identifying its various parts on the basis of different types of neurons and their concentrations. The most famous mapping system is that of the Broadmann's areas. Brain maps are important in that they help researchers and clinicians precisely identify the specific parts of the brain with which they are working. They are also used to identify parts of the cortex that may be associated with specific types of cognitive processes. Surgeons use these maps to guide brain operations.

Despite the fact that the cortex consists of "sheets" of neurons, much of it appears to function in small, vertically oriented columns (Filskov, Grimm, & Lewis, 1980). This columnar organization is most important for our understanding of the cortex's role in cognition. For example, it appears that sensory information is more or less projected through these "tubes" onto the cortex's surface and that each of the columns, microscopically miniscule in size, analyzes and records distinctly separate and specific bits of sensory information.

The cerebrum is not a solid mass. Rather it is divided into two (right and left) hemispheres. The cerebral hemispheres look very alike though the left one is generally slightly heavier and somewhat physically larger than the right in most people. More important than any structural differences between the two hemispheres are the different roles they play in cognition (we discuss these later in the chapter).

The two hemispheres, though separate from each other, are connected by a thick band of nerve tracts called the *corpus callosum*. This thick band physically connects the two hemispheres. It also brings them into constant communication with each other. The cerebral hemispheres also share information from lower brain centers.

This appears to be a good time and place to reacquaint our readers with the phenomenon of nervous system decussation or crossover. An understanding of this phenomenon helps us to understand better the distinct roles that the two hemispheres play in cognition.

Decussation is the process in which nerve tracts going to and from the cerebral cortex cross over from the original side of their origins. Sensory nerves from the body cross over in the spinal cord, and the cranial nerves do so in the brain stem. Thus, the sensory information from the left sides of the body and head are recorded in the right hemisphere, and that from the right sides is projected onto the left hemisphere (some variations in visual decussation are discussed later). In a similar way, motor neurons originating in the right cerebral hemisphere cross over in the brain stem to control the left side of the body while those originating in the left hemisphere decussate so as to control the right side of the body.

Each of the cerebral hemispheres is divided into five lobes. From front to back these are the frontal, parietal, temporal, insular, and occipital lobes. These lobes are not entirely separated or distinguishable from each other, either anatomically or physiologically.

The cerebral lobes have primary sensory zones, which receive information from our sense organs; primary motor zones, which activate specific musculatures in the body and head; and association zones, both sensory and motor, which integrate and interpret information from the primary zones with that from other sources.

Despite the common features, the lobes have some demonstrated specificities in respect to some of the basic cognitive-behavioral functions. The motor zone responsible for bodily movement, the primary motor cortex, is located in the frontal lobe. The parietal zone receives bodily sensations; the primary somesthetic zone is located in it. The primary auditory zone is located in the temporal lobe; the primary visual zone in the occipital lobe.

MAJOR FUNCTIONAL SYSTEMS OF THE NERVOUS SYSTEM

It was inevitable that as we studied the nervous system's anatomy, we also studied its functions. In this section we examine these functions more closely, from approaches that appear to be particularly pertinent to remedial and special education, that is, in terms of the nervous system's role as a transmitter of and interpreter of sensory information, as a transmitter and controller of information that results in motor behavior, and in terms of its central integrating functions, which are clearly essential to higher cognitive functioning.

Many remedial and rehabilitative activities with pupils are based on this trinity of functioning, which conceives us to be (1) sensory transducers, (2) generators of (motor) behavior, and (3) synthesizers and interpreters of informational inputs and outputs.

THE SENSORY SYSTEM

This functional division of the nervous system carries information into the nervous system from our general and special senses. The general senses are those that deal with general information from the body that is not dependent on specific senses such as touch, pressure, vibration, position, temperature, and pain. The special senses are the visual, auditory, gustatory, olfactory, and vestibular senses.

Remedial and special educators are concerned with both general and special senses categories, particularly those of touch and kinesthesis in the first, vision and audition in the second.

The Ascending Pathways

"The sensory system is composed of all of the sensory fibers leading from specific receptor organs to their final terminations at sensory cortical areas" (Gomez, 1978, p. 129). These fibers create the ascending pathways of the nervous system.

The ascending pathways, whether from the eye, ear, skin, muscles, follow the same common plan outlined in Figure 3–6. In our explanation of these pathways, as they proceed from sense organs to cortex, we write as if there were only single neurons at each level of the ascending pathway. In reality these pathways are made up of many such cells and their processes. Our presentation is based on Gomez's sequence (1978):

- There is a sense organ for each specific stimulus, e.g., the retina for visual stimuli, the organ of Corti for hearing stimuli, the vestibular organ for stimuli created by changes in position.
- The path from each sense organ to its cortical termination consists of at least three neurons.
- A stimulus impinging on a sense receptor is first registered by the nervous system at the level of the first or primary neuron that lies outside the central nervous system in special ganglia (groups of nerve cells), e.g., in the retina and organ of Corti. Stimulation of the sense organs creates an action potential in the primary neurons, which encode information about the stimulating event.
- Information is transmitted by the primary neuron to a second or secondary neuron in either the spinal cord or the lower levels of the brain—depending on whether spinal or cranial nerves are involved.
- The secondary neuron's axon crosses over (decussates) from the side from which it originated to the opposite side of its nervous system segment. It then ascends (with similar axons) into the thalamus.
- The secondary neuron's axon makes contact with a tertiary neuron in the thalamus, which as discussed can be considered the brain's relay station.
- The tertiary neuron's axon then passes together (with similar axons) in a thalamo-cortical radiation of fibers to terminate in the cerebral cortex's sensory projection areas.

How the Sensory System Functions

The nervous system must be able to transmit useful information about the physical world, both inside and outside the body, to the brain in order for cognition to take place. This is not simply a matter of reporting stimulation to the brain. Our senses are constantly being bombarded with stimuli. But stimulation by itself does not create information. Cognition

Figure 3–6 Ascending Pathways of the Sensory System

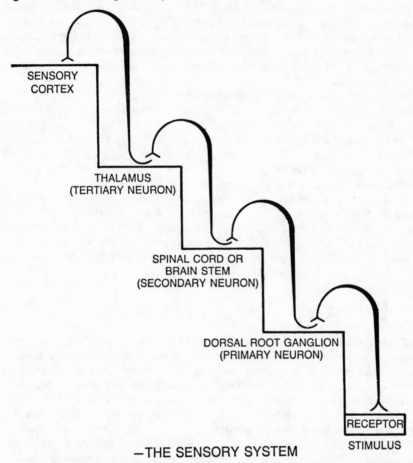

SENSORY CORTEX

THALAMUS
(TERTIARY NEURON)

SPINAL CORD OR
BRAIN STEM
(SECONDARY NEURON)

DORSAL ROOT GANGLION
(PRIMARY NEURON)

RECEPTOR
STIMULUS

—THE SENSORY SYSTEM

Source: Reprinted from *Common Neurologic and Language Disorders* by A.J. Gomez with permission of Center for Disorders of Communication, Medical Center Hospital of Vermont, © 1978.

cannot develop from it. Much of the stimulation we receive is meaningless; other parts of it cannot be interpreted; some of it is just plain "noise"—of auditory, visual, tactile kinesthetic nature—that detracts from what we should "know"; in other cases the stimulation is unclear or insufficient. Stimulation must somehow be controlled, managed, and monitored before it makes sense. A parent must hear the baby's cry over the noise of pots and pans in the kitchen and the sound of other children; an airplane pilot must screen out the reflections of the sky's sun on the windows of the aircraft in order to distinguish the reflections of another aircraft that may threaten collision. A policeman must be able to amplify the slight sounds of a burglar trying to slip away from a crime. Thus what we sense—hear, see, and feel—is not the result of raw stimulation. It is rather the product of nervous system selection and integration.

The processes of summation, inhibition, facilitation, convergence, and divergence were discussed earlier in this chapter. Phenomena like these, as well as specialized neuronal functions, play significant roles in turning raw stimulation into refined sensory information. They come into play as soon as our sense receptors are stimulated. And they continue to affect neural transmission at all levels of the ascending pathways—constantly clarifying, elaborating, and interpreting the information flow till it registers on the brain's cortex, i.e., comes into consciousness.

Special notation should be made regarding the nervous system's inhibitory functions. Cognition is as much a product of inhibition as it is of excitation, for selectivity and clarity in cognition depend on what we do not respond to. Combinations of excitatory and inhibitory influences exerted on neurons throughout the ascending pathways emphasize, indeed exaggerate, some aspects of the original stimulation while shutting out or minimizing others. All along the ascending pathways are both accentuation and denial of stimulus information. Both are essential to what we call *sensation* and ultimately to cognition.

In all of these functions the interrelatedness of all of the nervous system's structures is observed. Thus the sensory system is influenced by the motor system—and influences it in turn. For example, the amount of light coming into a pupil—which determines how much of a particular scene will be registered on the retina's ganglia—is controlled by the pupil's motor reactions. These in turn are controlled by neural centers in the brain stem and influenced by events in the cerebral cortex.

Special Neurons

Certain types of neurons in the various levels of the ascending pathways are specialized to respond to information about specific aspects of a stimulus. At one time it was believed that information received by our sense organs was projected directly onto the surface of the cortex after passing through the ascending pathways of the nervous system, much the same way that a motion picture camera projects images on a motion picture screen. We know that the cells in the ascending pathways modify this information as it is passed along. And within the cortex itself neuronal cells are arranged in what are called *hypercollumns* (Hubel & Wiesel, 1959), each cell of which acts as a feature extractor, and analyzes incoming information from the senses in respect to specific aspects such as movement, contrast, contours, sound, and pitch. Thus information from our senses appears to be analyzed and even catalogued before it finally projects onto the surface of the cortex.

THE MOTOR SYSTEM

Cognitive theorists are usually more interested in the nervous system's sensory aspects than in its motor side; cognition is traditionally considered as based on sensory information. The motor system's contributions are usually considered in terms of the information it provides through the senses, including the one that is specifically responsive to motor movement; the kinesthetic sense. However, the motor system's contribution to cognition is clearly beyond the provision of sensory inputs; for it is our movement through the physical world and our manipulations of physical objects that are responsible for much of cognitive learning. This fact has been recognized by educators throughout history. One of its most recent proponents has been Piaget. Within special education, Kephart (1971), Barsch

(1965, 1967a,b,c), and Getman and Hendrickson (1966) have written widely on the topic. Clearly we must pay the motor system some attention too.

Movement is the function of the motor system, writes Gomez (1978). And even simple movements are surprisingly complicated matters except perhaps at the simplest type of spinal reflex, e.g., when the tendon of the kneecap is lightly tapped by a hammer. Movement depends on posture, which is dependent on muscle tone. It must be coordinated in order to be effective. It has gross motor components and also fine motor components. Movement influences the sensory system and in turn is modified by the latter. The principles of hierarchical functioning that prevail for sensory information processing also prevail for motor information processing.

Descending Pathways

In our discussion of the sensory system (the ascending pathways of the nervous system) we moved from receptors, i.e., sense organs, to the cortex. It is appropriate that in discussing the motor system—the CNS's descending pathways—we describe it in reverse order, moving from cortex to effector (muscle) (see Figure 3–7). This motor system is typically divided into the higher motor and lower motor systems, the former comprising those parts of the brain and spinal cord that actually activate muscles.

The higher motor system is typically divided by neuroscientists into two separate components: the pyramidal and extrapyramidal. These two components are intimately involved with each other, both anatomically and functionally. The pyramidal system (so-called because its neurons look like pyramids) consists of the cortical motor cells that comprise the primary motor cortex. Some of the axons of these cells (the cortical-bulbar pyramidal tracts) terminate in the lower brain stem, making contact with the motor neurons of the cranial nerves that activate the muscles of the head and its sense organs. The axons of still other pyramidal neurons (the cortical-spinal tract) terminate in the spinal cord, where they control and activate the motor cells of the spinal nerves and cause muscular movements.

The pyramidal and extrapyramidal systems thus affect much the same motor neurons in the lower motor system. However, the path of the pyramidal system is a relatively direct one while the extrapyramidal system "cascades in synaptic relationships at various segmental levels" (Gomez, 1978, p. 133). Figure 3–7 presents the sequencing of events in the motor system, from cerebrum to muscular activation.

The pyramidal system is responsible for voluntary movement, i.e., those we associate with conscious willed activities that involve fine control. The motor activities of the extrapyramidal system are responsible for primitive and instinctual movements and those of a phasic nature that do not require direct attention, e.g., walking, chewing, and breathing.

CENTRAL INTEGRATION PROCESSING

Distinctions are made in neurology and neuropsychology between the transmission of information in the nervous system, both afferent and efferent, and the central integration of that information. The term *central integration processing* emphasizes the nervous system's role in managing, organizing, and controlling information, in a coordinated and directed fashion (Gomez, 1978). It also accentuates the nervous system's continuous activity; i.e., it is always, and at all times, processing information. What, however, does the word *central* imply?

Figure 3–7 Descending Pathways of the Sensory System

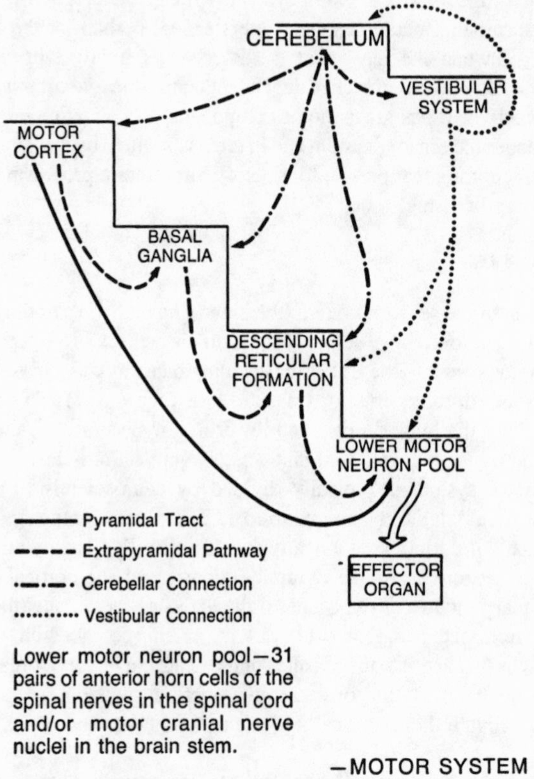
CEREBELLUM
VESTIBULAR SYSTEM
MOTOR CORTEX
BASAL GANGLIA
DESCENDING RETICULAR FORMATION
LOWER MOTOR NEURON POOL
EFFECTOR ORGAN
Pyramidal Tract
Extrapyramidal Pathway
Cerebellar Connection
Vestibular Connection
Lower motor neuron pool—31 pairs of anterior horn cells of the spinal nerves in the spinal cord and/or motor cranial nerve nuclei in the brain stem.
—MOTOR SYSTEM

Source: Reprinted from *Common Neurologic and Language Disorders* by A.J. Gomez with permission of Center for Disorders of Communication, Medical Center Hospital of Vermont, © 1978.

We have shown that information integration proceeds even at the single neuron level. However, when we talk about central integration processing, we are considering the activities of the nervous system as a system and more specifically the component known as the *central nervous system*: the spine and the brain, particularly the brain.

In our discussion of the sensory and motor systems we have examined the flow of information from receptor organ through the ascending pathways of the nervous system, and the transmission of motor impulses from brain and spine down the descending system to muscle effectors and glands. Nevertheless, it is the nervous system's integration of the information flow of the sensory and motor systems that constitutes the basis of what we ordinarily consider to be cognition.

Basic to the nervous system capacity for integration are those of its cells and regions that function in an association capacity. The word *association* in this case means just what it says, that is, association neurons in the nervous system whose major role is to associate, i.e., bring into relationships, the activities of other neurons.

Association cells are found at all levels of the nervous system. They increase in numbers and the complexity of relationships as we move up from the spine through the brain into the higher layers of the cortex.

Most of the neurons in the cortex (80 percent) are association neurons, e.g., internuncial ones. They do not have any direct sensory or motor roles. Their job appears rather to be the integration, interpretation, storage of information, and the utilization of that information to affect behavior. These neurons relate the various parts of the brain to each other. And they interpret the information processed at specific points of the brain within the broader contexts of information being processed elsewhere.

Earlier in this chapter we saw that all of the body's senses project their information to specific parts of the brain, i.e., primary sensory zones. Around these areas are secondary association zones that interpret the information received in the primary zones on the basis of previously learned (memory) information and from information that comes in from other parts of the brain. There are also outer association zones; these further extend the information range of the sensory zones. The outer zones overlap each other and as such fuse the information received from a number of senses.

The motor areas of the brain have similar zones. There are primary zones, secondary association ones, and so on; the outer motor and outer sensory association zones overlap each other or bring memory and motor information together.

The importance of the nervous system's associative activities can be understood from the standpoint of language. Specific parts of the cortex initially receive auditory signals. Other parts of the cortex specifically create the muscular innervations of throat and mouth muscles that create speech. Language emerges from these simple ingredients through the nervous system's associative mechanisms, which elaborate sensory and motor nerve impulses into complicated cognitive patterns.

THE RELATIONSHIP OF COGNITION TO NEUROLOGICAL FUNCTIONING

Our considerations to this point certainly help us to understand how the elements of the nervous system combine to work in cognition. But how does cognition actually come about?

This question cannot fully be answered any more than we can answer exactly how the universe works. We are still guessing. Our knowledge about the nervous system is expanding, but there are many unanswered questions. Some neurological scientists, e.g., Eccles (Popper & Eccles, 1977) and before him Sherrington (1906), believed that cognition can never be fully understood in terms of the physical functioning of the nervous system, that the mind somehow uses the brain and the rest of the nervous system but is yet something apart from it. This point of view corresponds with theological views of an immortal soul that is separate and distinct from the body.

Other neuroscientists believe that all cognitive functioning will in the end be entirely reduced to and explained by the nervous system and its functions, that it is just a matter of time till we are able to do so (Gerschwind, 1980). The debate continues.

Another area of debate, however, is unresolved. This concerns the degree to which the nervous system is preprogrammed by heredity and biology to produce certain types of cognitive activities. Are cognitive abilities and our behaviors basically innate, present at birth, or physically programmed to emerge at certain stages of development? Or are we what we are, and do we do what we do mostly on the basis of our learning experiences? B.F.

Skinner, the great behaviorist, has taken the latter position. He (1957) once tried to explain language entirely in terms of behavior in learning. His opinions were, however, challenged by psycholinguists like Chomsky (1957) and Lenneberg (1974), who have made a strong case for language being an innate ability that is made possible only because of the human nervous system's special characteristics.

Research tends to favor the view that there are certain biological formations related to cognitive characteristics within our nervous systems that are programmed or that affect cognitive functions at different times. Nevertheless, it is also true that experiences, including education, can modify the functioning of our nervous systems to a considerable degree.

What we do know beyond a shadow of a doubt is that all cognitive functioning relies on neurological functioning. Substances and experiences that improve or impair the efficiency of the latter also improve or impair cognition. Genetic defects, or developmental disabilities that damage specific parts of the nervous system, usually cause specific types of cognitive disability. Thus damage to specific parts of the cortex's occipital lobe (the visual cortex) damages our ability to perceive specific types of visual information. Damage to certain parts of the temporal lobe usually produces impaired ability to understand or produce speech. Damage to the amygdala and inferior portion of the temporal lobe can result in inability to remember experiences. So there is no doubt at all that whatever the exact relationship of cognition to the nervous system, the former is dependent on the latter.

ENCODING AND DECODING IN THE NERVOUS SYSTEM

At this point in our narrative we must wrestle with the question of how the stimulation of our receptor (sense) organs gets turned into information of the sort that we call *cognition*. We have used the term *wrestle* advisedly, for we surely cannot give any definitive answer.

What we do know is that the stimulation of our senses is translated into neural impulses and that the latter are elaborated into codes, thanks to the special physical properties of neurons and neuronal networks. Somehow cognition is associated with all of this. Those phenomena we call *perception, memory, reasoning, problem solving*, etc., are the consequence.

How does stimulation become cognition? The ancients believed that copies of the objects stimulating our sense organs somehow passed into our bodies as sensations and were recalled as images. The color blue, for example, went into our mind as "blue" and was stored in the form of that color. They did not know about neural impulses. We do know that our nervous system somehow takes the information impinging on our senses and reduces it to some sort of manageable codes that somehow make up cognition.

Some of these nerves are icons; that is, they resemble the stimulus, e.g., perceptions and images. Others may be analog ones, having direct physical relationships to the information coded though not reproducing the information in its original form. Music provides us with an example of how analog information is coded. In recording, musical information can be encoded in the form of little hills and valleys and irregularities scratched out in the grooves of phonograph disks or by rearranging metal molecules on a cassette tape.

Still another type of neural code used in cognition may resemble digital variety. The most complex types of written information—pictures, etc.—can be reduced by a computer to binary sequences of numbers 0s and 1s. Music can also be recorded on a digital basis; i.e., its sounds are translated into a series of digits that when decoded, recreate the original music. And there are cameras that can record visual images through digital coding. The utilization of codes to direct central motor behavior is easily understood on the basis of recent developments in robotics. In robotics, computers can code information from the environment and then decode it to direct machine-performed motor activities.

The holograph is still another way in which the nervous system may encode information. In holographic recording, the original form of the stimulus is broken into little fragments, which are stored in different molecules of the recording matter. Stimulation of any of these molecules is enough to create an image of the entire original stimulus. Neurologist Karl Pribam believes that this may be a major way that information is stored in the nervous system (1977, 1978).

Other neuroscientists believe that neural encoding of information may result from changes in the concentration of neurotransmitters in various neural tissues or through molecular changes in the neuron itself. Still others believe that changes in synaptic relationships are the basis of encoding. There may be a variety of different ways in which the nervous system codes information. But coding must exist in order for cognition to be managed by the nervous system.

LOCALIZATION OF COGNITIVE FUNCTIONS

Are different types of cognition located in different parts of the brain? Are different parts of the brain responsible for different types of cognition? These questions continue to be two of the oldest and most hotly debated in neuroscience.

We do know that motor and sensory functions of our bodies are precisely associated with specific parts of the cerebral cortex, that they are actually mapped out in our cortex. We can also trace the pathways between specific parts of the brain and our senses and muscles.

The disagreement concerns the so-called higher cognitive processes, i.e., those of perception, language, reasoning, problem solving, and memory; can these be neatly and precisely delegated to specific parts of the brain? Here the situation becomes controversial. There is no doubt that damage or excision (removal by surgery) of certain parts of the brain usually results in major damage to certain cognitive functions. Broca's area is a part of the cortex on the posterior margin of the frontal lobe. Damage to it almost always results in the loss or impairment of spoken speech. Similarly damage to Wernicke's area in the temporal lobe usually impairs the understanding of language. And such techniques as PETT are demonstrating that certain specific parts of the brain are more active than others during various kinds of cognitive activity.

However, there are still many unanswered questions. For one, there are many cases on record where parts of the brain have been damaged or removed; these parts were supposed to be essential for particular types of cognition yet the latter went on unimpaired. It is also a mistake to assume that because we damage a certain part of the brain and then find a particular type of cognition impaired, this part of the brain is specifically responsible for that type of cognition. Assuming this to be true is no more legitimate than to assume that a light switch creates light. Clearly there is more to the latter than a switch in an on position. So it is with the brain that even damage to a particular part of the brain impairs certain cognitive processes. This does not mean that the part is the only part responsible for other processes or that it is even the most important part for those processes. Luria, a major neurological psychologist, prefers to talk about neurons throughout different parts of the nervous system working together in functional systems to create particular cognitive activities. Disturb or damage any physical component of a system, and the whole system will not function effectively. Replace that physical component with another part of the nervous system, and we can restore the functional system to working order. There is evidence that this happens when individuals recover from brain injuries; i.e., they may do so by using parts of the brain that were previously not used in cognitive activities to carry on or replace the activity of parts irrevocably damaged (Luria, 1966).

The holographic storage theory suggested by Pribam also goes beyond the idea of simple localization. He (1977, 1978) suggests that information is holographically stored in specific parts of the brain, in fact over a variety of neural nuclei at different levels of the brain, allowing any part, when activated, to reproduce *all* of the information stored by other parts.

Still another "holistic" theory of brain functioning has been recently suggested by Johns and Schwartz (1978). They do not believe that cognitive activities can be conceived of as being assigned to specific parts of the brain. They believe rather that cognition should be understood as being comprised of electrochemical patterns involving large areas of the brain. An idea of how this might take place comes from television. The television screen is of uniform composition over its surface, and yet different patterns of information can be displayed on it at different times. Does the brain work this way too, with different cognitive activities represented by different brain patterns that come and go as our cognitive processes change? How can one explain memory this way? It is a repetition of the same pattern.

There are different ways of conceptualizing localization of cognition within the brain. Even when brain damage is a specifically localized cognitive defect, the defect is also likely to cause general cognitive impairments as well, e.g., a loss of ability to cope with new problems or to inhibit behavior indirectly, or perhaps a general dulling of all abilities.

Popular Views

Despite these reservations, remedial and special educators should become familiar with common ideas about the location of higher cognitive processes in the brain—even if they may not be altogether correct.

The frontal lobes of the cerebral hemispheres are usually assigned responsibilities for conscious thought, imagination, creative thinking, judgment, some aspects of memory, abstract thought, and control over emotions. In one of the frontal lobe's margins (the left in 90 percent of the population) is a small motor region important to spoken speech: Broca's area.

Damage to the frontal lobe has been associated with inability to recall facts that have just been learned as well as a loss of memory for such basic information as one's name and address. Individuals with damaged frontal lobes have been found to display poor judgment and a loss of the ability to engage in abstract thinking. When the latter happens, the individual may be able to think only in terms of the here and now and to deal with concrete objects; the person may have difficulties in seeing relationships and similarities and in formulating general ideas. If Broca's area specifically is affected, there are disturbances in spoken speech.

The parietal lobe responds with conscious awareness to bodily sensations. It also integrates motor and sensory information so as to guide voluntary behavior in meaningful ways. Impairments of the parietal lobe can result in disturbances of feeling, movement, and body image.

The temporal lobe is the auditory lobe. It receives auditory sensations and integrates and interprets them. Our receptive language centers are located here. Damage to the temporal lobe's primary auditory zone results in deafness. Damage to the secondary auditory association areas causes problems in the understanding of oral and written communication.

Visual functions are related to the occipital lobe, which receives fibers from the retina. Damage to the occipital lobe's primary visual zones can cause cortical blindness, i.e., an inability to see even though the eyes and the optic nerve are intact and functioning. If there is damage to its visual association zones, the individual may be able to see but be unable to recognize or understand what is being seen or have difficulties in visual recall and memory.

It should be remembered in all of this that all of the brain is in a real sense usually involved in the functioning of each of its parts. Furthermore, lower neurological centers affect the cognitive functions carried out by the higher centers so that damage to the former can impair the effectiveness of the latter.

CEREBRAL DOMINANCE

Cerebral dominance refers to the generally held conception that in normal adults and children (after a certain age) either the one or the other cerebral hemisphere becomes dominant over the other and generally speaking controls cognition. This belief appears to have developed in large part because the left hemisphere is dominant in respect to speech and language in most people and because most people are right-handed—the right hand being controlled by the left hemisphere. Cerebral dominance has been a popular theory. It received particular credibility in the 1930s through work carried out by Samuel Orton and his followers (1928).

According to Orton the left hemisphere is biologically dominant in most people, though in a few the right hemisphere is dominant. The important thing, as far as Orton was concerned, is that one hemisphere be dominant. This, he believed, makes normal cognitive functioning possible. If dominance is not established or is incomplete, cognitive confusion and disorganization are likely.

Orton wrote that in perceiving things the visual areas in the right and left brains create images that are exactly alike except for opposite orientations. Ordinarily the dominant hemisphere suppresses the images of the other hemisphere. If this doesn't happen, our minds may pick up images from both hemispheres and become confused. This may cause a student to reverse letters or the order of words in a sentence when reading. Or for that matter the student may not be able to tell correctly printed words from their reversals. Handwriting difficulties and problems in left and right orientation are other problems that can arise. Orton believed that dyslexia is created by lack of cerebral dominance.

More recently Silver and Hagin (1976) have emphasized that learning disabilities may be due to failure in dominance. Theodore Blau (1977) believes childhood schizophrenia can be explained in terms of dominance.

For a long while, in large part because of Orton, the left hemisphere was regarded in most cognitively well-organized people as being the master cerebral hemisphere. Then a series of research was carried out that suggested the idea of dominance may have led neuroscientists and educators to overlook the importance of right hemispheric functioning.

THE TWO HEMISPHERES

The left hemisphere has usually been credited with being the dominant or master hemisphere. This was largely on the basis of speech appearing to be localized there in the vast majority of people. The right hemisphere was considered a lesser, silent hemisphere whose purpose perhaps was largely that of providing a support system for the cognitive functioning of its left mate. For example, it is known that if the left hemisphere is damaged severely in early childhood, the right hemisphere is able to take over in respect to speech, though there is some loss of efficiency when this occurs (Teuber, 1974).

Gradually comparison of patients who had either left or right hemisphere damage began to increase our appreciation of the right hemisphere's role in cognition. Such research demonstrated that the left hemisphere is generally more essential to verbal abilities but that the right hemisphere is generally important for visual-motor and visual-spatial skills.

However, research done with individuals whose cognitive functions are impaired as a consequence of brain damage or surgical removal of brain tissue is rarely clear-cut for a variety of reasons. It is hard to isolate the effects of these procedures. Other brain structures besides the specific areas that are injured or incised may be affected, e.g., by shock, loss of blood supply, the damage to nerve fibers connecting the affected part of the brain with others. Also the cognitive processes that we observe after damage or tissue removal represent the efforts of the rest of the brain to function despite the losses it has incurred, i.e., to manage and compensate for its losses. Thus the information from such research was not sufficient to show how the cerebral hemispheres worked.

New techniques and new strategies of study and research and an explosion of both information and speculation appeared and are still resounding. A major breakthrough is the epochal work of Roger Sperry and his associates (Sperry, Gazzaniga, & Bogen, 1969). Sperry in the early 1950s suggested severing the corpus callosum in epilepsy-prone individuals to control the interhemispheric spread of the disease. This method, i.e., hemispherectomy, did in fact help control epilepsy to a considerable degree. But Sperry also discovered that sectioning, i.e., cutting through, the corpus callosum—as was some- times done to control the spread of epilepsy—separated the right and left hemispheres from each other in terms of their functioning. The corpus callosum is the largest nerve tract in the brain, and it is the one responsible for interchange of information between the two hemispheres. Severing it isolated the two halves of the brain and allowed them to be studied separately and distinctly from each other in terms of their cognitive processes. That is, severing the corpus callosum in effect seems to create two separate brains in terms of the cognitive performance of left and right hemispheres. Visual, tactual, auditory, olfactory, and kinesthetic stimuli and various questions, commands, and problems could be presented to either the right or left brains without the other one having any conscious knowledge about what was going on. It is true that even with the corpus callosum severed, the two halves of the brain still communicated to some degree through the lower brain components that remained unsevered. But generally speaking, they appeared to work separately, and it quickly became clear that the two hemispheres functioned in different ways cognitively. "Split brain" studies have cast much light on the differing cognitive roles that the two brain hemispheres play and have changed many earlier ideas about cerebral dominance. Now it appears that each hemisphere is dominant, though in different areas.

Another medical method of studying hemispheric differences that has helped confirm Sperry's work is the Wada method (Hiscock & Kinsbourne, 1980). In this method sodium amytal is injected into one cerebral hemisphere, temporarily paralyzing it. This allows the cognitive functions of the other one to be studied in relative isolation.

Noninvasive methods have also been used to study hemispheric differences. These have relied on visual, auditory, and tactile asymmetries in hemispheric processes (Hiscock & Kinsbourne, 1980). Though the two hemispheres communicate constantly with each other in normal individuals, there is neural decussation or crossover. This means, for example, that in normal individuals auditory and tactile information from the right side of the head and body are first projected to the left hemisphere and then passed through the corpus callosum to the right hemisphere. As a consequence the left hemisphere receives such right-side information first, i.e., before the right hemisphere. The right hemisphere receives left-side auditory information first.

In audition these asymmetries have been particularly exploited through the dichotic listening techniques developed by Kimura (1961, 1963, 1967). In dichotic listening, stereophonic headphones are put on a subject, and competing sounds are sent through each of the headphones. One type of sound arrives at the left ear at the very moment that a different sound arrives at the right ear. When the sounds are of a linguistic nature, e.g., words, nonsense syllables, and digits, the left ear is favored; i.e., normal adults or children report hearing the sort of information in their right ears prior to their left ears. On the other hand, nonlinguistic sounds like environmental sounds, musical chords, and aspects of loudness or softness fail to produce this right-ear advantage and indeed often yield a left-ear one (Hiscock & Kinsbourne, 1980).

The crossover phenomenon is also at work in tactile phenomena. Thus the tactile input from the index finger of the right hand projects to the left hemisphere and that from the right to the left hemisphere. By capitalizing on this, a right-finger advantage for recognizing three-dimensional nonsense shapes in normal people has been rejected (Kinsbourne, 1980).

In other experiments subjects have been asked to engage in motor activities with either left or right hands. They were given conflicting types of verbal directions at the same time. This was found to interfere more with the activities of the right hand than of the left. This was expected because both language and right-hand operations are left-brain controlled. The left brain has to split its operations, so to speak, to process both language and right-hand motor activities at the same time, if one disputed with the other, whereas the right hemisphere, which is relatively free of language responsibilities, would be less encumbered by conflicting verbal directions.

Visual decussation is quite different from auditory and tactile crossover and presents more problems in the study of left-right hemispheric differences. The visual information from both eyes simultaneously projects to both hemispheres. The crossover in the brain is accomplished on the basis of retinal splits. That is, nerve fibers from the retinal half of each eye that is closest to the nose project to the hemisphere on the same side as that eye, i.e., left retina to left hemisphere, right retina to right hemisphere. On the other hand the retinal half of each eye that is closest to the ear projects to the opposite, i.e., left retina to right hemisphere, right retina to left hemisphere. Thus stereographic vision is achieved.

It is obviously more difficult to make hemispheric distinctions on the basis of visual inputs. However, some success has been accomplished. Thus we are able to block off visually left-hemisphere or right-hemisphere parts of the retinas while stimulating the other halves. Or we can present flash stimuli so that they are seen in one part of the eye or another. Bryden and Herron thus found that verbal stimuli, e.g., words or letters, are more likely to be perceived under conditions of short exposure when flashed in the right-half visual field (left hemisphere) (Hiscock & Kinsbourne, 1980).

Hemispheric Differences in Cognition

For a while, in the excitement of the new insights provided by Sperry and associates, it became popular to talk about the left and right hemispheres as being two brains, separate and distinct from each other. This was partly due to the fact that much of the early research had been done with people whose cortexes had been split into two and truly separated.

Neuroscientists are now more cautious. They recognize that in normal people the two hemispheres are in continuous communication through the corpus callosum, that they constantly work together. For that matter the two hemispheres continue to communicate through subcortical associations in the thalamus even in patients in whom the corpus callosum has been fully severed.

Thus talk about right-brain education and attempts to train the different hemispheres as suggested by some educators are often useless. Are there, however, certain cognitive activities—cognitive processes—that are specifically dependent on the left hemisphere while others are specifically dependent on the right hemisphere?

The consensus of some of the more sophisticated researchers is that there is indeed specialization of a considerable degree and that this is present from early in life. Broadly speaking, it has been suggested that the right hemisphere tends to provide a general framework for cognition, while the left hemisphere processes the specific units to be integrated in that framework (Kinsbourne, 1983). There appear to be some more specific distinctions as well.

The left hemisphere appears to be more specialized for language functions than is the right. It is also able to deal better with sequential, linear types of information, i.e., symbolic information that is processed in a step-by-step progression or linear sequence. The left hemisphere appears to analyze information more effectively, systematically, and logically. It has indeed sometimes been described as the computer part of the brain. The right hemisphere on the other hand has been described as being better able than the left hemisphere to deal with holistic or parallel types of information. It is also more effective in coping with the general aspects of a problem. The recognition of faces is more dependent on the right hemisphere. The right hemisphere appears more responsive for artistic and creative and intuitive thinking. The left hemisphere works better symbolically while the right hemisphere processes nonverbal information more effectively than does the left hemisphere. It seems to play the dominant role in spatial and mechanical thinking.

The right hemisphere is generally attentive to the general shapes of words, while the left hemisphere sequentially deals with the letters and translates them into verbal symbols. The right hemisphere is sensitive to pitch, volume, the emotional characteristics of voices, and the aspects of certain vowels. The left hemisphere is responsive to consonants and decodes sound to create the acoustic codes that become language.

These distinctions are but some of the ones made between the functioning of the left and right brains. They have given rise to many speculations. It has been proposed that one of the differences between men and women is that the former are more left-brain dominant. Female sensitivity is attributed to more communication (through the corpus callosum) between the two hemispheres in women than in men. Some writers have written fancifully of the left hemisphere representing repressive modern industrialized civilization, while the right hemisphere stands for the artistic and creative aspects of humankind. In the speech that nominated Sperry for a Nobel prize (1981) it was proposed that the eastern world is right-brain oriented while the western world is a left-brain society and that this accounts for differences in life styles and the problems of communication between the east and west.

Much of this speculation will prove fanciful. Other speculation will probably never be proven one way or another. What does appear apparent, however, is that both brain halves partake in all cognitive functions but that one hemisphere or the other is also specialized to various degrees and in a sense controls certain cognitive functions. In most of us the left brain is lateralized for language from a rather early age. In fact it has been speculated that because the responsibilities for language are assumed by the left hemisphere early in life, other cognitive functions such as visual-motor ones are relegated to the right hemisphere.

Each hemisphere may be able to carry out the functions of the other in case of damage. Recovery of cognitive functioning after brain injury, in fact, may depend on different types of brain structures, in one way or the other, taking over for damaged ones. The period of development in which damage takes place is most important in this respect. Thus damage to the left hemisphere in an infant does not as significantly impair language functioning as in an older individual. In young children the language processes that cannot be supported by the left hemisphere can be shifted somewhat to the right one. There is, however, some loss in all abilities when this happens because of a crowding of cognitive processes in the undamaged hemisphere.

Some experts feel that our educational system tends to favor training of left-brain cognitive functions over right-brain. They recommend that this neglect be overcome by more emphasis in school on right-brain education, e.g., in art and music. A Bulgarian psychiatrist, Georgi Lozanov, has received publicity in this country for his method of Suggestopedia. This seeks to train the right brain through special methods while the left brain is being trained through regular education. While learning a foreign language (left-brain activity), a student will have to simultaneously listen to classical music (a right-brain activity). The pupils also learn to conjugate verbs via songs (involving both left and right brains simultaneously).

Are hemispheric differences responsible for specific types of learning problems? There is evidence that impairments of left-hemispheric functioning have devastating effects on language abilities, spoken and written, while those of the right hemisphere are more likely to disrupt spatial and manipulative skills. More specific problems have also been found. For example, Hecaen and Marcie compared right- and left-hemispheric lesions on a writing task. In the case of the right hemisphere, right-hemispheric injuries appear only marginally related to writing problems, affecting the interaction of letter strokes and resulting in the enlargement of the right-hand margin. In left-hemispheric lesions there seems to be a loss of continuity in writing words (Hiscock & Kinsbourne, 1980).

But can we attribute specific learning disabilities to left-brain–right-brain differences when both hemispheres are undamaged? For example, some learning disabilities may be due to over- or underdevelopment of one or the other of the hemispheres. The results have not been consistent (Satz, 1976). In fact some of the results have gone contrary to prediction. Poor readers do better in right-half retinal studies than do normal ones, when one would expect the opposite to be true if the left hemisphere is more important than the right one in reading. Reviews of cerebral lateralization and learning problems are available from Hiscock (1983); Kinsbourne (1983) and Hiscock and Kinsbourne (1980) make it clear that it is difficult to establish direct and reliable relationships between particular characteristics or functions of the brain and specific cognitive abilities and disabilities. This is also true for left-brain–right-brain distinctions. Nevertheless we will probably find more definitive relationships as we continue to study brain-behavior relationships. Our knowledge base about the latter is expanding at an ever more rapid rate.

Chapter 4

Intelligence

Intelligence has been one of the most important and influential of the cognitive constructs in both remedial and special education. With our long history of studying intelligence, and its derivative, the IQ, one might think that there would be some agreement as to what intelligence is, how we best go about assessing it, and what role it should play in education. Such, unfortunately, is not at all the case.

There have always been violent disagreements about this cognitive construct. Many of today's disputes were voiced in the early 1900s when the first popular test of intelligence appeared. Intelligence and the IQ were, are, and will continue to be controversial topics.

Many people would like to do away with the idea of intelligence altogether. Some of them believe that it is an outmoded concept that cannot be justified scientifically and that attempts to assess it lack educational and social value (Ebel, 1979; Lewontin, Steven, & Kamin, 1984). Some educators, psychologists, and sociologists believe that intelligence quotients and similar scores result in unfair estimates of people's abilities and thus in serious negative consequences, e.g., for children from minority groups (Garcia, 1981, Hilliard, 1979; Mercer, 1973; Mercer & Lewis, 1979). Some scholars believe that they are altogether racist in their implications (Kamin, 1974). Some educators have often criticized IQs as creating incomplete and misleading pictures of what handicapped individuals can do (Traver & Ellsworth, 1981). Teachers organizations such as the National Educational Association (NEA) criticize intelligence testing on the grounds that it doesn't provide useful guides to teachers and it is sometimes used to hold them accountable (unfairly) for their pupils' failures to achieve.

If this were not burden enough for any cognitive construct to bear, intelligence faces the additional problem that even among its supporters, i.e., those who strongly agree about the value of the concept, there are great disagreements as to what intelligence really consists and the best ways to go about evaluating it.

Yet the idea of intelligence and the efforts to assess it continue to engage the efforts of some of the finest minds in psychology and education and to receive general popular acceptance. How is this possible? One reason for this is simply that the construct has proven useful in many ways, e.g., in schools, hospitals, the armed services, for job selection. Whatever faults the critics have found with it, it continues to have practical utility. It gives us pretty good predictions as to how well people will do in school and in many other areas of life (Cooley, 1976; Cronbach & Snow, 1977; Jensen, 1979).

Another reason why intelligence has survived attacks on it as a construct is that it serves as a meaningful, explanatory term. It continues to be useful in explaining success and failure under a variety of circumstances. That is, it helps us to explain and to understand why some pupils in schools do better than others, why some individuals succeed in jobs while others fail. And it is this explanatory value of the construct that perhaps best explains why we continue to use it. Indeed we all have become so familiar with the term *intelligence* as an explanation that almost everybody uses the term on an everyday basis—even those critics who would like to do away with the idea of intelligence altogether.

A third reason for the persistence of this much debated and controversial cognitive construct—intelligence—is the possibility that it stands for personal qualities that are real and important to our lives (Anastasi, 1983). So that even if it is not fully understood at the present time (which is generally agreed by all) and even if it is often misused (which is also often agreed), it still seems worthy of our study and consideration. In particular, intelligence in its various forms seems to us to be a cognitive construct of considerable importance for remedial and special educators, and it is from the standpoint of its being a cognitive construct that we approach it in this chapter.

THE STUDY OF INTELLIGENCE

The reader is probably acutely aware of the fact that we have not as yet provided any definitions of intelligence. This avoidance has been intentional. We want first to provide an appropriate perspective for our study of the topic before proceeding to a consideration of its definitions. Definitions are provided later. For the meanwhile, readers should rely on their own ideas of what intelligence is to guide them. In its most basic and most frequently used sense, intelligence is a commonsense construct, i.e., one that corresponds with what people generally think about people's abilities.

Intelligence As a Label for Intelligent Behavior

Let us begin our approach to the study of intelligence by conceding that it is, first of all, a descriptive term. That is, it is a name that identifies observable behaviors that we call *intelligent*, i.e., "observable portion[s] of the individual's overall behavior, behavior produced in the context of the everyday natural environment, as well as with . . . intelligence tests and in laboratory situations" (Charlesworth, 1976, p. 148). These include behaviors that result in high grades on a social studies test or on the *SAT*s. They also include behaviors that one chess player uses to checkmate another and allow some individuals to succeed in business while their competitors fail. Such are the types of behaviors that we might call intelligent because they succeed with problems. It is obvious that people differ to the degree in which they engage in such intelligent behaviors; i.e., some demonstrate more of them, and others less.

Some behavioral scientists would limit the use of intelligence, both as a term and an explanation, to such descriptions. Thus Chein (1945) contended, "No psychologist has ever observed *intelligence*: many have observed intelligent behavior" (p. 111). It is "an attribute of behavior, not an attribute of a person" (p. 120). In other words he advises us not to think of intelligence as something that characterizes an individual or belongs to a person but rather as a descriptive label that identifies certain types of behavior. Along these lines we can talk about a person demonstrating generally intelligent behavior, i.e., as being successful in dealing with a broad range of problems and in a variety of situations. We can also talk about individuals demonstrating specific types of observable intelligent behavior, i.e., as being able to solve certain types of problems, in certain types of situations—but not doing well with other types of problems or in other situations.

Intelligence As a Comparison of Individuals

Another way of studying intelligence is in terms of comparisons made between individuals. Intelligence usually implies that someone is able to do better (or worse) than others in certain ways (Conger, 1959; Jensen, 1979). We almost always think of intelligence in a comparative way. Some cognitive scientists have observed that our modern usage of the idea of intelligence could never have developed except through comparing people with each other. In this way it is quite different from other cognitive constructs like those of learning and memory. We can study a pupil in isolation when learning. For example, we can see how long it takes the student to learn a list of spelling words, to become competent in solving trigonometry problems, or to tie shoe laces neatly. We can also study a single person's memory efforts in recalling a memorized paragraph or in identifying something seen in the past. However, intelligence is almost always studied in terms of someone being more or less intelligent or having more or less intelligence as compared to others, though the comparisons we make are not always conscious ones. And, of course, tests of intelligence compare people.

Intelligence As a Cognitive Explanation

We have observed that intelligence can be discussed in behavioral terms and that it implies comparison. Beyond these two aspects, *intelligence*, of course, is also a term used to identify hypothetical inner qualities in an individual, i.e., potentials, capacities, abilities, that are presumed to account for individual differences in achievement (intelligent behavior). The following definition by Conger (1959) makes this point very well: "intelligence is not a thing in any tangible sense. We cannot see it, touch it or hear it. It is purely a hypothetical construct, a scientific fiction, like the concept of force in physics. We invent it because it helps us explain and predict behavior" (Robinson & Robinson, 1976, pp. 14–15).

Intelligence, as a hypothetical cognitive construct that presumably causes or is otherwise responsible for intelligent behavior, and for differences in people's achievements, is the focus of this particular chapter. An important consideration along these lines is that we typically consider intelligence to represent cognitive capacities, abilities, or potentials, that are stable and persist over time; i.e., we consider intelligence as a more or less constant property of an individual. This issue of stability and persistence over time is an important one. Intelligence is not a hit-and-miss or now-and-then characteristic of individuals. Almost anyone can occasionally behave in an intelligent way. We would not, however, consider the individual as being really intelligent or having good intelligence unless consistently able to carry out such behaviors. Similarly on any given occasion any person may appear severely deficient in intelligence—even if quite intelligent. It would be a grave error to infer strengths or weaknesses in intelligence on the basis of a single or occasional observation—or test.

Intelligence, then, as a cognitive construct is usually interpreted as being an enduring characteristic, property, or trait of the individual. We can also study intelligence from the standpoint of its ongoing processes, e.g., in terms of the cognitive processes a pupil engages in, when dealing with particular situations requiring intelligent behavior (Neisser, 1976; Sternberg, 1981). In such studies we are interested in intelligence as an activity rather than as a structure or property of the mind. There has been increasing interest in this type of approach.

PROBLEMS IN ASSESSING INTELLIGENCE

Many of the controversies that confront remedial and special educators when they discuss intelligence are not over the construct itself but rather over the means we use to assess it. Many scientists and practitioners believe that the construct of intelligence is a meaningful one but disagree violently about current ways of evaluating its existence and operations. Almost always the controversies concern the use of tests to assess intelligence (or IQ, which has come to be a synonym in many people's minds for intelligence).

Many legitimate objections have been raised about the use of intelligence tests, e.g., to assess the ability of minority groups on the basis of tests developed for white, middle-class populations, which may cover items that are not familiar to the members of minority groups (Garcia, 1981; Hilliard, 1979). Other objections contend that intelligence tests are too strongly influenced by environmental factors and the kind of schooling an individual receives to provide a fair estimate of true ability. Indeed, some important researchers feel that the whole idea of intelligence tests should be abandoned on such grounds while others keep trying to develop tests that are "culture fair" (Cattell, 1979; Mercer & Lewis, 1979) and still others try to estimate ability from behavioral estimates (Fogelman, 1974). This chapter is not primarily concerned with the issues of testing intelligence. However, we cannot altogether separate the issues of assessing intelligence from other ones involving the construct.

HISTORICAL UNDERSTANDING OF INTELLIGENCE

The word *intelligence* is derived from the Latin term *inter legere*, which means to bring together. It was introduced into the English language in the fourteenth century and defined at that time as the faculty, i.e., ability, of understanding (Frank, 1976). Latin and English interpretations of the construct still have these connotations.

However, it was not until the nineteenth century, when Charles Darwin's theory of evolution became a dominant force within western science, that British psychologist Herbert Spencer (1820–1903) redefined intelligence in the form that was to guide modern developments. Spencer conceived of intelligence as being a special cognitive force that organisms (animals as well as humans) utilize to adapt to the demands of their environments. He described it as developing to higher and higher levels through evolution and as being used competitively, i.e., to determine survival of the fittest. Different species differ in intelligence. And within each species, there are intraspecies differences; its membership manifests intelligence in different degrees.

This original interpretation of intelligence, i.e., in terms of adaptation, is still very much with us. Thus Wechsler (1944) has explained the results obtained from his tests in terms of adaptation.

Sir Francis Galton (1822–1911), another British psychologist, developed Spencer's idea (Mann, 1979). Galton tried to find out why some individuals were successful while others failed, and he developed a variety of tests to study people's abilities for this purpose.

Galton's investigations took place at a time when there were two major views of the mind. One was that it is composed of innate separate faculties (abilities) such as perception, memory, judgment, imagination, and reasoning. The other view was that the mind consists of many distinct tiny mental elements derived from sensations (created by our modalities and muscles) that become associated with each other so as to form the mind and all of its components. Galton took the latter position. His tests thus focused on sensory and motor responses. He believed that the more mental elements one is able to associate together, the brighter that individual is; the mentally retarded are deficient in the associations they can make.

According to Galton the associations formed between elementary mental elements are developed into various specific abilities. However, in their sum they also constitute general ability. It is this general ability, he believed, that is crucial to success or failure in life. He identified it as intelligence.

Subsequent researchers sought to assess intelligence in a variety of ways. Many used sensory and motor tests, as did Galton earlier. But these did not prove useful. They couldn't predict success in school or on the job. Other researchers tried to test specific faculties (abilities) such as perception, memory, reasoning, judgment. Their efforts, too, were in vain (Mann, 1979).

The first true breakthrough in practical intelligence testing came with Alfred Binet (1857–1911), who with his associates developed a test of general ability that was successful in terms of predicting academic achievement. Binet approached intelligence from the standpoint of it being comprised of and representing an amalgam of a number of higher abilities such as memory, reasoning, judgment. And he measured these abilities, and through them intelligence, using a variety of complex questions, problems, and puzzles that were arranged in order of difficulty and according to age. Depending on the number of items a person passed, the higher that person's mental level is. Later investigators substituted the term *mental age* for mental level, and in 1914 a German psychologist by the name of Stern came up with the idea of dividing the "mental age" that someone achieved on a test by chronological age. He called this index the intelligence quotient, IQ (Anastasi, 1976).

Binet's theories concerning the nature of intelligence constantly kept changing. He never satisfactorily explained what his tests measured though he kept trying to do so until his untimely death at the age of 52. But he had succeeded in developing a test that worked, that could help school authorities determine with reasonable successes who would succeed or fail in school, and that assisted them in grouping children for instruction.

Many investigators, psychologists, and others disagreed with Binet's approach to intelligence from the very first. Some developed competitive techniques. However, thanks in large part to the excellent adaptation of Binet's method for American use by Terman and Merrill (Terman, 1917), Binet-type tests became the standard of the world for mental assessment over many decades. Indeed the *Stanford-Binet Test* (Terman and Merrill's version of Binet's test) only recently lost its leadership in the realm of childhood assessment to the *Wechsler Scales*.

Binet-type tests not only were successful. They popularized the idea of general intelligence and the idea of ascertaining aptitudes and abilities in school and elsewhere.

Until World War I intelligence tests were usually administered on an individual basis. During the war, however, the U.S. Army asked American psychologists to develop group intelligence tests for army recruits (Anastasi, 1976). The success of those tests (Alpha, verbal; Beta, nonverbal) encouraged the widespread use of ability tests of all sorts. Today, when ability testing of all sorts is commonplace, it is worth remembering that they all can trace their ancestry to those Alpha and Beta tests, and to Binet and Galton before them. For those interested in learning more about intelligence tests, there is a good general text by Sattler (1982).

DEFINITIONS OF INTELLIGENCE

But what is intelligence? What are we talking about when we say one individual is more or less intelligent than another? What do intelligence tests measure? We are ready to confront this question. We do so first by considering a variety of definitions that have been given as to what intelligence is, or at least as to what it is that intelligence tests measure. We draw on older definitions since they stem from a time when great efforts were made to define intelligence. There has been little agreement as to the best way to define it.

Dictionary-Type Definitions

Pieron (1926) defines *intelligence* as a capacity to understand easily (Frank, 1976), and McNemar (1964), as encompassing the fact that individuals differ in their ability to learn, to comprehend, and to understand.

Intelligence As Ability to Learn

Some theorists have defined *intelligence* in terms of the ability to learn, i.e., considering IQs for example as estimates of educability (Robinson & Robinson, 1976). Binet (& Simon, 1908) suggests that "it was the capacity to learn," while Pieron (1926) sees it as the capacity to understand easily. McNemar (1964) describes the construct as encompassing the fact that individuals differ in their ability to learn. Woodrow (1921) describes it as an acquiring capacity.

Knowledge Definitions

Knowledge definitions equate intelligence in some ways with the acquiring of information or identify it with information already achieved—thus, Henmon's (1921) description of intelligence as a "capacity for knowledge and knowledge possessed" (p. 195).

Adaptive Definitions of Intelligence

We have already discussed the fact that *intelligence*, with its strong Darwinian roots, is often described in adaptive terms. In fact, most theories of intelligence agree that it has adaptive characteristics. Binet and Simon in 1905 provided a definition revealing these: "It seems to us that in intelligence there is a fundamental faculty, the alteration or the lack of which is of the utmost importance for practical life. This faculty is judgment, otherwise called good sense, practical sense, initiative, the faculty of adapting oneself to circumstances" (Robinson & Robinson, 1976, p. 5).

More recently David Wechsler (1944), of the *Wechsler Intelligence Scales*, gave a somewhat similar definition: "Intelligence is the aggregate or global capacity of the individual to act purposefully, to think rationally, and to deal effectively with his environment" (p. 3). Similarly, Stern (1914) equates intelligence with the capacity for adaptation while

Fischer (1969) notes that "intelligence refers to the effectiveness, relative to age, peers, of the individual's approach to situations in which competence is highly regarded by the culture" (p. 669).

Identification of Intelligence with Specific Cognitive Characteristics

As we have seen, Binet strongly identifies intelligence (in one of his definitions) with a particular cognitive ability: judgment. Still others have tried to be more specific in terms limiting intelligence to identification with specific types of cognitive processes. Terman (1916) believes that it is in large part identifiable with abstract thinking. Hagerty defines intelligence as the ability to deal with novelty. Garrett (1946) defines it as the capacity to utilize symbols (Thorndike et al., 1921).

Omnibus Definitions

There have been a variety of multifaceted definitions. Peterson (1922) offers the following definition of intelligence: "Intelligence refers . . . to one's ability to be affected by a wide range of circumstances and to delay reaction to them while the significant elements are selected out and weighed with respect to their bearing on the attainment of any particular end" (p. 388).

Freeman (1925) gives the following definition:

> Intelligence may be regarded as the capacity for successful adjustment by means of those traits which we ordinarily call intellectual. These traits involve such capacities as quickness of learning, quickness of apprehension, the ability to solve new problems and the ability to perform tasks generally recognized as presenting intellectual difficulties because they involve ingenuity, originality, the grasp of complicated relationships, or the recognization of remote associations. (p. 258)

Stoddard (1941) suggests the following comprehensive definition:

> Intelligence is the ability to understand activities that are characterized by (1) difficulty, (2) complexity, (3) abstractness, (4) economy, (5) adaptiveness to a goal, (6) social value, and (7) the emergence of originals, and to maintain such activities under conditions that demand concentration of energy and a resistance to emotional attitudes. (p. 255)

Many other definitions are available, including those by Piaget (Chapter 6) and information-processing theorists (Chapter 7)—but none with which everybody would agree. It is for this reason perhaps that Boring (1923) suggests that "intelligence is what the [intelligence] tests measure" (p. 260). And Thurstone (1924) advises (at one period of his career) that we be content simply to know that the term has practical work: "There is considerable difference of opinions as to what intelligence really is, but we still use the term as long as it is demonstrably satisfactory for definite practical purposes. We use electricity for practical purposes even though we have been uncertain as to its ultimate nature, and it is so with intelligence tests" (p. xiv).

PSYCHOMETRIC THEORIES OF INTELLIGENCE

There is still no consensus as to the nature of intelligence. However, this does not mean that we should discontinue our efforts to define (and refine) the construct, particularly when these efforts may make it more effective for practical ends. The most important of such efforts has resulted in what we may call *psychometric theories of intelligence* since they have developed from the study of tests and test results. These theories not only strongly influence the interpretation of intelligence tests today; they also significantly affect many areas of academic evaluation.

Factor Analysis

Psychometric theories of intelligence usually depend heavily on the theories, methods, and results of factor analysis. Thus, to understand these psychometric theories, we must first understand a little about factor analysis.

The principal objective of factor analysis is to simplify the data obtained from observations (these observations—in the case of intelligence—usually being test results). Put another way, factor analysis tries to explain data in the simplest term that makes sense. For example, let us assume that we give 20 different reading tests to a particular group of pupils. Do these tests all measure different types of reading ability? Or do some of the tests measure the same ability? Factor analysis can help us answer this question. By applying it to the results from these tests we are able to determine whether one, several, or many factors, i.e., abilities, explain the results of our reading tests.

In its simplest forms, factor analysis proceeds as follows: a number of different tests (it could be 100 or more) are given to the same group of subjects. The scores from these tests are then placed in a correlation matrix that shows how the results from each of these tests correlate with the others (see Table 4–1). When tests correlate positively and strongly enough with each other, they can be said to share in a common factor. Their sharing in that factor is expressed statistically by the square root of their correlation, i.e., its variance; this variance has proven extremely useful in "sorting out the contribution of different factors [to] . . . test performance" (Anastasi, 1976, p. 72). The higher the square root is, the greater the variance that tests have in common and the more those tests can be presumed to share in a common factor. When, however, tests correlate only slightly in a positive direction, correlate negatively, or do not correlate at all, they are judged as *not* sharing in a common factor.

In general we may distinguish three types of factors: specific, group, and general. A *specific factor* is one that is identified with (let us say, is present in) one test but not in any of the others that we are studying. A *group factor* is present in more than one test but not in all of the tests. A *general factor* is one that is present in all of the tests studied. (See Figure 4–1.)

Several things are important to keep in mind about factor analysis. First, there is no single best way of factor analyzing data. In fact there are many disagreements as to the methods to be employed and the ways that we should interpret their results.

Second, the factors that one obtains from factor analysis, the kinds, and numbers of them, and the importance that we attach to them, depend very much on the particular factor analysis that is used in carrying out a study. The same test may be shown to be highly specific in its factor composition, to represent a group factor, or to be identified with a

Table 4–1 Correlation Matrix for Nine Aptitude Tests (Given to Pilots)

		1	2	3	4	Tests 5	6	7	8	9
1			.38	.55	.06	−.04	.05	.07	.05	.08
2		.38		.36	.40	.28	.40	.11	.15	.13
3		.55	.36		.10	.01	.18	.13	.12	.10
4		.06	.40	.10		.32	.60	.04	.06	.13
5		−.04	.28	.01	.32		.35	.08	.13	.11
6		.05	.40	.18	.60	.35		.01	.06	.07
7		.07	.11	.13	.04	.08	.01		.45	.32
8		.05	.15	.12	.06	.13	.06	.45		.32
9		.08	.13	.10	.13	.11	.07	.32	.32	

Nature of the tests:

1. AAF Vocabulary (a multiple-choice synonym test)
2. Technical Vocabulary (composed of terms such as an aircraft pilot learns)
3. Reading Comprehension (based on short paragraphs of material such as a pilot student has to read)
4. Tool Functions (on knowledge of uses of common tools)
5. Biographical Data Blank (Pilot) (containing items regarding past experiences, emphasizing mechanical experiences)
6. Mechanical Information (mostly about knowledge of automotive equipment and repairs)
7. Spatial Orientation I (requires rapid matching of aerial photographs)
8. Speed of Identification (requires rapid matching of outline drawings of airplanes)
9. Pattern Assembly (a paper form-board type of test)

Source: Reprinted from *The Nature of Human Intelligence* by J.P. Guilford with permission of McGraw-Hill Book Company, © 1967.

general one, depending on the factor analytic methods employed—and the interpretations given to the factors. Let us show how this can happen.

The more similar the tests in a particular test battery are to each other, the more highly they correlate, and the more clearly they load on (share in) a general factor. The more diverse the tests are in a particular battery, the less chance that a general factor will emerge from factor analysis, and the more chance that specific factors (each identified with a single test) will appear. Or let us say that we make up our battery with tests that group in different ways; e.g., some tests are of a mathematical nature, others of a verbal nature, and still others of a visual-spatial nature. In this case our factor analysis will most likely reveal multiple group factors, one of which might be called a *mathematical factor* (ability), another a *verbal factor* (ability), and still another a *visual-spatial factor*.

Actually the same test, depending on its placement in a particular type of battery, can be identified with general, group, or specific factors. The identical test can thus yield a general factor if it is included in a small battery of homogeneous tests, produce a group factor if the original battery becomes part of another larger more heterogeneous battery, and produce a specific factor if it is placed in a battery with tests of an entirely different nature.

Furthermore, depending on the particular factor analytic method used, any particular test shown can be identified with one, some, or all varieties of factors. Thus, one part of a test's variance can be identified with a general factor, showing it has something in common with all other tests in a particular test battery; other parts with several group factors, thus showing

Figure 4–1 Factor Patterns

(general factor heavily shaded; group factor lightly shaded)

  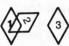

| All factors
unique | General and
unique factors | Group and
unique factors | General,
group, and
unique factors |

It is also possible to have general and group, but no unique (specific) factors; group factors alone; or a general factor alone. These are unlikely.

Source: Reprinted from *Essentials of Psychological Testing* (3rd Ed.) by Lee J. Cronbach, p. 313, with permission of Harper & Row Publishers, Inc. Copyright 1949 by Harper & Row Publishers, Inc. Copyright 1960, 1970 by Lee J. Cronbach.

that the test assesses a number of separate "group" abilities as well; and, finally, one part with a specific factor that indicates it is also measuring something unique. Figure 4–1 shows some of the possibilities that can occur when we break up the variance of any numerical operation test on the basis of its correlations with other tests in a correlation matrix.

Different factor analytic approaches usually seek to emphasize the importance of one or the other of the different types of factors, depending on the researcher's theoretical or methodological preferences. Much of the disagreement in factor analysis stems from the disagreements about how factor analysis should be done and how the factors should be interpreted. Thus it is possible to emphasize a general factor through one type of factor analysis and to show group and specific factors as being of minimal importance (Spearman, 1927), to show the general factor as being of secondary importance and quite subordinate to group factors (Thurstone, 1948), or to show that everything can be reduced to specific factors (1936a, 1936b, 1938).

If these disagreements aren't enough, another set of problems arises when one tries to name the factors. Unfortunately factor names are not always precise. In fact the same factor can be identified by a number of different names—all of them plausible sounding but each suggesting different meanings. Obviously if we wish to use these factors to guide test interpretations or to guide instructional practices, the name-calling problem is a serious one.

What Are Factors?

What do factors represent? Do they represent properties of the mind that we can use to explain intelligence? A number of theorists believe that their factors are manifestations of actual cognitive structures or processes that cause behavior and that in various ways are manifestations of the brain's activities (Burt, 1949). Other theorists have been more modest. They make the point that factors are essentially statistical in nature and should not be regarded as anything more than a convenient way of organizing test results. Thus, distinguished factor analyst Philip Vernon (1969) tells us that "primarily it is a formal way of classifying and interpreting test performances" (p. 22).

How should the readers of this book regard factors? Anna Anastasi (1976) says they should be regarded as "descriptive . . . simply an expression of correlation among behavior measures . . . and not as underlying entities or causal factors" (p. 376). Remedial and special educators should judge them as hypothetical constructs from the standpoint of their practical utility under specific conditions. Such a position neither minimizes the contributions of factor analysis to the study of intelligence nor overestimates what factors truly mean. With this in mind we are ready to review some of the major psychometric theories of intelligence, most of which were developed on the basis of factor analytic studies.

THE TWO-FACTOR THEORY OF INTELLIGENCE

Charles Spearman (1904, 1914, 1927) originated factor analysis. He can also be said to have brought the term *intelligence* formally into modern psychology, although its beginnings, as we have seen, are found in Francis Galton's work and Binet was to make it popular.

Spearman had first applied his version of factor analysis to the results of a number of tests he had given to schoolchildren. He found all the tests positively correlated with one another. From this he concluded that they shared a common characteristic. This he called g for general ability. He also found that each of the tests seemed to measure something very specific, i.e., some characteristic altogether distinct from that assessed by the other tests. This type of "ability" he called s. His statement concerning these findings was as follows: "The observed facts indicate that all branches of intellectual activity have in common one fundamental function (or group of functions) whereas the remaining or specific elements of the activity seem in every case to be wholly different from that in all others."

From this basis he developed his two-factor theory of intelligence. Spearman (1927) observed that various tasks (tests included) differ in the amount of g that they share. He refused to identify this g exactly with intelligence, since he considered the latter term to be too vague and confused for precise scientific use. He regarded g as a form of mental energy that was related to the ability to perform the major intellectual operations identified with intelligence.

We need not consider Spearman's theories of cognition in any depth. What is of most interest to us is his conceptualization of a general mental factor that accounts for intelligent behavior. Indeed it is this general factor g that Spearman regarded as his major contribution to science. He was not interested in the specific factors he discovered, beyond specifying their role in explaining test performances. Specific factors, identified by s, are task specific, e.g., simply representative of what particular tests measure of themselves and nothing more, whereas he believed that g is the ultimate explanation of human ability.

The existence of a general ability factor is usually supported by factor analytic approaches including some that significantly depart from Spearman's original methods. This general ability factor is usually identified with or as g in a number of theories of intelligence.

Does the g truly represent some form of mental energy? Does it too stand for "general" intelligence? Some theorists think it does (Cattell, 1971). Others simply have defined g as a statistical measure that shows most ability tests are positively correlated with each other— and nothing more (Burt, 1949). In this chapter we use the term g and general intelligence interchangeably at times and regard it as a hypothetical construct, "an inferred property . . . a disposition of the individual" (Charlesworth, 1976, p. 148).

In Spearman's days, as now, many disagreed with the idea of general mental ability. They did so either by denying its existence altogether or simply by considering it to represent an average or sum of a number of separate and distinct abilities—and thus to be an imprecise and crude measure of many abilities. Nevertheless Spearman's idea gave intelligence testing the theoretical underpinnings that it badly needed. Most intelligence tests of general ability now, as then, are made up of test items that are highly intercorrelated, i.e., load on a general factor. This is true for the *Stanford-Binet Tests* that were deliberately constructed to produce measures of general ability. It is also true of *Wechsler Scales*, whose subtests are presumed to measure more specific types of abilities; they too are saturated with *g*. It is even true of tests like the *Illinois Test of Psycholinguistic Abilities (ITPA)*, which seeks to assess specific psycholinguistic abilities (Brody & Brody, 1967). For criticisms of Spearman's theory, however, read Guilford (1967) and Vernon (1969, 1981). For the most recent view of *g*, Vernon's review in the *Journal of Special Education* (1983) is a must. Some cognitive theorists saw all abilities as very specific. Thus Edward Thorndike (1926) insisted that intelligence is made up of literally countless specific abilities or "common elements" of cognition, which when functioning all together, make up general intelligence. He believed these common elements are created by bonds or connections (associations) formed between neurons in the brain. Such a theory, incidentally, has received support from a number of neurological researchers (see Chapter 3). IQ tests, Thorndike said, simply provide an opportunity for the expression of all of the (specific) common elements.

Since these common elements could also work in various groups, Thorndike (1926) identified three different types of intelligence that could be tested: (1) abstract—ability to deal with ideas and symbols, (2) mechanical—ability to deal with mechanical objects, and (3) social ability—ability to deal with individual and attitudes.

Nevertheless, no matter how we approach intelligence or test it, whether in general, group, or specific terms, Thorndike insisted that we are dealing with the same types of common elements. Higher cognitive processes according to Thorndike are constituted on the same basis as lower ones; just more common elements are involved. A person with higher intellectual abilities differs from one with less ability in "the last analysis of having not a new type of psychological process but simply a larger number of connections of the ordinary sort" (p. 450).

Thorndike was not a factor analyst. His theories of intelligence were based on his learning experiments. Nevertheless his theories were supported by the later factor analytic studies of Geoffrey Thomson (1948) who developed the sampling theory of intelligence. Like Thorndike, Thomson believed that the mind is composed of many separate, distinct, and independent abilities that are joined together by mental bonds. They thus form groups of overlapping factors (abilities) that are common to some tests and not to others. Typical among these groups are ones that make up verbal ability, number ability, spatial, cognitive speed, and so on.

If we, however, take samples of all of these bonds working together, we obtain measures of general ability. In other words general intelligence tests simply sample the overall kinds and numbers of bonds that the mind has formed; i.e., they sample common bonds between the multitude of separate abilities that create cognition. The more general a test is, the wider the number of common bonds being sampled. The narrower a test is, the fewer common bonds that it samples.

Intelligence is a consequence of bonds. Some people (the more intelligent) are rich in bonds while others (less intelligent) are poor in bonds. Unlike Spearman, Thomson was not a hereditarian and he believed that education could positively affect intelligence by creating more bonds.

It is obvious that Thomson's theory of intelligence greatly resembled Thorndike's as to the nature of intelligence. Like Thorndike he believed that the underlying abilities that make up what we call *intelligence* are very tiny and very specific. Like Thorndike his theory provides an interpretation of general ability in terms of many independent specific ones; like Thorndike he also contributed to what today are known as *multiple-factor theories of abilities*.

MULTIPLE-FACTOR THEORIES

Spearman discovered what are now called *group factors* in his later factor analytic work, but he tended to disregard them because they didn't fit into his two-factor theory. Group factor theories of mental ability began in earnest with American psychologist T.L. Kelley, who rejected both the idea of general ability and the attribution of intelligence to a multitude of tiny bonds. Kelley believed cognitive operations could fundamentally be explained by a small number of group factors, each of which is common to certain types of tests but not to others. These group factors working together, he believed, constitute what is called *intelligence* (1928).

Kelley's work was advanced by Louis Thurstone (1936a, 1936b, 1938, 1940, 1944, 1948), who formulated new methods of factor analysis to extract these groups from the test correlation matrices and in the process created what came to be known as the *multiple-factor theory of intelligence*.

Thurstone was dead set against the idea of general ability and sought to do away with it. He proposed that all cognitive behavior, and specifically that associated with intelligence, is made up of what he called *primary mental abilities*, which are identified by group factors. He originally identified nine primary mental abilities as enough to explain intelligence for all practical purposes—though other primary abilities could also be distinguished. These nine primary factors are (1) *S*—spatial, (2) *P*—perceptual, (3) *N*—numerical, (4) *V*—verbal relations, (5) *W*—words, (6) *M*—memory, (7) *I*—induction, (8) *R*—arithmetic reasoning, and (9) *D*—deduction. Further research found Thurstone reducing and changing the factors to seven: (1) verbal comprehension, (2) word fluency, (3) number, (4) space, (5) associative reasoning, (6) perceptual speech, and (7) general reasoning (Anastasi, 1983).

Thurstone and his associates developed tests they believe to represent best these primary mental abilities; i.e., the tests were saturated with these. They used these tests to create what have come to be known as PMA (primary mental abilities) intelligence tests (Anastasi, 1983). Thurstone's method represented a breakthrough in psychometric theory and was critical to the later development of differential aptitude tests of all sorts, i.e., batteries of tests designed to measure a variety of broad cognitive and personality traits, the results from which could be organized into test profiles, etc. His work paved the way for the differential assessment of abilities in psychology and education.

Thurstone's first test of primary mental abilities was developed with college students. He followed this effort with primary mental ability batteries for high school, then junior high school, and then elementary school. Later tests were developed for preschool children. His wife Gwen Thelma Thurstone used these latter tests after World War II to identify specific learning strengths and weaknesses in culturally deprived preschoolers and to develop special programs of remediation on their basis (Mann, 1979).

Despite Thurstone's attempts to banish the general ability factor altogether, it kept appearing in his statistical analyses. Nevertheless, unlike Spearman, whose methods of factor analysis first revealed the general factors and then went on to define group and specific factors, Thurstone's methods always revealed *g* as a leftover factor, i.e., a second-order factor, after he had identified the primary abilities, i.e., group factors, that accounted for test performances.

Primary Mental Abilities

How many primary mental abilities (factors) are there and how many should we bother measuring? It depends on how one wishes to define *primary* and the methods of factor analysis employed to obtain them. Thurstone concerned himself with relatively few—the ones he believed are most important to academic success. Guilford identified as many as 120. Actually, depending on the tasks employed, and the ways we analyze them, we can produce an almost infinite list of so-called primary factors or abilities. But most of them will prove of little practical value in terms of their identifying aspects of cognition that are worthwhile.

In other words, if an ability is so unique that it doesn't relate to any other type of ability or activity, it is probably a useless curiosity. If we are to concern ourselves with primary mental abilities, they must be broad enough to identify significant areas of human behavior. Horn believes that no more than 30 independent primary factors can be considered as established by research up to this point. He (1978b) observes that each is a

> kind of intelligence on its own in the sense that the aspects of thinking represented by the factor can be seen to be interesting and worthwhile in its own right . . . and that individuals who do well in the area of functioning represented by any particular factor . . . do not, in general, do as well in the thinking . . . represented by other factors. (p. 61)

However, he also states that so many factors are too many to be useful and that we should reduce them to 6 to 10 second-order broader factors, i.e., factors obtained by performing a factor analysis of such primary mental abilities. In other words we should perform factor analyses on the factors we obtain from an original factor analysis. As stated, there are many ways to go in factor analysis.

To conclude our review of multiple factors, we should observe that just as Spearman's theory of *g* strongly supports intelligence testing today, so does Thurstone's theory of primary mental abilities provide much of the scientific basis for efforts to identify specific abilities and disabilities. It has thus been of great importance to remedial and special education.

HIERARCHICAL THEORIES OF INTELLIGENCE

Hierarchical conceptualizations of intelligence have not affected remedial and special education as strongly as have general and multiple-factor theories. This may partly be due to the fact that they have not appeared as readily applicable to remedial or special education situations. However, they do make good sense and they have proven themselves flexible enough to permit wide application (Humphreys, 1981).

Two particular theories of hierarchical intelligence are briefly discussed. Both are based on factor analysis. The first is that of Cyril Burt (1949) and the second by Phillip Vernon (1961). Both are British educational psychologists whose theories can be viewed from one standpoint as elaborations of Spearman's pioneering investigations and from another a reconciliation of general and multiple-factor theories.

According to Burt, a general factor takes part in all intellectual operations. However, group abilities equivalent more or less to Thurstone's primary mental abilities further account for cognitive achievement in a number of broad though less distinctly circumscribed areas. Then there are specific factors that are interpretable in terms of the cognitive activities required for specific tests or tasks or ones that are very similar. The performance of any ordinary task (test) is thus likely to be multidimensional in terms of the operations of intelligence, with a general factor, special group factors, and finally a number of specific factors explaining it.

Vernon's theory is an extension of Burt's. Figure 4–2 shows an early model of it; Figure 4–3 shows a later, more refined one that breaks group factors down still further into major and minor ones.

In Vernon's theory a test of intelligence first of all assesses the g factor; then two major group factors; then minor, more specialized group factors; and finally a number of specific factors, i.e., identified with individual tests or behaviors. To use Vernon's (1969) own phraseology, the mind can be conceived of as some sort of a branching cognitive tree. More precisely, the g factor in Vernon's model accounts for the greatest amount of cognition variance. The remainder is partly accounted for, in different degrees, by two broad (group) cognitive components, both sharing in g but having special types of characteristics of their own, these being a verbal education factor ($v{:}ed$) and a spatial practical one ($k{:}m$). A lesser share of cognition is then further explained by the operation of more specialized (though still broad) group cognitive components, such as fluency (f), number (n), induction (i), and perceptual speed (s). At a still lower level, cognitive activity influences only specialized

Figure 4–2 Sketch of a Possible Hierarchy of Abilities

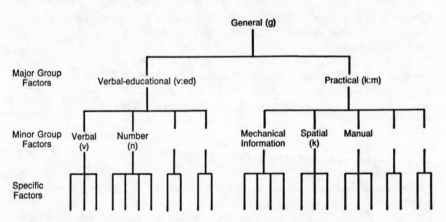

Source: Reprinted from *The Structure of Human Abilities* by P.E. Vernon with permission of John Wiley & Sons, Inc., © 1950.

Figure 4–3 Presumed Main General and Group Factors Underlying Tests
Relevant to Educational and Vocational Achievements

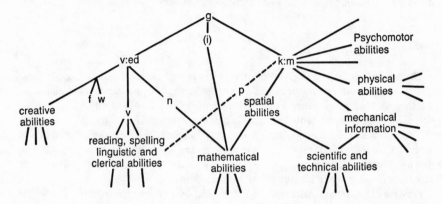

Source: Reprinted from *Intelligence and Cultural Environment* by P.E. Vernon with permission of
Methuen Inc., © 1969.

skill areas such as in music. Finally, "at the bottom of the hierarchy are the specific . . .
factors which underlie high or low performances in a particular test, but tell us nothing more
about ability at anything else" (1969, p. 22).

Hierarchical models appear to make eminent sense in explaining how intelligence is expressed. Certainly a general intellectual factor appears to be operating in almost everything
we do, but we can also observe the influences of more and more specialized abilities. An
artist and a sculptor both may be stronger than a writer in *k:m* but differ from each other in
the further differentiation of that group ability; one sculptor may differ from another in that
limited area. In the last 10 years there have been attempts to reconsider differing views of
intelligence such as general and multiple factor ones within a hierarchical framework.

TRIADIC THEORY OF INTELLIGENCE

One theory of hierarchical intelligence has had considerable influence in the United
States: Cattell's (1971) triadic or investment theory of intelligence, in which a distinction is
made between fluid and crystallized intelligence. This theory uses factor analytic information but goes far beyond it to speculate about the nature of intelligence. It has both biological
(organismic) and social-cultural (learning motivational) aspects. It is clearly hierarchical,
proceeding from general to relatively specific abilities (Brody & Brody, 1976).

Capacities

The capacities are identified by Cattell as the most general of cognitive abilities. They
relate to and reflect the general structural properties of the *entire* brain. They influence
almost all cognitive activities. The most general of all of the capacities is *g* (otherwise
known as *fluid intelligence*). This is identified with the brain's general structural capacity. It

is genetically determined though environmentally influenced. The other capacities (less general than g) are g_s (speed capacity) and g_r (retrieval capacity). These are identified with the brain's functional characteristics, perhaps its chemical properties (Brody & Brody, 1976).

Provincials

The provincials are a second (lower order) class of abilities identified by Cattell. These reflect and are associated with local (as opposed to general) brain structures and functions, and they are thus more restricted in terms of cognitive operations and influences. Capacities, identified as they are with the brain's general structure and functions, can be expected to influence almost all behavior. But provincials, which are cognitive powers identified with specific parts of the brain, express themselves in more specific types of behaviors. There is thus a p_v (visual perceptual power), p_a (auditory power), p_t (tactile power), and p_c (cerebellar power), e.g., as in kinesthetic-balance performances.

Provincials, like the capacities, are determined by the genetic characteristics of the nervous system but are environmentally influenced.

Agencies

The agencies represent the investment of an individual's cognitive capacities and provincial powers in particular types of skills. The nature of the investments is determined by the effects of the individual's life experiences on the capacities and provincials. Playing important roles in this investment are the social reinforcements provided by the individual's environment, e.g., home, neighborhood, and school, as well as personal motivations.

The most general and best known of the agencies is crystallized intelligence (g_c). Its influences are readily identified. There are other more specific agencies. These are expressed in narrower types of intellectual skills, ones that are much the same as Thurstone's primary mental abilities, e.g., g_v and s, verbal and spatial abilities, respectively.

The agencies are split into two classes. One is called *aids* or *acquired* cognitive skills and can be interpreted as intellectual algorithms, i.e., general principles that have been learned and that have fairly broad applicability in a variety of problem situations. The other set of agencies are the *proficiencies*. These represent specialized types of skills that address specific purposes, i.e., a foreign language one learns to become an international business person or the skills that an orthodontist may require to adjust teeth (Brody & Brody, 1976).

The triadic theory is presented in schematic model form in Figure 4–4. The various cognitive levels and their components interact consistently. Also, g_c (crystallized intelligence) is a product of other agencies and acts on those agencies. For critical assessments of this theory see Brody and Brody (1976).

FACET THEORIES OF INTELLIGENCE

Some theorists have tried to describe *intelligence* in terms of its different aspects or facets (Anastasi, 1983). They do so because they believe that such theories best explain the complicated nature of human ability. The most prominent example of this approach, and one that has been most influential in special education, is Guilford's structure of intellect model in which human cognition is conceptualized in a cubelike scheme.

Figure 4–4 The Triadic Theory

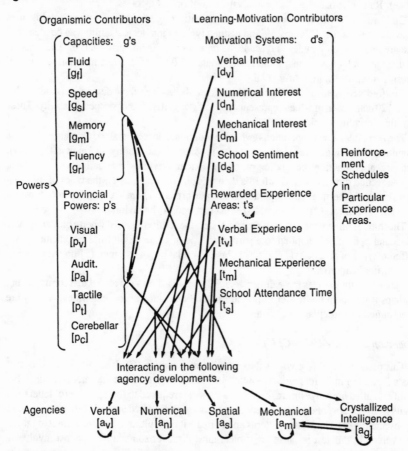

The arrows indicate direction of influence and contribution to (cognitive) growth. Thus, verbal ability, a_v, receives contributions from the capacities, g's, the powers, p's, a motivational factor, d_v, and a reinforcement in an experience area, t_v. To avoid complication of the diagram not all individual but only class connections are made. The semicircular arrows below the agencies indicate their self-development capacities as "aids."

Source: Reprinted from *Abilities: Their Structure, Growth, and Action* by R.B. Cattell with permission, © 1971.

The Structure of Intellect Model

The structure of intellect (SI) theory of intelligence was developed by Guilford and has been the subject of more than 20 years of research. It is quite different from the others in this chapter (Guilford, 1967; Guilford & Hoepfner, 1971). For one, while Guilford used factor analysis to support his theory, he did so in an after-the-fact manner. He didn't develop his theories as a result of his factor analytic work (as did, for example, Spearman and Thurstone). Rather he has used factor analysis to confirm his theories.

Guilford has gone far beyond Thurstone in criticizing the idea of general intelligence. Indeed he insists that 120 separate and distinct types of intellectual ability can be identified and are relevant to everyday and academic types of intelligent performance. And whereas Thurstone finally agreed that *g* did exist, though he downgraded its importance, Guilford doesn't accept the notion of *g* at all.

Guilford's SI model of intelligence classifies abilities along three distinct dimensions that yield 120 cells, each of which represents a specific cognitive factor or specific ability. These abilities are quite specific.

The first dimension is operations (what the individual does mentally). Operations include cognition (knowing), memory, divergent production (an ability to think differently), convergent production (generation of logical conclusions), and evaluation.

The second dimension in Guilford's theory is one of content, i.e., the types of information on which the intellect's operations are performed. There are four distinct types of content: (1) figural, (2) symbolic, (3) semantic, and (4) behavioral.

The third SI dimension is that of products, i.e., the results obtained when a particular type of mental operation is applied to a particular type of content. Guilford has identified six different types of products: (1) unit, (2) class, (3) relation, (4) system, (5) transformation, and (6) implications.

Table 4–2 summarizes these dimensions. Figure 4–5 shows the model that forms a cube. Perhaps it will help the reader to provide several examples of these abilities, as they are exemplified in particular tasks or tests.

Cognition of Figure Units (CFU)

This particular ability involves the operation of cognition (C). It involves a content that has a figure (F) in it. Its product is a unit (U) of some sort. A test that measures the CFU ability is called *hidden print*. In this test the subject is required to form pictures of letters and digits from patterns of dots. A variety of other dots are scattered around these patterns so as to obscure the digit and letter patterns and to make it difficult to recognize them. Cognition is involved in this test because the subject must discover something. The test involves a visual figure (figures in other modality areas can also be used). The response to the test (its product) produces a unit; i.e., the subject must identify a particular digit or letter.

Table 4–2 Symbols Used in Guilford's Model

Operation	Content	Product
C—cognition	F—figural	U—unit
M—memory	S—symbolic	C—class
D—divergent production	M—semantic	R—relation
N—convergent production	B—behavioral	S—system
E—evaluation		T—transformation
		I—implication

Figure 4–5 Guilford Model of the Structure of the Intellect

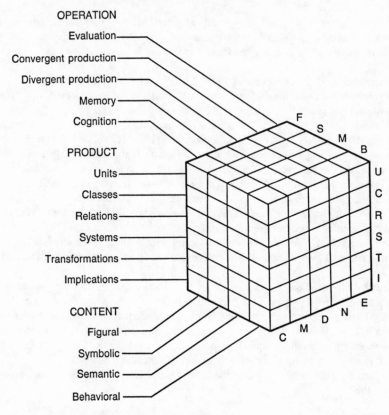

Source: Reprinted from *The Nature of Human Intelligence* by J.P. Guilford with permission of McGraw-Hill Book Company, © 1967.

Evaluation of Semantic Transformation (EST)

One particular SI test in which this ability is manifested is "Story Titles." Here the subject reviews a very short story and then is required to select a title that best names the story. The cognitive operation here is one of evaluative judgment (E). The content is semantic (S) since it is meaningful. The product from the application of evaluative judgment to the semantic content is a transformation (t); i.e., the subject must change (transform) the meaning of the content into a title.

Guilford and his associates claim that they have actually identified 98 separate and distinct factors so far through special tests, confirming the SI model (Guilford, 1967; Guilford & Hoepfner, 1971). Guilford believes that more of these factors will be identified and measured in due course.

Criticisms have been raised about the way that Guilford has "found" his specific abilities (Brody & Brody, 1976) and about their actual usefulness. But Guilford (1979) is extremely confident that his conceptualization of abilities is correct.

JENSEN'S TWO-LEVEL THEORY

The two-level theory of intelligence is not as prominent as it was when it created an enormous stir in educational and psychological circles (1969). Still the two-level theory commands our attention; it clearly has some implications for remedial and special educators.

Jensen introduced the constructs of Level I and Level II abilities to account for the differences he found on the test performance of low- and middle-class socioeconomic status (SES) white, black, and Mexican-American pupils. Level I abilities are simple, basic ones, associative in nature, involving "the neural registration and consolidation of stimulus inputs and the formation of associations" (1969, pp. 110–111). They are responsible for associating, registering, and storing information and are also called on in simple recognition of information or its rote recall. Tasks involving Level I abilities include the recitation of digits in the order in which they are heard and rote memory learning of all sorts.

Level II abilities are more complex and advanced in nature than Level I abilities. They are responsible for higher intellectual activities. They are thus the basis for the transformation of past learning experiences and their generalization to new situations. They are called on in problem solving, abstract thinking, reasoning, etc. We usually identify intelligence with the operation Level II abilities. And indeed most intelligence tests emphasize Level II thinking.

Jensen hypothesized that Level I and Level II abilities are genetically determined and develop more or less separately from each other. Further, he has found that children who have low IQs (but are not learning disabled) often have adequate Level I abilities but are deficient in Level II ones. He has also suggested that children from lower socioeconomic classes in general and minority pupils in particular are likely to be deficient in Level II skills. It is obvious why his theories have aroused so much controversy.

An excellent review and critique of the Level I/Level II theory has been provided by Vernon (1981).

IMPLICATIONS OF INTELLIGENCE THEORIES

In this particular section of our chapter we examine some of the implications of the theories of intelligence just reviewed. We do so only briefly, because the topic is well covered in other books, i.e., by Sattler for general implications (1982), by Robinson and Robinson in respect to the mentally retarded (1976), by Lerner for the learning disabled (1981), and by Sabatino and Miller for other handicaps (1978). Our intention in this quick review is to provide a general framework for later, deeper study. Most of our attention incidentally is devoted to general intelligence since this is the particular intelligence construct that remedial and special educators are most likely to encounter.

Implications of General Intelligence Theories

Within this section we consider some of the implications that the theories of general intelligence—that we identify with *g*—hold for remedial and special education. However, let us make some things clear before we proceed.

First, we want to observe that it is quite appropriate to employ the construct of general intelligence for some purposes while using other conceptualizations of intelligence, e.g., those of separate mental abilities, for others. We recommend that our readers proceed in this way. The idea of general intelligence will prove useful under certain circumstances but irrelevant at other times. We should use the construct when and if it helps us understand a child better and assist in the education. We should use other conceptualizations of intelligence when they are more meaningful. Sometimes we may want to ignore intelligence altogether, e.g., when we actually proceed to instruct a child.

While estimates of general intelligence cannot tell us the whole story, i.e., give us a comprehensive picture of a child's potential or abilities, this doesn't detract from their usefulness. We will find estimates of *g* useful for many purposes in school. This is true even though, as we all know, children of the same age who appear similar in respect to general intelligence, e.g., have identical IQs, and on further study usually reveal quite different combinations of specific abilities, e.g., auditory discrimination, hand-eye coordination, memory.

We must at all times be sensitive to the possible abuses that can result from the misinterpretation of measures of general ability. But we should also be aware of the biases that many people have against the construct. Let us specifically consider some of the biases against the IQ and IQ testing since general ability in most people's minds is usually identified with the IQ as it is evaluated through tests.

Among some of the major criticisms raised against IQ testing are the following: They cause teachers to lower their expectations for certain types of children and thus teach them less effectively; they discriminate against minorities; they disproportionately load classes for the mentally retarded with black, Hispanic, and other children of non-white, middle-class backgrounds; they label children as being mentally inadequate and inferior, thus damaging their self-concepts; they exclude individuals from higher education and job opportunities (Garcia, 1981; Hilliard, 1979). There is some support for all of these complaints. Nevertheless, the negative effects of IQ testing can be shown, on closer examination, to be grossly exaggerated.

Much of the criticism of IQ results from the resentment that people have against the idea that we can or should characterize people who may include our children or ourselves as less intellectually able or adequate. Most of us can accept the idea that we are weak or less able in respect to particular types of ability. A poet is not usually upset when he is told that he is deficient in mathematical abilities. An engineer is not usually bothered if she is considered somewhat deficient in written verbal skills. Most of us are tolerant of the fact that we have poor memories—as long as we can convince ourselves that we are bright otherwise. IQ tests, however, appear to grade us in terms of our total worth as persons—which naturally makes us uncomfortable. And it is the derogatory implications of low IQ scores that, more than anything else, arouse people's hostility towards IQs and the idea of general mental ability.

Nevertheless IQ tests by themselves rarely are responsible for identifying a child as mentally retarded or for excluding someone from attending college or from a desired job. Also overlooked is the fact that IQ tests frequently identify children as intellectually competent even when their parents or teachers believe otherwise. And if IQ tests are partly responsible for assigning a pupil to a special class or otherwise identifying a pupil as needing special services, what is wrong with that—if the pupil is helped by so doing. In this respect IQ tests were originally responsible for identifying gifted children; indeed, the entire idea of giftedness developed from intelligence testing.

Beyond all this, and perhaps most important of all, IQs and other measures of *g* (*SAT*s, *GRE*s, etc.) almost always predict performances in school better than other types of assessments (Charlesworth, 1976). They also predict performances for a variety of jobs—from salesmanship to engineering—quite well. This seems to be due to the fact that success in school or employment depends on a multitude of factors subsumed under the concept of g, and the latter is what IQ tests and other general ability tests assess better than any other types of tests. As psychologist Samuel Messick (1976) observed, "Diagnosing each ability separately doesn't help much, because life doesn't present challenges to only one ability at a time" (p. 1041). The Japanese rely heavily on general ability tests for personnel selection; this may account for their employees' low job-failure rate.

To conclude, IQ tests (and other tests of g) are imperfect, they are often interpreted incorrectly, and they may be used in ways that are injurious to particular individuals. Nevertheless they predict overall achievement in school and elsewhere better than almost any other type of evaluation approach.

For an interesting and constructive set of articles on assessment, including reviews of general ability and its assessment, we recommend a special issue of *The American Psychologist* (Glaser & Bond, 1981).

Meaning of g to Educators

For the rest of this section we discuss the construct of general intelligence (symbolized as g) as it explains the "covariation (or correlation) of individual differences in performance in a wide variety of situations" (Jensen, 1979, p. 82). And we accept the premise that IQs provide a reasonably valid means of assessing this cognitive construct.

Let us first observe that teachers will not find g important in all types of school situations. For example, it will not play a particularly important role in situations requiring muscular strength and endurance, sensory responses, rapid reaction times, or simple rote memory. It will, however, be found of considerable importance in circumstances that present complex problems or require abstract reasoning or judgment. This means that g is important for all but the most routinized and stereotyped of academic learning situations (Jensen, 1979).

Tests that are loaded with g include the *Stanford-Binet* and *Wechsler Intelligence* scales; the test items in these scales are usually quite complex. Other tests loaded with g are the *SAT* and *GRE* and the standardized tests used to assess candidates for admission to professional schools. Aptitude and achievement tests of all sorts, too, are typically loaded with g, particularly at higher grade levels. All scholastic achievement is correlated with g after the age of five.

More specifically, g is likely to play an important role in learning tasks that are complex and require comprehension and judgment; demand the pupil to put forth conscious mental efforts; are spaced in ways that permit the pupil time to think through problems; are hierarchical in nature; i.e., the learning of later items in a task sequence depends on the learning of earlier ones; involve meaningful materials; require transfer from one situation to new and somewhat different ones; and involve the acquisition of new types of skills rather than the improvement of earlier acquired ones (Jensen, 1979).

Specific Uses for Remedial and Special Educators for IQ Tests

Some of the specific uses that remedial and special educators may find for IQ tests (which measure g) include grouping individuals according to their general overall ability; determining whether academic difficulties are attributable to general limitations in mental capacity; determining school readiness; determining whether a child is intellectually capable of doing accelerated work in school; determining giftedness; making general prognoses about the chances of recovering from different emotional and cognitive disabilities; e.g., IQs are good predictors of children being able to recover from autism in later life (Goldfarb et al., 1978); deciding whether various types of cognitive training or interventions do in fact improve pupils' overall abilities (Head Start programs have used IQ tests for this purpose, as have projects seeking to accelerate the intellectual ability of retarded pupils) (Garber & Heber, 1973, 1978); predicting pupils' chances of responding to remedial education; the better the IQ, the better the chance that the pupil who is behind academically will respond to remediation (Anastasi, 1982); and predicting the chances of a pupil doing well in later college placement and skilled or professional employment (Jensen, 1979).

Implications of Multiunit Theories of Intelligence

As we have seen, Thorndike and Thomson conceived of the mind as composed of a multitude of tiny identical cognitive units. Working together, these units determine overall ability. Working in groups they create differentiated special abilities. Educational efforts that increase the numbers of these cognitive units or shape their organization effectively should have beneficial effects. A number of remedial programs and special education programs seem to reflect this philosophy, even if their promoters are unaware of any particular theory of intelligence. Among these are many enrichment programs such as Head Start and infant stimulation and reading programs such as the neurological impress variety (Heckelman, 1968). These methods in many ways proceed on the basis of the more the better in so far as improving overall cognition is concerned. As seen in Chapter 2, there may well be a legitimate basis for such an approach in the sense that increased experiences seem to stimulate the brain's growth (Rosenzweig, 1981).

Implications of Multiple-Factor Theories of Intelligence

Thurstone's tests of primary mental abilities have not proven useful in assessing abilities for practical purposes of school placement and academic predictions. This is partly because the tests were flawed. It is also partly due to the fact that tests of so-called primary abilities just don't predict school achievement as well as general ability tests do (Anastasi, 1976).

Thurstone's work, however, laid the groundwork in many ways for the modern learning disabilities movement. His influence is seen throughout Chapter 5, which is concerned with specific abilities.

Implications of Hierarchical Theories of Intelligence

That intelligence works hierarchically seems to be supported by our commonsense understanding of how abilities are organized as well as by modern sophisticated research. If nothing else, it appears to be a useful way for remedial and special educators to consider the ways in which intelligence is applied.

We certainly appear to find evidence that abilities are hierarchically organized in school. Thus, we can usually distinguish pupils who are generally more or less intelligent (g). We also can distinguish between those who are academically inclined ($v:ed$) and the more vocationally, i.e., practically, inclined ($k:m$). Among the academically inclined are some who are more verbally adept than others and those for whom mathematical skills are their forte. Among the practically inclined are those with differing types of mechanical or vocational skills.

School systems in Great Britain and in the United States have sometimes divided schooling for various pupils on the basis of such hierarchical distinctions. Some of our more prominent tests seem to adhere to the idea of hierarchically organized abilities. Thus the *Wechsler Intelligence* offers a full-scale IQ, which is a measure of *g*; verbal and performance scales, IQs that approximate *v:ed* and *k:m*; subtests within the verbal and performance scales that when factor analyzed cluster into broad group abilities; various subtests that are often interpreted as representing narrower group abilities; and finally specific test items that may represent *s*.

With hierarchical interpretations of intelligence becoming more popular (Anastasi, 1983), they will increasingly be applied to learning problems.

Implications of the Triadic Theory of Intelligence

Cattell and Horn (Cattell, 1971; Cattell & Horn, 1981; Horn, 1979a, 1979b) have elaborated the triadic theory of intelligence in a number of ways in their research writings. Horn has extended it to meet the demands of more recent cognitive research. The part of the original theory, however, that has come to hold the most interest for educators is its conceptualization of fluid and crystallized intelligence.

Fluid intelligence (g_f), as we have seen, is supposed to represent "raw" natural biological intelligence, i.e., cognitive ability that is not affected to any great degree by experience, schooling, etc. To use Cattell's (1979) words, it is called fluid "because it flows with unrestricted expression into . . . all areas of intellectual endeavor" (p. 5). Presumably if we can effectively assess g_f, we would have a measure of pupils' "true" general abilities and know what those pupils are potentially capable of intellectually, without the effects of experience or school getting in the way. All tests are to various degrees dependent on the testees' learning experiences. Are there some tests that may nevertheless minimize these, so that we can still measure fluid intelligence? Cattell and Horn believe that *Raven's Progressive Matrices* do this to some degree, i.e., are reasonably culture free. Cattell himself (1979) has worked for years to develop his own culture-fair test that can effectively measure g_f, and he claims considerable success in so doing.

Cattell's test, however, has not been widely used in educational settings within the United States. Indeed culture-fair tests, generally speaking, have not yet become popular; this is in large part due to the fact that they haven't predicted school achievement very well to date.

Nevertheless the distinction between fluid intelligence and crystallized intelligence, i.e., that part of the natural general intelligence that has been crystallized out of past experiences (including culture and school), seems to be a useful one. For example, it explains why a ghetto child can appear so abysmally slow in school in respect to school achievement but be able to do so well in the everyday world. As Horn (1979b) puts it, "The fluid intelligence factor represents a kind of good thinking that people seem to have in mind when they say things like 'he isn't very well educated but he's smart' " (pp. 62–63).

Crystallized intelligence (g_c) on the other hand is book learning. It represents learning that has developed from past experiences. Whereas fluid intelligence ("natural smartness") declines with age, crystallized intelligence is more enduring and can even increase with age.

It is one reason why older people still behave intelligently, indeed can display wisdom despite declines in natural cognitive ability.

Cattell and Horn believe that ill health and brain injuries can reduce the amount of fluid intelligence at children's disposal. Teachers, thus, may not be able to rely on spontaneous self-directed learning from such children.

Actually pupils (and everyone else) solve most problems in school and elsewhere using both g_f and g_c in varying proportions. One pupil may solve a mathematical problem by personally reasoning it through (strong evidence of g_f). Another may do so by applying a principle (algorithm) he has been taught (strong evidence of g_c).

By proper observations of their pupils and effective interpretations of tests—e.g., *Raven's Progressive Matrices* provide a good measure of g_f while vocabulary tests provide an effective assessment of g_c—teachers may be able to tailor regular or remedial education to their pupils more effectively. The g_f g_c distinctions may prove to be important to educators.

Implications of Structure of Intellect Theory

Guilford's structure of intellect model of intelligence has been extremely influential in remedial and special education, particularly in gifted education, since the divergent cognitive operations distinguished in the model seem to have particularly important implications for gifted pupils (Guilford, 1979).

One reason that Guilford's theories and claims have continued to be popular is because the idea of 120 separate and distinct cognitive abilities has great appeal to educators concerned with cognitive development and remediation. Guilford, despite much criticism has not waivered in his belief that SI theory can be used to improve intelligence. He believes that it is possible to correct "imbalances in education" and to encourage and remediate cognition by educationally addressing the specific abilities revealed by the SI model. Indeed, he (1967) states, "the map of the territory is well laid out; the results to be achieved are clear" (p. 41).

There are two ways he suggests to achieve these results. The first is that of indirect approaches,

> mainly through the teaching of ordinary courses of instruction. One avenue is through curriculum construction; by choosing to give courses that provide opportunities for exercising various SI functions. Each course content under consideration can be examined in light of the SI model to see what its potential could be for exercising those functions. (1967, p. 41)

The second is that of direct approaches. And this represents efforts to train specifically the intellectual abilities revealed by his model. Efforts along these lines have been made with cognitively handicapped pupils by Meeker (1975). Renzulli (1973) has utilized the SI model to guide the training of gifted and creative pupils. Similarly, the Creative Education Foundation, centered at the University of Buffalo, has claimed to train some 30 SI abilities successfully (Reese, Parnes, Treffinger, & Kaltsounis, 1976).

Guilford (1979) envisions the day when high school pupils will take courses about SI functions so that they will be better prepared to train their own children cognitively and when even television programs will exercise SI abilities in children.

Implications of the Level I/Level II Theory of Intelligence

Jensen's Level I and Level II functions cannot be separated in anyone's everyday performance, though the proportions of each at work in any given activity can be expected to differ. A certain minimal level of effective operation of Level I abilities is necessary for Level II abilities to function effectively. However, a pupil who is quite adequate in Level I functions will nevertheless have trouble with most conceptual work in school and have difficulty in coping with higher academics.

There are clear implications for remedial and special education in Jensen's theories. First of all, one should perhaps teach pupils according to their strengths and weaknesses as revealed in terms of Level I/Level II distinctions. Thus if a pupil is quite deficient in Level II abilities, we might have to teach by more repetition (rote learning) and by emphasizing memory work. If, however, a pupil is strong in Level II abilities, we can perhaps skip a variety of the basic instructional steps with that student (if the Level I skills are adequate) because we can assume that the student will nevertheless catch on. Additionally we can assume that Level II deficiencies are probably prominent in slow learners and mentally retarded pupils, while Level I deficiencies may be at the bottom of many remedial problems and learning disabilities in children who appear to be otherwise intelligent, i.e., high in Level II abilities.

OTHER APPROACHES TO INTELLIGENCE

All intelligence tests provide means of estimating a pupil's learning potential in the sense that IQ scores, mental age, etc., can predict with considerable success how well a pupil will learn. However, such tests have often been criticized for appearing to suggest that intelligence is a fixed, static process or set of processes that cannot be improved much. Furthermore, they do not truly reveal a pupil's potential for further intellectual development; IQ scores, for example, have been lambasted over and over as too simple, narrow, and static in nature to provide good estimates for cognitive approvement (Ebel, 1979; Feuerstein, Rand, & Hoffman, 1979; Feuerstein et al., 1981).

In the 1970s, a particular approach to assessing and training cognitive abilities was identified with the name of learning potential. In a nutshell this involves giving unfamiliar problems to pupils and then seeing how much coaching they need to solve the problems.

Current interest in learning potential has a rather extensive history. In the Soviet Union, where standard IQ tests have always been viewed suspiciously (as a capitalist tool of exploitation), psychologist L.S. Vigotsky conceived of intellectual development in terms other than IQ or mental age. He sought rather to determine how much improvement a child could achieve on various tests if given proper training. From this he estimated the child's "zone of potential intellectual development." His estimates were based on the number of prompts that were needed to help children solve problems of various difficulties. Using his method, one would find, for example, that learning disabled pupils respond better to prompts than do brain-injured or moderately retarded children (Rice, 1979).

In the United States there have been several approaches to the study of learning potential. Milton Budoff (Budoff, Meskin, & Harrison, 1971) developed one of the better known of these some years ago. The best known current researcher in the field, however, is Reuven Feuerstein.

Feuerstein, an Israeli clinical psychologist, coaches his pupils to determine their learning potential on tests and tasks that appear to be minimally affected by school achievement or cultural background (which Cattell and his associates would suggest tap fluid intelligence). One of these tests is the *Raven Progressive Matrices* which requires the completion of various matrices in which most of the parts have already been filled according to a certain sequence or pattern. Another test he uses is the *Organization of Dots* test, in which the pupil must draw lines between specific groups of dots that create geometric shapes amid a mass of other dots. Still another test he uses is the *Stencil Design Test*. Here the pupil is presented a drawing of a design composed out of two superimposed stencils. The child then must identify the separate stencils from a range of stencil shapes (Rice, 1979).

To assess a pupil's learning potential, according to Feuerstein's approach, the examiner first administers pretests, of the sort discussed, to obtain baseline scores. The examiner then teaches the pupil the principles and skills involved in the test. The pupil is then tested again to see if performance has improved. More coaching is given in the event of failure until the pupil succeeds or reaches the stage where the student apparently is incapable of succeeding. In such assessment the pupil is introduced to increasingly more difficult tests. The pupil's learning potential is defined in terms of the ability to modify and improve performances on these tests after coaching (Feuerstein, Rand, & Hoffman, 1979; Feuerstein et al., 1981).

Kaufman Assessment Battery for Children

Remedial and special educators are likely to become familiar with the *Kaufman Assessment Battery for Children (K-ABC)* in the 1980s (Kaufman & Kaufman, 1983). This highly publicized instrument is the result of a sophisticated test development process. It has been hailed by its publishers as a revolutionary approach to children's abilities. It is claimed to assess two types of cognitive processing: simultaneous and serial (see Chapter 6) and to distinguish cognitive ability (process) from achievement (product). The *K-ABC* also offers measures of learning potential. It is supposed to provide a basis for cognitive academic training and remediation. For a comprehensive and critical assessment see the Reynolds and Miller special issue of the *Journal of Special Education* (1984).

Nonpsychometric Approaches to Intelligence

Much recent research on intelligence has been carried out on a nonpsychometric basis, i.e., through experiments and other types of research, into the types of processes that go on during intelligent behavior, i.e., when a pupil responds to a stimulus, solves a problem, or makes a decision. Sternberg (1981, Sternberg & Wagner, 1984) is one of the more important contributors. Much of his research is based on information-processing theories (reviewed in Chapter 7). This important research does not yet have major implications for educational programming and remediation.

Componential Analysis

We would like to call attention to one of the more promising of these approaches, called *process analysis* or *componential analysis of intelligence*. Robert Sternberg (1980) of Yale is one of the most prominent researchers in this type of study, which seeks to determine the distinct steps, or components, in intellectual functioning and the ways in which these are applied in intelligent behavior. He studies the methods people use to solve different types of problems and the stages they go through along the way. Sternberg (1981a, 1981b) believes that this type of approach will eventually enable teachers to determine strengths and deficiencies in intellectual functioning and to develop ways of accelerating the former and correcting the latter.

Piagetian Views on Intelligence

Jean Piaget, a Swiss psychologist, has developed still another nonpsychometric approach to intelligence. (Chapter 6 is devoted almost entirely to his work.) However, standardized intelligence tests based on his theories (Uzigris & Hunt, 1975) have not been too useful.

Finally, developments in neuroscience are suggesting new ways to conceptualize intelligence and to assess it. Some psychologists and neurologists are trying to assess intelligence directly, i.e., in terms of brain functioning. There have been efforts to use evoked brain potentials for this purpose. Edward Beck, one of the pioneers in such procedures, believes that tests of evoked potential can produce a sort of fingerprint of the brain (Rice, 1979). However, neurological tests of any sort have not proven themselves able to predict school success with anything close to the success of traditional intelligence tests. Nor have they proven useful to this point in educational programming.

Gardner's Seven Multiple Intelligences

Howard Gardner (1983), a psychologist who has long been interested in creativity, believes that humans have seven independent intelligences. Each of these intelligences is supposed to be controlled by a specific part of the brain. Two of them—the ability to use language and the ability to reason logically or mathematically—are the intelligences that we usually assess with intelligence tests. Gardner believes that other intelligences are also important and are being neglected. These encompass musical skills, spatial skills (involved in analyzing the visual world), bodily and kinesthetic talents that govern such behaviors as dancing, interpersonal skills such as those used by salespersons and politicians, and intrapersonal skills that respond to one's own thoughts and feelings. Though the seven intelligences work together in various ways, they also work in isolation; indeed each is supposed to have its own separate memory. Gardner believes that each of the seven intelligences develops and matures at different rates.

There is some similarity between Gardner's conceptualizations and those of factor theories. Thurstone (1938, 1940, 1948), for example, dealt with different types of intelligence, primary mental abilities. In addition, some tests that while not necessarily identified as intelligence tests, measure specific types of "intelligences." For example, *Seashore Measures of Musical Talents* (1919–60) has long been recognized as an excellent test of musical ability.

Gardner's idea of different neurological centers for his seven intelligences has some support from neurological theory (Chapter 3) but is still quite speculative. What his theory does nicely is to explain the phenomenon of *idiot savants*, i.e., wise idiots. It has always puzzled the science and the public alike how certain individuals who appear to be grossly mentally retarded when it comes to most things can show unusual ability in narrow areas such as number work, art, or music. Gardner's explanation is that one of the seven intelligences in such individuals is still intact and well developed, even though the others may not have developed properly or have been impaired.

TRAINING OF INTELLIGENCE

Can one improve intelligence? A recent issue of the *Journal of Special Education* was devoted to this topic (Miller, 1981). This is a long-argued issue. Binet, the father of the intelligence test, believed that it could be done. However, it later was believed that intelligence is an inherited property of the mind that cannot be altered much by experiences or education. Among the recent representatives of this type of thinking are Jensen (1969). Eysenck (1973), and Burt (1955). They agree that general mental ability is indeed benefited by good health and that it can be enriched through education. However, they also believe that it is basically a stable trait (or set of traits) that can't be improved much through special education or training. Jensen (1979) advises that schools recognize and live with this "fact" and that they adjust curricula accordingly rather than continue efforts to improve their pupils' cognitive abilities.

On the other hand there has been a wave of optimism in the 1960s and 1970s to the effect that intelligence can indeed be improved. The book *Intelligence and Experience* by J. McVickers Hunt (1961) claimed to prove that intelligence wasn't fixed at all and that its growth depended on early experiences. In 1975 popular psychology writer Maya Pines presented a very optimistic picture about such training, while neuropsychologists have found that proper environmental experiences and education actually accelerate and increase the growth of brain processes (Rosenzweig, 1981).

There are different ways to approach this training of intelligence. Some of these may result in IQ score gains without any real improvement in intelligence. It is possible that others may actually improve intelligence itself (Anastasi, 1982).

Training in Test-Taking Orientation

There is little doubt that a pupil's orientation toward taking an IQ test will affect performance on the test. Some pupils are anxious and tend to block. Others don't know the rules of test taking and make blunders that result in low IQ scores, i.e., ones that do not truly reflect their abilities. Test-coaching schools can assist pupils to develop better test-taking abilities and to learn more effective ways of taking tests. Such training can thus help to raise IQs. It cannot, however, be considered to improve intelligence itself (Anastasi, 1982).

Test Coaching

A second way of improving IQ test scores (or the scores of other broad cognitive assessment instruments like the *SAT*s) is intensive short-term mass drill on items similar to the test that the individual will take. Well-constructed general ability tests employ test items that are not easily improved on by such drill. However, there is no doubt that such drill does result in IQ gains. Once again, however, it is not likely that such training actually improves intelligence (Anastasi, 1982).

Training of Cognitive Skills

Here the intent is to train cognition or intelligence directly. Anastasi (1982), a distinguished psychometrician and an early critic of many cognitive training approaches, has come to the conclusion that "contrary to the still prevalent popular notion regarding the fixity of the I.Q., there is a rapidly growing body of evidence that the behavior domain sampled by tests of academic intelligence or scholastic aptitude is responsive to training" (p. 1089).

In the 1960s and 1970s there was an upsurge of programs attempting to improve intelligence of the type that appears to be significant to academic achievement. These were developed largely in the United States and Israel, where large minority populations were having difficulty in adjusting to the majority culture. Most programs were directed to infancy and preschool levels. These programs yielded promising results. Other programs designed for school-age children also produced promising results (Anastasi, 1982). Investigations working with older pupils, in whom the chances of improving intelligence would seem limited, e.g., college students and professional school applicants, also report good results (Anastasi, 1982). These investigations don't just report significant improvements on scholastic aptitude or IQ tests. They also report improvements in academic achievement. A number of programs aimed at improving cognitive ability have been tried with the educable mentally retarded pupils, with generally positive results reported (Borkowski & Cavenaugh, 1979; Sternberg, 1981).

Sabatino, Miller, and Schmidt (1981) have extensively reviewed the topic "Can Intelligence Be Altered through Cognitive Training?" And the conclusion concerning the handicapped was "yes, products such as intelligence can be increased with handicapped persons if delivered as a meaningful intervention" (p. 159). Sabatino and his associates observe, however, that such training must be continuous, unlike that required for normal children, that indeed "learning cognitive processing may [have to be] . . . a life long experience for them" (p. 140).

Feuerstein, too, has developed remedial programs to develop a child's learning potential and to thus improve cognitive abilities. His training procedures are based on his assessment methods. He recommends that specialists identify the particular kinds of cognitive processes that cause pupils the most difficulty in solving learning potential test problems and then provide specific coaching to improve them. His remedial program is called *instrumental enrichment intervention* (Feuerstein et al., 1981).

In instrumental enrichment intervention a pupil who appears deficient in cognitive abilities is given a series of increasingly demanding tasks similar to those assessed by learning potential tests and taught how to solve them. Exercises involve the organizations of dots, perceptual orientation in space, numerical progression, temporal relationships, etc. Feuerstein claims that he has and is able to correct deficient cognitive functioning and to improve achievement drastically in schools in many pupils who had been or would ordinarily be diagnosed as hopelessly mentally retarded according to the scores obtained on traditional intelligence tests. He is a severe critic of the latter, which he says ignore the dynamic quality of learning.

Feuerstein's results have been viewed with considerable enthusiasm by some knowledgeable experts in the field of intelligence. And his efforts ought to be lauded as provocative approaches toward helping pupils improve their intellectual abilities. However, many of the students he has worked with seem to have been culturally deprived or poorly educated rather than mentally retarded. Such individuals are likely to do poorly on intelligence tests but can respond well intellectually when given individual attention. Further research is needed to clarify some of the questions raised about Feuerstein's approach.

A Final Note about Training Intelligence

Many questions must be answered before we can decide whether it is possible to improve intelligence significantly through training. Nevertheless, regardless of whether one is optimistic or pessimistic over the possibilities that general intelligence can be improved, almost all theorists agree that people can learn to use better what abilities they do possess.

SUMMATION

This chapter has given a broad overview of the cognitive processes that are subsumed under the name of intelligence. As we have seen, intelligence can be conceptualized both in broad general terms and in very specific ones. There is a great deal of disagreement as to the actual nature of intelligence and indeed whether it is a hypothetical construct worth retaining at all. Furthermore, there are major controversies over its assessment.

At the same time, there is still great interest in this topic. A new journal called *Intelligence* appeared in 1977. A number of recent books are trying to develop new perspectives on the topic (Resnick, 1976), while new research and theories are proceeding at a very rapid rate (Sternberg, 1981a, 1981b).

Intelligence does have a place in remedial and special education. Its study can be intellectually stimulating to remedial and special educators, giving them new ideas and insights about the pupils. The measures of intelligence can be usefully employed to help programs for remedial pupils.

However, the term IQ should be abandoned; it arouses too much anxiety and hostility. It also has derogatory implications for people who achieve low scores. Other terms can be used in its place, which do not claim to sum up a person's worth within a single number. *Academic ability* (AA), *school-related ability* (ARA), and *school achievement index* (SAI) are some.

Our readers should dismiss the idea that intelligence is a fixed quality that characterizes an individual, once and for all, throughout an entire lifetime. There indeed is considerable stability to our assessments of intelligence for groups of individuals. However, there is also ample evidence that any single individual can drastically gain (or lose), e.g., in terms of IQ points, from one examination to another. This is one good reason for using more than one test to assess anyone's intelligence.

The fascination with intelligence is international. Venezuela actually created a post of Minister of Intelligence. This minister is expected to seek out new ways to improve and upgrade the intelligence of the Venezuelan people. This is but one indication of the continuing interest the construct of intelligence has. It is here to stay, and special education can assist pupils by guiding their teachers in their making of placement and instructional decisions.

Chapter 5

Specific Cognitive Abilities

Interest in the study, diagnosis, and remediation of specific cognitive abilities, i.e., perceptual abilities, attention, memory, actually goes back many centuries (Mann, 1979). Its modern impetus, however, appears to come from efforts made to differentiate intelligence along the lines of separate and distinct cognitive abilities. The modern learning disabilities (LD) movement received much of its inspiration from such efforts. This is acknowledged by Hallahan and Cruickshank (1973), who in their review of the LD movement stated:

> [The movement] . . . from a theory of a unified general intelligence factor "g" to a more refined group factor, and finally to specific ability theories helped to provide a ripe climate for the development of learning disability theory. Since the concept of specific abilities and disabilities can be considered a *sine qua non* of learning disability theory, the historical trend within mental measurement theory to concern for identification of specific abilities assumes tremendous importance. (p. 88)

Specific cognitive abilities are indeed useful hypothetical constructs for educators to use in the diagnosis and remediation of learning problems (Sabatino, Miller, & Schmidt, 1981). But is there any reason to concern ourselves with these abilities outside the study of intelligence? After all, even the *Stanford-Binet Scale*, perhaps the most general of all general intelligence tests, has been differentiated along the lines of separate and distinct abilities for diagnostic and remedial purposes (Meeker, 1965; Meeker & Meeker, 1973; Vallett, 1964). Other, now more popular tests, like the *Wechsler Scales*, provide a number of component scores (besides estimates of general ability), which easily lend themselves to this purpose (Kaufman, 1979). Why not deal with specific cognitive abilities within the framework of intelligence? Actually the decision as to whether to do so is entirely arbitrary. We can and do in fact often study specific cognitive processes within the broader framework of intelligence.

There are good reasons, however, why we may choose to study many specific cognitive abilities apart from their association with intelligence. For one, most intelligence theories and assessment approaches are selective in terms of the cognitive abilities (processes) that they address. That is, they usually select for study and assessment those specific abilities that appear to have the most predictive value as far as school and academic achievement is concerned. They minimally concern themselves with and even neglect other important cognitive abilities or do not evaluate them in sufficient detail for purposes of instruction or remediation. It is for such reasons that we may choose to study specific cognitive processes (abilities) apart from the study of intelligence.

This is the way, indeed, that the fields of remedial education and learning disabilities seem to have oriented themselves toward the assessment of specific cognitive processes. Many tests of specific abilities are given to supplement traditional IQ tests (or general aptitude and achievement tests) on the basis that information about their strengths and weaknesses can guide education and remediation. Thus such tests as the Marianne Frostig *Developmental Test of Visual Perception* (Frostig, Maslow, Lefever, & Whittlesey, 1964) became popular not because intelligence tests did not assess visual perception extensively but because they didn't assess it in precise enough ways as far as certain remedial and learning disability specialists were concerned.

A similar situation confronts us in the study of language processes. The Binet and Wechsler tests certainly do not neglect language. Some scholars believe that language's role in intelligent behavior has been overemphasized (Thurstone, 1948; Piaget 1950). Intelligence tests, however, do not specifically assess language processes *as* language or at least they don't do it in ways satisfactory to remedial and learning disability specialists who wish to assess language in ways that have precise implications for training and remediation. Consequently a number of special language tests have been developed to meet the specific needs of remedial and special education (Sabatino & Miller, 1978).

Still other tests of specific abilities appear to be required to assess cognitive areas that are almost entirely ignored by traditional intelligence tests, such as those of gross motor or sensorimotor abilities. It is on this basis that tests such as the *Bruninks-Oseretsky Tests of Motor Proficiency* (Bruninks, 1971), the *Southern California Sensory Integration Tests* (Ayres, 1972b), and the *Purdue Perceptual-Motor Survey* (Roach & Kephart, 1966) were created.

There is still another reason for interest in specific cognitive abilities outside the framework of intelligence. This is concern with what have been called *component* or *basic cognitive abilities* (Lerner, 1981).

That is, some remedial and learning disability theorists consider certain specific cognitive abilities to be the building blocks (components) of the cognitive abilities assessed by traditional intelligence tests or creating as it were the (basic) foundations for the later development of academic types of intelligence. Kirk's psycholinguistic abilities and Frostig's developmental perceptual abilities express both these perspectives. They direct attention to cognitive abilities (or processes) other than those assessed by traditional intelligence tests.

To sum up, current interest in specific cognitive processes (abilities) has a number of roots in century-old efforts to isolate and assess and train specific cognitive abilities, including those of perception, motor functioning, and language; psychometric theories that identify specific ability components in intelligence; efforts to assess and train specific abilities that are not adequately assessed by traditional intelligence tests for educational or remedial purposes; and attempts to study abilities that are essential in various ways to the development of the abilities traditionally assessed by intelligence tests.

Because many of the prominent modern theories of specific cognitive abilities have developed within the contexts of remedial and special education—and apart from studies of intelligence—their interpretations of cognition vary somewhat from those of the psychometric variety that we reviewed in Chapter 4. They also differ because, unlike intelligence theories that seek to understand and explain how individuals vary in ability, specific ability theories were developed to meet clinical and remedial needs. This is clearly revealed in the definitions of specific abilities now reviewed.

DEFINITIONS OF SPECIFIC COGNITIVE ABILITIES

Definitions of specific abilities are reviewed from the standpoint of several authors so that the reader can appreciate the different ways in which cognitive specificity can be conceived. We should like to observe first that the term *ability* is often used interchangeably and imprecisely with other terms, e.g., *capacity, skill, process, system, behavior,* and *function.*

Lerner

Lerner's (1981) excellent text on learning disabilities defines specific abilities or processes from a number of standpoints. In one broad definition, she states that "the term cognitive abilities refers to a collection of mental skills that are essential human functions. They enable one to be aware, to think, to conceptualize, to use abstractions, to reason, to criticize, and to be creative" (p. 159).

She (1981) also defines specific abilities in terms of what she calls a *components of mental functioning* approach to cognition—not to be confused with the cognitive components of Sternberg's component theory of intelligence; *basic psychological processes;* and a *cognitive processing approach.*

Lerner (1981) observes that components of mental functioning approaches to cognition stress the "multidimensional abilities (and consequent disabilities) of mental functioning" (p. 168). The remedial implications are explicit in her next statement:

> One implication of this approach is that a child may perform well in some respects and poorly in others. As testing instruments are developed to measure subabilities [translate as specific abilities] the teacher is able to compare performance in various subskills [again translate as specific abilities] and note disparities. Moreover, along with the diagnostic tools to identify subareas of mental function [specific abilities], methods of teaching to build these are generated. (p. 168)

Lerner also observes that "the approach to remediation often associated with learning disabilities is that of cognitive processing . . . [which] refers to the child's abilities in processing information, perceptual modalities . . . or pathways of learning" (p. 140). These abilities are basic psychological processes.

Lerner's distinctions help us to understand both the nature of specific ability concepts most prevalent today, and their importance to remedial and special education cognition consisting of a number of separate abilities or subabilities. A pupil may be strong in respect to one ability and weak in respect to others. There are also methods of teaching and remediation that develop or correct or compensate for disabilities.

In discussing specific abilities as basic psychological processes, Lerner (1981) makes the point that we have raised earlier in this chapter, i.e., that specific abilities are often regarded as basic to general intellectual functioning and academic performance. She observes that "there are a variety of differing (sometimes conflicting) theories" and "models of specific cognitive abilities," but that "all of them specify underlying processing abilities, such as auditory processing, visual processing, kinaesthetic and tactile processing, memory abilities, language abilities, and so forth. Moreover, each of these processing abilities is further subdivided" (p. 170).

In other words specific ability approaches study those cognitive abilities that are basic to, or underlie, other abilities, e.g., such as assessed by intelligence tests. They also assume that we can break up various cognitive abilities areas, such as auditory processing, visual processing, memory and language abilities, into even more specific subabilities.

Johnson

Johnson (1981) provides us with still another definitional approach to specific cognitive abilities, observing that "a psychological process [specific ability] is an independent structure that analyzes information received by the brain in a specific way" (p. 89). Like Lerner, Johnson places specific abilities into a remedial framework: "The diagnostic remedial method, also called the process method, makes three basic assumptions: each individual has a set of independent psychological processes; psychological processes can be revealed by psychological tests; children with learning disabilities have specific dysfunctions in one or more of these processes" (p. 89).

Johnson (1981) provides us with a useful illustration of how these basic independent processes (or abilities) may operate during a particular academic task. He does so from the standpoint of a child naming pictures in a coloring book: The child first sees the picture (visual reception process). The child associates the picture with one that was previously seen (visual memory). The child matches the recognized visual images with the appropriate auditory word (visual-auditory integration). This requires that the child remember the verbal name of the image (auditory memory). The child then says the word aloud (verbal expression).

Johnson and Morasky

In their 1980 book on learning disabilities Johnson and Morasky try to avoid using the terms *cognition* and *specific abilities* altogether by taking a behavioral approach to specific abilities. The book doesn't even list the term *cognition* in its index. Johnson and Morasky, however, write about "basic processes," "systems and behaviors," which appear to be synonymous with what we call *specific cognitive abilities*. Johnson and Morasky do agree that specific process theories focus on isolated and narrow areas of functioning, and these areas are usually considered to be priority areas. At one point in this book they describe a "basic process" approach. This is described as usually involving a

> Sequential developmental focus . . . mostly on a single or narrow process
> rather than an orientation to all development. In most single basic process theories
> or programs there is a fundamental assumption that the system or component of
> the system being studied is a *priority* prerequisite to other behaviors. The search is
> for a single or limited set of systems that are basic in the organism when it comes
> to learning behaviors. (p. 88)

They (1980) define processes elsewhere in the context of remediation, *Basic processes*. Aspects that focus on underlying etiology, upon behavior and systems prerequisite to the removal of current learning problem behaviors and to the elicitation of normal behaviors.

Emphasis is typically upon a single system or process sometimes arbitrarily elected as 'basic'" (p. 83).

Other Definitions

Torgeson (1979) is a well-known learning disabilities scholar who tries to "behaviorize" specific cognitive abilities in his definition: "Processes are constituted of specific covert behaviors, which transform and manipulate information between the time it enters as a stimulus and the time a response to it is selected" (p. 516).

Fass (1981) on the other hand provides a *task* definition of specific cognitive abilities: "Visual processing consists of a number of visual perceptual tasks that are involved in receiving, organizing, and interpreting visual stimuli" (p. 86). Fass also defines a *specific ability* as the ability to do something specifically which is a nice way of "operationalizing" abilities. Thus, "*visual discrimination* involves the ability to recognize the similarities and differences among items" (p. 87).

These definitions make the point again that cognition may be defined and studied in a number of different ways. Whether it helps to equate cognition with behavior, systems, and tasks in the ways that Johnson and Morasky, Torgeson, and Fass have done is a matter of debate (Ledwidge, 1978).

THE NATURE OF SPECIFIC ABILITIES

This particular section might well be titled "Where Do All Those Abilities Come From?" This question is facetious, to be sure. At the same time it must be asked and answered if we are to understand the nature of specific cognitive processes and their role in remedial and special education.

The truth is that an incredible number of specific cognitive abilities have been identified as important to human development, learning, academic achievement, social adjustment, etc. (Mann, 1979). How were they discovered—and why should educators (or anyone else) be concerned with them?

The beginnings of interest in specific abilities date far back. It was evident centuries ago, as now, that humans engage in a variety of significantly different activities, ranging from levels required to biologically survive, e.g., breathing and digestion, to psychological ones, i.e., perceiving, remembering, solving problems, and making judgments. Some philosophers, psychologists, and educators believed that these activities were caused by the exercise of inner powers or abilities. Thus they described people as being able to perceive objects visually because they have the ability of visual perception, to remember because of their memory abilities, to think because of their reasoning abilities. Differences in people's ability to perceive, remember, think, were then attributed to strengths and weaknesses in these inner abilities. A person who can't visually distinguish things "obviously" has poor visual perceptual abilities. One who can recall information with a high degree of accuracy has a good memory. If the person makes bad judgments, it is because of poor reasoning ability. An individual attending persistently to a task has good powers of attention and concentration.

It is on such a basis that theories of specific cognitive abilities first developed from observations of people's behavior, from attempts to explain their behaviors on the basis of inner abilities or powers, and by explaining differences in their behaviors by differences in these abilities or powers.

Perception, memory, judgment, and reasoning were popular cognitive processes from the time of the ancient Greeks well into the twentieth century. They are still among the most popular of ability areas. Attention became popular in the sixth century AD. Motor abilities became prominent (in the cognitive sense) during the eighteenth century. Once neurologists demonstrated that the nervous system was composed of sensory, motor, and association neurons in differing proportions, perceptual-motor abilities became extraordinarily popular. The philosophies and training practices of such well-known special education pioneers as Sequin and Montessori reveal this. In a similar fashion, when neurologists found that specific parts of the brain served different purposes in language reception and expression, a variety of "new" language abilities were created (Mann, 1979).

At the beginning of the twentieth century, when compulsory education mandated that schools educate handicapped pupils, educators looked for cognitive explanations of the latter's academic difficulties. Guided by the neurological and psychological theories of the day, they found them. Since auditory, visual, and perceptual imagery and memory abilities appeared to be the ones most critical to the acquisition of reading and other academic skills, tests were devised to assess these abilities, and techniques were created to train them. Modern aptitude tests and remedial assessment procedures have their roots in these early practices.

Throughout history, efforts have been made to train and correct specific abilities in order to improve them when they are "normal," to correct them when they appear to be impaired, to use "able" abilities when others are weak or disabled, and to make curricular adjustments based on the strengths and weaknesses of specific abilities. Present ideas about ability or process training are not new altogether. This does not mean that our modern theories and methods are antiquated relics. It does mean that we must examine and consider their claims in light of what we have learned.

The specific abilities that modern remedial and special educators are likely to encounter have been hypothesized because they seem to explain pupils' learning and learning failures reasonably. For example, visual-motor coordination is a cognitive process or ability that one might "reasonably" expect to be involved in handwriting; good auditory skills seem to be required for reading; visual-spatial abilities are "obviously" involved in geometry.

A number of specific ability theories are derived from neurology, e.g., Ayre's (1975) theories of sensory integration and Orton-Gillingham's (1973) language approaches. Still others have developed on the basis of specialized psychological theories. Thus the *ITPA* was founded, theoretically, on Osgood's S-R language model (Kirk, McCarthy, & Kirk, 1971), while Frostig's (Frostig & Horne, 1967) visual perceptual theories took some of their inspiration from Gestalt psychology. Some specific abilities are justified by factor analysis, e.g., Kaufman's "ability" interpretations of the *Wechsler Scales* (1955).

All specific abilities represent in various degrees the conceptions of particular theorists as to how the mind works to create behavior. They are also likely to represent someone's special interests and beliefs. Thus Kephart's (1971) motor theories were certainly inspired by his background in physical education, while Kirk's (1940, 1968) *ITPA* model received its impetus from his interest in the reading problems of cognitively handicapped pupils.

Do these theories, and the testing and remedial methods accompanying them, help us to understand how our pupils learn (or fail to learn)? Do they help us teach better or remediate problems more effectively? These are the grounds on which we must ultimately judge them. So, having answered the question "Where do all those abilities come from?" we should perhaps ask and try to answer another one: "Should those abilities stay around?" The answer is yes if they are useful, no if they are not. And this leads to another question: "How does one decide?" There are no easy answers.

SPECIFICITY OF SPECIFIC

How specific must a cognitive ability be in order to be considered specific? This is not a facetious question but rather a serious concern. We are helped to understand and answer this question by our earlier study of intelligence in Chapter 4. There we found that literally countless specific cognitive abilities could be "discovered" depending on the nature of the behaviors studied, the evaluation instruments employed, the statistical analyses done, and the purpose for which particular abilities were being studied.

We also discussed that specific cognitive abilities can be grouped together to form broader, though still quite distinct, specific cognitive abilities and that the latter can be further grouped to form yet broader but specific abilities. Thus language can be studied from the standpoint of a number of very basic skills; it may be studied as two major ability groups: receptive and expressive; or it may be studied as a unitary language ability. Specificity is a matter of definition. We will explain some broad, as well as some very narrow, areas of functioning, as representing the operations of specific abilities.

Students of cognitive processes must become used to ambiguities and inconsistencies. That is one of the prices we must pay when dealing with hypothetical constructs in psychology and education. These constructs are not as firmly anchored in external data as are those of the physical sciences. We find this to be particularly true for specific cognitive ability constructs that have been influenced by many different specialized terminologies, theoretical biases, and personal whims.

As shown in this chapter, specific (cognitive) abilities are sometimes identified as behaviors, processes, structures, systems, and even terms of tasks. Such a looseness in descriptions can cause confusion regarding the nature of specific abilities. Thus Johnson and Morasky describe the *Illinois Test of Psycholinguistic Abilities (ITPA)* as a deficit behavior approach to learning disabilities. Nevertheless the *ITPA* clearly deals with specific abilities. Readers must maintain a consistent framework of reference throughout this chapter in order to avoid confusion by conflicting terms and explanations. A number of criteria can help us make this determination.

The first criterion for specific cognitive abilities is that each of them implies "inner" (nonobservable, i.e., hypothetical) characteristics that are distinctly different from those of others. The second is that specific ability approaches are typically oriented to determining adequacies, i.e., strengths and weaknesses, in relatively narrow areas of cognitive functioning. These areas are studied, diagnosed, and remediated on grounds that they are stable though modifiable; they explain the same types of behaviors in a variety of situations, i.e., are generalizable; and they are essential to key areas of school learning and performance.

Different Types of Specific Cognitive Processes

Specific ability theories can be classified along a number of dimensions. Some share several dimensions.

Neurology

Some types of specific abilities are clearly neurological in their implications (Delacato, 1966a, 1966b; Ayres, 1975). Others are related by theorists to the nervous system though their relationships are not explained to any great degree (Kephart, 1971; Myklebust, 1973). For still others the nervous system is ignored (Frostig & Horne, 1967) or written off as irrelevant (Kirk & Kirk, 1971).

Modalities

Specific abilities are quite frequently classified in terms of specific modalities, sensory or motor. A good number of investigators have gone this route, studying various perceptual and motor abilities with different degrees of specificity and in varying degrees of combination (Barsch, 1965, 1967a, 1967b, 1967c). Modality approaches to specific abilities are often anchored in neurological theory as the working structures of the nervous system consist of sensory and motor and association neurons. The Orton-Gillingham (Orton, 1928, 1973) approach is one of these, as are Silver & Hagin's (1976) theories and techniques. But just as often modality approaches are justified by psychological theories that do not have neurological implications. Thus Frostig (Frostig & Horne, 1967) drew many of her inspirations from Gestalt psychology, while Sabatino (1973, 1974) utilized concepts of central processing, and Fernald (1943) applied notions of multisensory learning—all on the basis of psychological theories.

Language

Some specific ability theories focus on language. Because language is inevitably tied to sensory inputs and motor outputs, language ability theories often emphasize sensory modalities (Wepman, 1958; Kirk & Kirk, 1971; Orton, 1973). Some theorists, however, try to distinguish and separate language from perception (Vellutino, 1974). A number of language theories have a strong neurological indebtedness. This is to be expected because many of those who work with language do so within medical settings (Wepman, 1958). Other theorists base their theories entirely on psychological theories (Kirk & Kirk, 1971).

Academic Skills

A number of specific abilities have been proposed to make sense of academic achievement and difficulties (Otto & Smith, 1980). *The Durrell Analysis of Reading Difficulty* (Durrell, 1955) and the *Gates-MiKillop Reading Diagnostic Tests* (1962) include auditory blending and discrimination tests. Spelling remediation approaches often emphasized visual auditory remediation approaches (Hildreth, 1955). Mathematics remediation has also taken a specific ability approach on occasion (Johnson & Myklebust, 1967).

Attention and Memory

Cognitive areas like attention and memory have also been studied in terms of constituting specific abilities. The digit span tests used in intelligence tests scales (such as the *Wechsler* and the *Stanford-Binet*) are popular ways of assessing these abilities. The *Detroit Test of Learning Aptitudes* has also been used for this purpose (Baker & Leland, 1935). Special tests have also been developed, e.g., the *Revised Visual Retention Test* (Benton, 1963) and the Graham and Kendall (1960) *Memory-for-Design* tests. The greatest amount of recent interest in these areas, however, has been expressed within the framework of information-processing systems (Chapter 7).

Imagination

In the past, reproductive imagination (imagery) was frequently implicated in reading and spelling (Hildreth, 1955). This is less true in modern approaches. Getman (1965), however, gives imagery a distinct place in his Visual Motor Model. Imagery can also be assessed directly and indirectly, through tests of perception and memory, many of which presume the

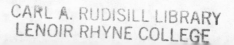

functioning of imagery, e.g., the *Revised Visual Retention Test* (Benton, 1963). There has also been a strong revival of interest in imagery in recent years within cognitive psychology and educational research (Greeno, 1978, 1980; Paivio, 1979; Pressley, 1977). But this is not usually in terms of imagery being conceptualized as a type of specific ability.

Creative Imagination

Creative imagination is a particular favorite of instructors concerned with the education of the gifted and talented (Renzulli, 1973). We have already discussed the applications of Guilford's SI abilities to the study of abilities relevant to giftedness and creativity.

Higher Cognitive Processes

The higher cognitive processes have not received much attention in terms of a specific ability focus. There are good reasons for this. Most of what we call *higher cognitive abilities* are assessed adequately by intelligence, academic aptitude, and academic achievement tests. These tests evaluate pupils' abilities to organize ideas, comprehend, use abstractions, reason, etc. Some of them, e.g., the *Wechsler Intelligence Scale for Children*, have also been used diagnostically to identify higher cognitive abilities and disabilities needing special attention, i.e., in teaching and remediation (Kaufman, 1979). Information-processing theorists have also shown a great deal of interest in analyzing higher cognitive processes (Chapter 7).

DISTINCTIONS BETWEEN DEVELOPMENTAL ABILITY AND BASIC PROCESS APPROACHES

Distinctions are sometimes made between developmental and maturational ability approaches and those of the basic process type. As Lerner (1981) describes it, psychologists and educators taking a developmental or maturational approach are concerned with "the sequential growth" and "progression of [all] cognitive abilities under appropriate conditions" (p. 160). In contrast, psychologists and educators taking a basic process approach are prone to concern themselves with a specific type or set of abilities, e.g., perceptual or language ones. They assume that particular abilities have priority in respect to others in teaching, training—and remediation. Their "search is for a single or limited set of systems [i.e., ability or abilities] that are basic . . . when it comes to learning behaviors. There is the assumption of some type of functional priority" for these in learning (Johnson & Morasky, 1980, p. 88).

Developmental theorists are likely to view cognitive problems differently than do basic process theorists. They view such problems as resulting from "maturational lags" rather than from specific disabilities. They "hypothesize that children with learning disorders are not so different from children without them. It is more a matter of *timing* than an actual difference in abilities. They assume a temporary developmental lag in the maturation of certain abilities and skills" (Lerner, 1981, p. 160).

In other words, developmental theorists are concerned with the overall general development of a child's abilities. They conceive of cognitive disorders (other than those caused by specific neurological disabilities) as being a matter of uneven development or maturation rather than as representing deficits in, or impairments of, specific cognitive abilities. They often recommend that a child be given more time to mature as a way of encouraging cognitive improvement because they believe that further maturation can overcome many learning problems. Where they intervene with remediation, they are prone to emphasize activities that encourage general cognitive growth—to help all of the child's abilities to develop evenly.

In contrast, basic process theorists believe that the development of certain abilities is basic to the development of others. They are likely to recommend that these abilities receive priority in training or remediation and also that they should be trained separately from others. Thus, some basic process theorists would advocate that motor training or remediation precede training or remediation and that perceptual training and remediation precede language training and remediation. Whereas developmental theorists are likely to assess all aspects of a child's cognitive functioning, and to do so from a developmental point of view, basic process theorists usually focus on the precise identification of particular, specific abilities in isolation from others.

The distinctions between developmental abilities and basic process (abilities) approaches hold up only partly. Thus Piaget's theories (Chapter 6) must be regarded as developmental in nature. Yet Piaget too writes in terms of basic processes and theorizes that the development of some processes should precede the development of others. And developmental remedial specialists sometimes recommend direct attention to specific learning problems. On the other hand many of the so-called basic process approaches appear to be broad and developmental in numerous ways. Kirk's language test, the *ITPA*, assesses perceptual as well as language modalities (Paraskenopoulos & Kirk, 1965). And the language training and remediation program most closely associated with the *ITPA* (Minskoff, Wiseman, & Minskoff, 1972) trains perceptual modalities as well as oral language decoding and encoding. Similarly Frostig (1967, 1968, 1974) sought to assess and remediate a variety of cognitive functions, though her name is most often associated with perceptual abilities, and she considered her work to be developmental in nature.

The distinctions between developmental and basic process theories become less distinct when we examine one of the remediation premises espoused by developmental theorists. When a child is found to have a learning problem, developmental theorists recommend that the remedial specialist retrace the child's steps in development until a baseline of effective functioning is found (Lerner, 1981). After this baseline is reached, remediation of the problem is to proceed in such a way as to assist the child to develop "through and past the problem-solving stage, in a normal fashion . . . to a level of appropriate functioning" (Johnson & Morasky, 1980, p. 85).

Yet basic process trainers often take the same approach. Frostig trainers (1967, 1974) begin perceptual training at the level at which the child can cope perceptually and then proceed developmentally upward "through and past the problem-solving stage." Similarly Kirk (1968) has suggested that a major reason for learning disabilities may be a maturational lag in a particular ability area. This lag causes the child to avoid or minimize activities involving the ability. As a result, this ability doesn't develop effectively, and a specific disability is caused. Remedial efforts are to be directed toward developing the deficient ability at an age-appropriate level.

Are we at an impasse in all of this? Can no clear distinctions be made between developmental and basic process approaches? As is so often the case in life, and science, we must be satisfied with approximations.

As compared to basic process theorists, developmental theorists do in fact more strongly emphasize the general development of cognitive functioning, e.g., Gesell and Amatruda (1974). They also stress more strongly the importance of maturation and enriched learning opportunities for helping children to develop and improve cognitively. They are less concerned with tests of specific abilities and with specific remedial approaches.

As compared to developmental theorists, process theorists are more likely to focus on one or several types of specific abilities for training or remediation at particular times. Their approach is likely to be narrower and to attempt greater precision. They are more likely than developmental theorists to intervene directly in a child's learning problems rather than to wait for time and nature to make improvements.

How do developmental and basic process theories fit into our considerations in this chapter? Some developmental and basic process theories can be considered as specific ability theories, while others do not. Thus we do not consider Piaget's developmental cognitive theory (Chapter 6) to be a specific ability approach. But neither do we consider information-processing theories, which might be considered to be a type of basic process orientation to cognition, to constitute a specific ability approach. Our decision as to what constitutes specific ability types of approaches is based on the criteria we established earlier, which we now restate in somewhat different terms.

Specific ability approaches are oriented to determining adequacies, strengths, and weaknesses in circumscribed areas of cognitive functioning. These are studied, diagnosed, and remediated on grounds that they are stable though modifiable; they are essential to key areas of learning and school achievement, they are usually identified with particular scales or tests, and most of them deal with abilities as if they are a collection of separate and distinct cognitive powers, each of which controls, or otherwise determines, specific types of behavior. Readers desiring more comprehensive information about them will find Lerner's (1981) text an excellent guide.

NEUROLOGICAL ABILITY THEORIES

As discussed, a number of specific cognitive theories attempt to establish links between cognitive processes and the nervous system (Ayres, 1972a; Myklebust, 1973; Kephart, 1971). One of the most ambitious of these attempts is the neurological organization theory of Doman and Delacato (Delacato, 1966a,b; Doman, Spitz, Zuchman, Delacato, & Doman, 1967). The cognitive processes it deals with are specifically identified with as brain levels.

The theory presumes that when normal children mature, they pass through a number of developmental stages, each of which is characterized by increasingly advanced levels of neurological organization or brain levels. In a normal child there is a progression from brain stem levels to those of cortical functioning.

According to Doman and Delacato, the following brain levels are to be delineated for study and training: spinal cord-medulla level, pons levels, midbrain level, early cortex level, and cortical hemispheric dominance. A child's cognitive competency and the type of cognitive-behavioral performances the child is capable of depend on the particular brain levels achieved. The functioning of lower brain levels must be mastered and consolidated before that of higher levels can be successfully accomplished.

Children suffering from uneven cognitive development, i.e., learning-disabled, brain-injured, retarded, etc., reveal unsystematic or faulty progressions in their development of the functions associated with one or the other of these brain levels. A pupil may have reached an age when higher brain levels should dominate cognitive functioning. Indeed the pupil may have even developed some abilities appropriate for this age. But unless the pupil has previously mastered all of the functions associated with earlier brain levels, the child will not be cognitively competent; there will be cognitive and behavioral deficits and deficiencies of various kinds.

Doman-Delacato remedial treatment approaches were designed to help a child organize or reorganize neurological levels so as to become progressively competent at all brain levels, proceeding from the lowest to highest. Their remedial techniques and treatments are essentially carried out in the form of motor activities appropriate to each brain level. Thus a child is "patterned" motorically, through passive manipulation of limbs and other parts of the body in order to help develop brain stem capacities. The child is then taught to creep and crawl to encourage the development of midbrain structures. Laterality training develops correct left-right hemisphere cortical controls, etc.

In respect to the latter, Delacato (1966) suggests that piano playing in preschool years be discouraged because the use of both hands tends to activate both brain halves and may thus hinder the development of left hemispheric dominance. In a similar vein children at one time were discouraged from playing as two-gun cowboys since double draws also activate both hemispheres. Sometimes parents were advised that children's left arms be tied down or that they sleep in certain postures, once again to assist in the development of the left-hemisphere dominance. Doman-Delacato's theories and methods have been controversial (Freeman, 1967), but they also have many supporters.

Doman-Delacato's neurological organization theory is both neurological and developmental. We identify it as being a specific cognitive ability theory, first, to indicate that the nervous system, when conceptualized in certain ways, can be conceived in specific ability terms; second, because the brain level approaches accentuate specific types of training.

MOTOR ABILITY THEORIES

It is questionable as to whether we should identify any type of specific ability strictly as a motor theory. Most theories that focus on motor abilities usually do so in conjunction with perceptual ones; indeed they sometimes involve language and other higher cognitive abilities. In similar fashion, many specific ability theories identified as perceptual or language frequently have motor components. The Doman-Delacato approach, which we earlier classified as neurological, can also be classified as a motor theory because its training efforts are very motoric, though directed to the improvement of specific (hypothetical) neurological components. Similarly the theories to be discussed as motor theories have neurological and perceptual implications. We have designated them as *motor* because of the singular importance they assign to the motor system in cognition.

We have selected the theories of Newell Kephart (1960, 1971), Raymond Barsch (1967a,b), and Bryan Cratty (1967, 1969a, 1969b, 1971) as exemplars of motor theories. As so often can be expected, these theories are reflections of the people who developed them. Kephart was a psychologist who had a strong physical education background. Ayres is an occupational therapist. Cratty is a physical educator. While their theories also attend to perception, their major focus (most of us would agree) is on motor activities, on the premise that gross motor abilities are basic to the development and the expression of cognition. We consider them to be of specific ability nature because in one way or the other they emphasize the development and remediation of separate and distinct cognitive components.

Newell Kephart

Kephart's motor theory was first explained in depth in his book *The Slow Learner in the Classroom* (1960, 1971), one of the earliest of modern books devoted to learning disabilities. Its basic premise is that "higher [cognitive] activities [are] dependent upon the basic structure of the muscular activity upon which they are built. Higher level mental processes develop out of and after adequate development of the motor system: . . . [and that] it is logical to assume that all behavior is basically motor, that the prerequisites of any kind of behavior are muscular and motor responses" (1971, p. 79).

It is equally logical to assume that the prerequisites of cognition are muscular and motor abilities. Apropos of Kephart's definition, Johnson and Morasky (1980) observe that "motor should be considered to mean an internalized neurophysiological event that relates to . . . external movement . . . [and] . . . bodily involvement" (p. 108).

Kephart's theory of cognition presumes that cognition develops hierarchically and sequentially. This is fitting because he was influenced by Piaget's theories (Chapter 6). According to Kephart, cognition is created from layers of abilities that develop in a fixed sequence as the child matures. Each subsequent layer builds on earlier ones. Within each layer, special types of abilities should develop in an orderly fashion.

Basic Movement Pattern

More specifically Kephart believed that cognitive development begins with the sequential emergence of basic movement patterns in the following order: posture, laterality, directionality, and body image. These are fundamental, in respect both to later motor adequacy and to the development of higher cognitive abilities.

Basic Motor Generalizations

Once the child's basic movement patterns have been established, basic motor generalizations can proceed. They too develop in a sequential fashion—if the child is growing normally. Balance and posture constitute the first of these generalizations. A child must be able to maintain the body in a stable and controlled fashion in order to develop more advanced motor functions. Locomotion (the ability to move about) develops in conjunction with walking, running, jumping, and skipping. Contact, the third motor generalization, involves the motor abilities of reaching, grasping, and releasing. Receipt and propulsion, the fourth of the generalizations, are involved in catching and throwing, pulling and pushing, lifting, and similar activities. Basic motor generalizations enable the child to develop an understanding of objects and situations and their relationship. They must be properly established in order for higher cognitive development to proceed properly.

Perceptual Motor Matches

As children obtain information through motor activities, they also observe the perceptual features of their world by investigating things through their senses. A great deal of perceptual data is thus accumulated. But it must be integrated with previously learned motor information (basic motor generalizations) in order to become meaningful. That is, children's perceptual data must be matched and integrated with their motor information. It is only thus children can develop accurate and stable perceptions. Perceptual motor matches, for example, enable children to form stable, accurate perceptions of things that often look quite different from various angles, distances, etc. Children who fail to develop effective perceptual motor matches are unable to collate perceptual and motor data properly. The consequence of such failure is cognitive maldevelopment, i.e., the development of a number of uncoordinated "splinter" skills and an inability to achieve at higher cognitive levels. In short, perceptual motor matches stabilize and validate perceptual information by relating the latter to motor information; this is essential for full and efficient cognitive functioning.

According to Kephart, learning disabilities may result from failures at any of the levels we have discussed, i.e., from failure to develop properly basic motor patterns, or motor generalizations, or because of ineffective perceptual motor matches. Kephart also believed that proper training or remedial exercises can prevent or overcome problems in this area.

Barsch

In his book *Achieving Perceptual Motor Experiences*, Barsch (1967a) states that "the organism is designed for movement" (p. 327). And movement efficiency was the goal he set for the developmental-remedial program called *movigenics*, which he devised to help children develop cognitively. He also believes perception is important, particularly when joined with movement; indeed he describes language as being a *visual spatial phenomenon* (p. 367). He advises that three basic components must be attended to in remediation: (1) postural-transport orientations, (2) perceptocognitive models, and (3) degrees of freedom, i.e., bilaterality, rhythm, flexibility, and motor planning. These are emphasized in Barsch's movigenic curriculum, which, while originally intended for use with normal children, has been adapted to the needs of children with learning problems and disabilities.

Cratty

Bryan Cratty has written a variety of books and manuals about the training of motor abilities. A physical educator, Cratty's exercises to train or improve motor abilities have a distinct physical education flavor. His training activities can be divided into those concerning perception of the body and its position in space, locomotion, ability, strength, endurance and flexibility, catching and throwing balls, manual skills, movement and thinking.

While critical of what he called "movement messiahs," he also believes that motor activities play a significant role in the development of cognition. In order to do this, they must, however, be associated in various ways with higher cognitive processes (Lerner, 1981). Beyond that he views motor training as providing opportunities for the improvement of cognitive functioning. Participation in games is valued as a means of developing and reinforcing higher thinking because the participants learn to use rules and to use language within specified contexts and because the high motivational states created by games reinforce cognitive learning.

PERCEPTUAL MOTOR THEORIES

The theories that we have chosen to classify as perceptual motor are really quite motoric in their orientation. In one of these theories, that of Ayres (1972a, 1975), considerable attention is devoted to such fundamental motor phenomena as tonic neck reflexes, muscle tones, the ability to contract antagonistic muscles at the same time, while Knickerbocker in a book inspired by Ayres, *A Holistic Approach to the Treatment of Learning Disorders* (1980) devotes a great deal of discussion to neuromotor processes. Nevertheless, the theories in this section also emphasize perceptual processes; they are in particular visually oriented. And that is why we have classified them as perceptual motor. The representative theorists whom we have chosen to review as representing the perceptual motor position are Ayres (1972a, 1972b, 1975) and Getman (1965).

Ayres

Jean Ayres is one of the most neurological and motoric of perceptual motor theorists. This is an expression, perhaps, of her background in occupational therapy. She has developed a number of tests including the *Southern California Perceptual Motor Test* and the *California Motor Accuracy Test*. She has also developed a number of remedial procedures. These are more likely to be used by occupational therapists (in hospitals and clinics) than by remedial and special educators in school. She has presented her theories in the book *Sensory Integration and Learning Disorders* (1972a). The objective of her sensory integrative approach is "to enhance the brain's ability to learn how to do things." She distinguishes her approach to learning problems on the basis that it doesn't try to teach specific skills of any kind but rather "enhances" the brain's ability to do them. "For if the brain develops the capacity to perceive, remember and motor plan" its abilities can be applied "towards mastery of all academic and other tasks" (p. 5).

As observed, Ayres' theories and methods are directed in great part to gross motor functions. Thus her *Southern California Sensory Integration Tests (SCSIT)* (1972b) have items that assess imitation of postures, bilateral motor coordination, position in space, standing balance, etc. She is, however, also concerned with fine motor abilities and specific types of perceptual processes, e.g., tactile perception.

Ayres theorizes that effective sensory integration is essential to normal learning and that disturbances in that integration are likely to cause learning disabilities. It follows that training to improve sensory integration will also help to remediate learning disorders.

Getman

Gerald Getman's theory of a visuomotor complex is an ambitious one. His visuomotor complex extends from a base in what he calls "innate response systems" to a summit of higher cognitive abilities (see Figure 5–1). Getman's theory and the developmental and remediation practices that he and others have developed on its basis are strongly motoric. This is to be expected in light of Getman's optometric background. Optometrists, much more than ophthalmologists (their medical counterparts), are interested in the training and retraining of the motor aspects of visual functioning. For example, orthoptics is an optometric method that was developed to improve visual acuity by training individuals to make flexible ocular movements. Furthermore, Getman was closely affiliated with the Gesell Institute, which strongly emphasizes the study of motor development. Getman's affiliation with the Gesell Institute also seems to account for the developmental framework within which he has cast his theory.

Getman is a pioneer in what is known as *vision training*. This training is not done from a standpoint of visual acuity, which is simply a matter of light patterns reaching the retina. It is rather carried out to improve a child's basic visuomotor learning schemes. He believes

Figure 5–1 Visuomotor Complex

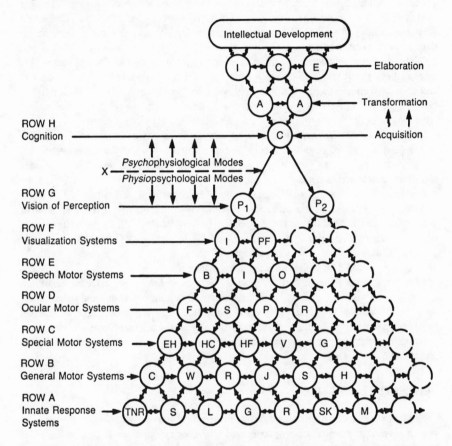

Source: Reprinted from "The Visuomotor Complex in the Acquisition of Learning Skills" by G.N. Getman in *Learning Disorders*, vol. 1, p. 60 with permission of Special Child Publications, © 1965.

that the successful development of these visuomotor learning schemes is essential for learning of all sorts, including that of an academic nature.

The motoric nature of Getman's theory is clearly revealed in the developmental levels of his visuomotor complex model. Each level of the model emerges from and builds on earlier ones (see Figure 5–1).

The innate response system is largely composed of reflexive motoric units. Some of these are linked to the visuomotor complex and visual responses. The general motor system is one of gross components, i.e., location and mobility skills such as creeping, walking, running, jumping, skipping, and hopping.

The special motor system builds on the cognitive abilities developed in two earlier levels. It involves a variety of hand/hand, hand/foot, and hand/eye relations; it also includes voice and gestures.

The ocular motor system, a still more advanced system, involves the development of cognitive abilities that respond to the movement and coordination of the eyes. Then the speech motor system emerges at a level of cognitive development in which visual and language abilities interact (like Barsch, Getman believes that speech-motor patterns are dependent on visual abilities).

With advancing development, the visualization system emerges. The abilities at this level make it possible to recall visually previous sensory experiences, i.e., objects and scenes in the form of images. The system provides for both immediate visualization (when one can picture something present but not actually seen) and past-future visualization, which involves the review of past and the preview of future visual events.

The next system in Getman's visual motor complex is vision, or perception. This system represents the level of cognition where perception actually takes place, i.e., when we actually perceive things. It consists of a number of perceptual abilities. It also includes significant motor components.

Cognition is the next level in Getman's model of cognitive functioning. At this level, higher cognitive processes take place. They are made possible because of the integration of perceptual information achieved at the preceding (vision) level. Intellectual development in its highest senses is now possible. The child's mind is now capable of interrelating different perceptions and of transforming and elaborating perceptual information. And it is finally able to develop and deal with abstractions and principles.

Like many other specific ability theorists, Getman believes that effective cognition depends on the basis of foundation abilities, particularly visual perceptual and visual motor ones. Weaknesses and deficiencies in visual perceptual and visual motor development can be expected to result in a variety of learning disorders and academic failures. Getman and other optometric vision trainers seek to improve, remediate, and normalize deficient visual and visual motor abilities.

PERCEPTUAL ABILITIES

Readers who may have felt uncomfortable when we discussed neurological, motor, and perceptual motor theories as being concerned with specific cognitive abilities should feel more at ease in reviewing the literature on what we call *perceptual abilities*. Because perceptual abilities have been particular favorites for remedial and special educators, we discuss this in some detail.

Definitions of perception abound. A common one is that perception involves the identification or recognition of sensory data and the extraction of meaningful information from these data about what is being perceived. Some theorists conceive of perceptual data as an early step in information processing. Specific ability theorists are likely to consider it as constituting a set of fundamental cognitive abilities.

The importance of perception's role in cognition has been stressed throughout the centuries. Philosophers, psychologists, and neurologists and educators at different times (including our own era) have recognized that the input from our senses is fundamental to cognition (Mann, 1979).

Historical Background

Perceptual abilities have been distinguished as separate and distinct from other cognitive abilities from antiquity onward. The ancient Greeks and Romans distinguished five senses:

sight, hearing, smell, touch, and taste. The list grew to seven in the nineteenth century when kinesthetic and alimentary senses were added. Each sense was interpreted as involving separate and distinct perceptual systems, each of which was composed of a number of subabilities. Educators began to emphasize the importance of learning through the sense and of using methods that teach to the strongest perceptual areas. Thus, in the early decades of this century, pupils were being classified as audiles and visiles and taught on this basis (Mann, 1979). Remedial specialists, like Fernald (1943), stressed the inclusion of tactile kinesthetic teaching to bolster visual and auditory senses. Perceptual training was going on well before the Civil War.

Visual perception has always been favored above all areas of perception, both in cognitive theory and in special and remedial education circles. Auditory perception has been the second most intensively studied perceptual ability system.

The kinesthetic senses have long been thought to contribute to thinking and to support visual and auditory learning. The same may be said for the tactile sense, which is sometimes assessed and trained in a way undifferentiated from kinesthesis, while at other times dealt with separately. The motor and perceptual-motor theorists reviewed earlier in this chapter have certainly not neglected it. Ayres (1972a) in fact has distinguished a characteristic among learning disabled pupils that she feels may play an important role in their problems. She calls it "tactile defensiveness."

Smell and taste in their day have been assessed and trained as specific abilities or ability groupings. In fact such training still goes on in Montessori and certain special education circles. It has not received much attention from remedial teachers.

Visual Perception

There has been and continues to be a great amount of research into visual perception. Visual perception as a phenomenon to be researched and explained should, however, be distinguished from visual perception conceived of as a particular ability or set of abilities that can be assessed and trained. It is this latter type of hypothesized visual perception that has been stressed by Kephart, Ayres, Barsch, and Getman, and it is this latter type of perception that remedial and special educators are most likely to encounter in their work.

Frostig's notions, theories, tests, and training approaches (together with the *ITPA*) dominated the modern field of learning disabilities in its early day (Frostig & Horne, 1967; Frostig et al., 1964). Other visual perceptual approaches have also been popular. Some perceptual approaches such as Frostig's consider visual perception as a set of specific abilities. Others, for example the *Bender-Gestalt* (Bender, 1938), focus on a particular aspect of visual perception, e.g., the visuomotor aspect. Still others attend to perception in a general sense, e.g., the *Motor Free Test of Visual Perception* (Colarusso & Hammill, 1972).

Marianne Frostig, above all, made visual perception popular in recent times. Her methods promised to help pupils develop or correct cognitive skills that are essential to school success. Perception, from Frostig's standpoint, is differentiated into a number of specific (perceptual) subabilities that are critical to academic success.

Let us examine her *Developmental Test of Visual Perception (DTVP)* (Frostig et al., 1964) to understand how she conceived of visual perception. The *DTVP* has five subtests: (1) visual motor coordination, the ability to coordinate vision with movements of the body, specifically the hand; (2) figure-ground perception, the ability to focus on the most critical aspects of a visual scene, putting the other aspects (perceptually) into the background; (3)

perceptual constancy, the ability to perceive objects as being the same; (4) perception of position, the ability to recognize forms in various positions; and (5) perception of spatial relationships, the ability to perceive objects in relationships to each other and to the observer. These are the perceptual abilities that she believed most important to later academic learning. They are ones that she also found to present the most problems for neurologically impaired children. Training or remediating these perceptual abilities, she claimed, would improve and correct, or even overcome, a child's learning difficulties.

The popularity of Frostig's programs has in large part been due to their ready adaptation to classroom settings. The *DTVP* is a paper-and-pencil test suitable for group administration. Frostig's training exercises, designed to develop or correct deficit perceptual areas, are available in convenient work sheet format and are easily administered, thus more popular in schools than those of Barsch and Getman. She (1969) also developed a program for gross perceptual motor development, but it never became as popular as her original perceptual training program, perhaps because it does not lend itself readily to classroom use.

Auditory Perception

Relative to visual perception, auditory perception was a relatively neglected specific ability (or abilities) in the early years of educational assessment, though a number of early reading tests did make an effort to evaluate its contributions to the learning process. One reason for this relative neglect is that classroom teachers found auditory perception more difficult to assess than visual perception, given the limitations imposed by paper-and-pencil tests and classroom contexts.

Among the early instruments, other than those of a reading nature, used to assess auditory perception specifically were the *Detroit Tests of Learning Aptitude* (1935) and Wepman's *Auditory Discrimination Tests* (1958). In the early 1970s, interest in auditory perception showed a great increase. This was in large part due to the technological advances that made it possible to assess auditory perception with both greater ease and scientific accuracy. The advent of the cassette tape recorder, for example, enabled classroom teachers to assess language and auditory processing more readily. And new specialized educational tests, some discussed in this section, were also developed.

Sabatino (1973) in *The First Review of Special Education* addressed the topic of auditory perception in a review of the literature up to the late 1960s. He observed ''that late 1969 and 1970 showed a tremendous increase in interest in auditory perception, research assessment and training in auditory skills'' (p. 75). Some of this work included Sabatino's own approach to auditory perception from an information-processing point of view (Sabatino, 1973, 1974) and the *Illinois Test of Psycholinguistic Abilities (ITPA)*. The *Goldman-Fristoe-Woodcock Auditory Skills Battery* (1976) is one of the most recent efforts to address auditory perception as consisting of separate abilities.

Tactile and Kinesthetic Abilities

The tactile and kinesthetic sense modalities together constitute what is called the *haptic system*. The haptic senses have not altogether been neglected in special education training. Many motor and perceptual motor training programs either directly or indirectly assess and train tactile and kinesthetic abilities, e.g., Ayres (1972a, 1972b) and Kephart (1971). In remedial education, there was an early emphasis by Gates, Monroe, and others (Mann, 1979). The Fernald   VAKT (visual-auditory-kinesthetic-tactual) remedial program stresses the use of tactile and kinesthetic training to support and strengthen the functioning of weak or deficient visual and auditory modalities in academic learning (1943). The Orton-Gillingham remedial methods also stress such training (1973), as does Kephart's work.

A distinction should be made between the ways that remedial and special education approach the haptic senses. Remedial educators are likely to use tactile and kinesthetic modalities to strengthen and support other abilities. Special educators are likely to try to train or remediate their functioning through a variety of methods including tactile-motor training exercises, and the use of sandpaper forms and cutouts (Frostig, 1974; Getman & Hendrickson, 1966).

Smell and Taste

There has not been sufficient interest in either smell or taste as abilities to be assessed or trained for educational purposes to justify consideration here.

Crossmodal Perception and Perceptual Integration

The idea behind crossmodal perception and perceptual integration is the switching or conversion of information from one modality system to information in another one. This is presumed to be necessary for such tasks as reading, in which visual information is also transformed into an auditory (language) code somewhere in the nervous system, or for that matter in terms of simple touching, when haptic sensations can create the visual image of an object. That such switching does happen has been substantiated in many research efforts. Presumably, inability to engage in crossmodality or modality integration activities results in learning disabilities.

Herbert Birch was a major researcher in crossmodality work (Birch & Belmont, 1963, 1965; Birch & Telford, 1963). Ayres (1975) and Chalfant and Scheffelin (1969) have emphasized its importance. Frostig (1969) advocates exercises in crossmodality training. Johnson and Myklebust (1969) have emphasized the importance of visual auditory information conversion in reading.

Language

Language too can be studied from the standpoint of being constituted from a number of separate and distinct abilities.

There are a variety of oral language tests and oral language training programs. The best example of assessing and training language from the standpoint of separate and distinct abilities of specific abilities has emerged from the *Illinois Test of Psycholinguistic Abilities* (Kirk et al., 1971), which together with the Frostig approach dominated the early 1970s in the field of learning disabilities.

The *ITPA*

The *ITPA* and *ITPA* training activities are based on a language model developed by a behaviorist (Osgood), which may account for its being described as a deficit behavior or task approach to learning disabilities by Johnson and Morasky (1980). Indeed the *ITPA* language model (see Figure 5–2) can also claim membership as a type of information-

Figure 5–2 *ITPA* Three-Dimensional Model

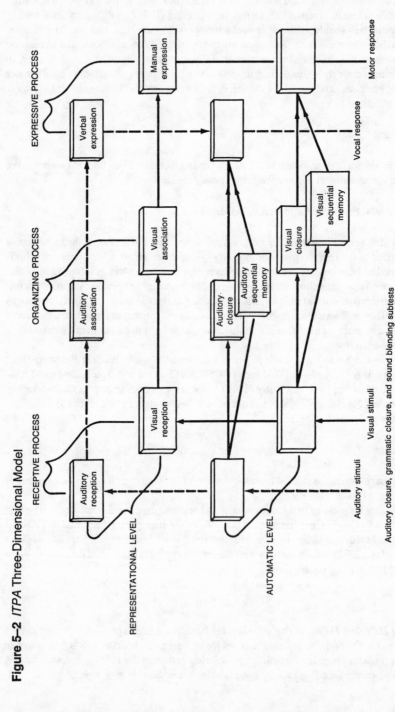

Source: Reprinted from *Illinois Test of Psycholinguistic Abilities*, revised edition, examiner's manual, by S. Kirk, J. McCarthy, and W. Kirk, by permission of University of Illinois Press, 1968.

processing model (see Chapter 7). The way it is actually used, however, is a classical example of the specific ability approach.

The subtests of the *ITPA* are supposed to assess separate abilities. The subtests are supposed to assess language according to channels of communication, i.e., the various modalities receiving information; psycholinguistic processes: receptive processes managing information inputs and expressive processes managing the output of information; organizing processes, i.e., engaged in internal manipulation of language inputs and linguistic abilities; and finally organization levels, which include automatic and representational language components, the first concerned with automatic habits, the latter with symbolic functioning.

The *ITPA* has a strong modality emphasis. Indeed it can be criticized on the grounds that it seems to assess the modalities more than language. An examination of the *ITPA*'s subtest titles substantiates this criticism in part. Channels of communication are assessed through tests of visual perception and auditory reception. The organizing abilities assessed include the receptive abilities of visual association and auditory association and the expressive abilities of verbal expression and motor expression. The automatic representation level is specifically assessed through tests of visual sequential memory, auditory sequential memory, visual closure, auditory closure, grammatical closure, and sound blending. The *ITPA* does not assess the symbolic expressive level components of Osgood's theory.

A number of training programs have been developed to train *ITPA* psycholinguistic abilities (Bush & Giles, 1969; Minskoff et al., 1972). For an in-depth critical assessment see Newcomer and Hammill (1976).

Myklebust

Another important approach to specific language abilities has been developed by Helmut Myklebust (1973), who created an extensive language theory that claims roots in neurology—as suggested by his use of the term *psychoneurological*. It is a most ambitious theory that extends into all areas of academic skill acquisition, including written language, an area in which specific ability efforts have generally been neglectful.

Myklebust's theories are committed to the premise that the brain functions in both general and special ways to make language possible. Myklebust believes that the perceptual modalities, visual, auditory and tactile, etc.—and their integration—are fundamental to language and all other cognitive systems.

Myklebust deals with specific cognitive abilities in three major categories: (1) intrasensory, utilizing brain processes primarily dealing with a single sensory system, e.g., vision; (2) interneurosensory, i.e., involving more than one brain system; and (3) interactive, which involves all systems (Gearhart, 1973).

It is quickly apparent when viewing Myklebust's theory in its fundamentals that perceptual (motor) and crossmodal factors are critical ones. Thus Myklebust interprets dyslexia to be an interneurosensory learning disability, one in which there is an inability to associate visual images with the sound of words. He regards agnosias as examples of an inability to interpret or express motorically information received through sensory channels. He attributes failures in complex areas of language functioning to failures in inner language resulting from an inability to integrate the experiences of the brain's different systems; as a consequence the brain is unable to transfer information readily and efficiently from one perceptual motor system to another.

Omnibus Abilities

A number of specific ability programs cover a large number of abilities that are presumed basic to learning and school achievement. They are often appealing because they seem to make sense—they look reasonable and right (e.g., Vallett, 1967), but the user should carefully examine the grounds on which their claims rest before applying them.

REMEDIATION OF SPECIFIC ABILITIES

If one takes the position that specific abilities are important to learning and that specific disabilities result in learning failures, then clearly remedial and special educators should take responsibility for assessing specific abilities and for remediating those that are deficient. Most specific abilities (strengths and deficits) are assessed by tests. We do not discuss the issues or the problems in assessing specific abilities here. There was a time when this would have been important. They are, however, discussed in many books on assessment, e.g., Sabatino and Miller (1978) and Salvia and Ysseldyke (1981). Most books on learning disabilities devote considerable space to their consideration.

We, however, briefly discuss several of the issues and problems of intervention and remediation via specific ability approaches. We do so first from the standpoint of process training and then from the perspective of aptitude-treatment interaction.

PROCESS TRAINING

Proponents of process training believe that certain specific abilities must function adequately in order for normal learning and school performance to go on. A specific disability may devastate a child's learning and result in school failure. It is presumed that various types of intervention and remediation develop, correct, or remediate deficient specific abilities and disabilities (Lerner, 1981, p. 171). Let us examine some general types of process training.

Training of Deficient Specific Abilities

An ability may be deficient because it is undeveloped (not matured properly), weak because of uneven development or because the child has overemphasized the use of other specific abilities, or deficient because of neurological impairments or some type of unusual environmental deprivations, e.g., deprivation of adequate visual experiences. Training efforts to correct specific ability deficits (disabilities) are usually developmentally oriented in the sense that training begins at a level where the child's specific ability is functioning adequately (which may be low) and tries to train or remediate the ability so that it becomes mature or stronger. Specific exercises are often used for this purpose. The idea is to eliminate or at least minimize the disability—to remove the dis from the *ability*.

Teaching through a Preferred Specific Ability

If one or several child's specific abilities are weak or impaired, it is possible that the child may show special strengths in regard to other abilities. Such abilities can be considered *preferred ones*. Teaching to preferred abilities takes advantage of the child's strong abilities and avoids weak ones. The idea is to circumvent the specific abilities that are weak. Thus, a child with strong visual abilities but deficient auditory ones might be provided a reading program that minimizes phonics training and emphasizes whole word recognition.

Combined Approaches

The combined approaches usually slant teaching to preferred abilities. At the same time they provide training or remediation of specific disabilities.

Use of Strong Abilities To Support Weak Ones

Using strong abilities to support weak ones is a time-honored practice. That is, the instructor relies on strong abilities to support deficiencies when instructing a pupil. Many multisensory approaches proceed on this basis. Fernald (1943), for example, used tactile kinesthetic supports for learning when a pupil's visual or auditory abilities were found deficient.

Does process training of any kind work? There have been great debates on this subject. We reserve comment until the close of this chapter.

APTITUDE-TREATMENT INTERACTION

One of education's most enduring attempts is to match instruction to pupils' special characteristics or needs. It is an appealing idea that one type of instruction is appropriate for a particular type of pupil, another type of interaction for another type. Many efforts have been devoted to developing instructional and remedial approaches along the lines of this idea, i.e., adapted to special pupil characteristics such as high and low verbal ability, strong auditory and weak visual abilities.

The effort to validate this type of approach has been identified as aptitude-treatment interaction. Many of the arguments in support of the diagnostic-descriptive approach to remediation (which has taken a position that certain types of intervention are appropriate for specific types of problems) are based on the presumption that valid aptitude-treatment interactions can be found and that such ATIs are educationally meaningful.

Let us review a definition of aptitude-treatment interaction. Gage and Berliner (1979) define it in the following way: [an ATI] "is a situation that occurs when students high in one characteristic [often a specific ability] learn better when taught by one method ['treatment'] while students lower in that characteristic [perhaps having a disability in respect to the characteristic] learn better by another method" (p. 184).

This is one particular form of ATI—we might call it a *high-low ability type*. There are others. The important thing to note about the ATI is that it presumes that pupils who are strong in one type of characteristic, or weak in another, will do better with certain types of instruction as opposed to other types.

Figures 5–3 through 5–5 show hypothetical examples of research into different types of instruction using an ATI model. The pupils in these examples have been classified as being strong or weak in *ITPA* sound-blending ability (as assessed by the *ITPA*). The ATI effort here is one that attempts to match teaching methods to the pupil's differences in sound-blending ability.

In the first hypothetical example (Figure 5–3) pupils high in sound-blending ability do better than low sound-blending ability pupils in both phonics and visual types of instruc-

Figure 5–3 Nonsignificant Interaction between Two Levels of Ability and Two Alternative Instructional Methods of Teaching Word Recognition

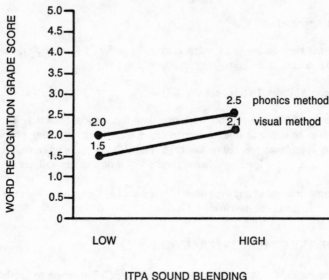

tions. Both high- and low-ability pupils, however, do better in phonics instruction than they do in the visual instruction. There is no aptitude-treatment interaction. In the second hypothetical example (Figure 5–4) there is a significant ATI. High sound-blending ability pupils do much worse in visual instruction than do low sound-blending ability pupils. The results suggest that we should try to avoid visual training with high sound-blending pupils altogether. However, both high and low sound-blending ability pupils do better in reading when phonics training is used than they do through visual instruction. We may be better off if we use phonics training with both groups.

The final example (Figure 5–5) presents a sort of ideal ATI situation. It shows the treatment lines actually crossing. On the basis of this interaction high sound-blending pupils should be taught by a phonics method while low sound-blending ability pupils should be taught by visual methods.

ATI research has been carried out in all sorts of areas. It has studied the ways that various .ypes of instruction relate to different levels of ability or different types of learning styles. ATI research has also studied the match of instruction to strengths and weaknesses in specific ability areas. Their results, on occasion, have been encouraging. Overall, however, they have been inconclusive and cannot be regarded as substantiating the usefulness of any specific types of intervention to correct any specific learning disability or to take advantage of particular strong abilities (Ysseldyke & Algozzine, 1982; Arter & Jenkins, 1979). One reason for this is the dominance once again of general ability factors, which limit the influence of more narrow ability factors or pupil characteristics when it comes to instruction (Messick, 1976). ATI research, however, continues and may yet provide some support for the use of specific ability approaches to instruction and remediation.

Figure 5–4 Hypothetical Significant Interaction between Two Levels of Sound-Blending Ability and Two Alternative Methods of Teaching Word Recognition

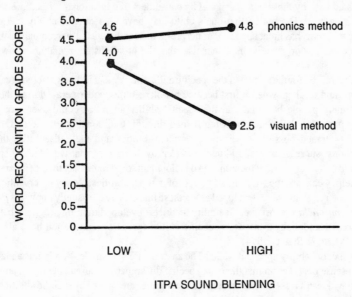

Figure 5–5 Hypothetical Significant Interaction between Two Levels of Sound-Blending Ability and Two Alternative Instructional Methods of Teaching Word Recognition

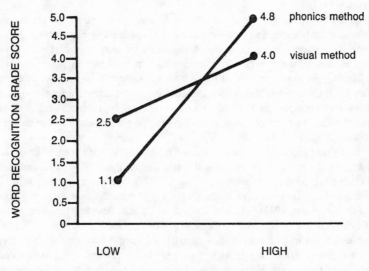

OBSERVATIONS ABOUT SPECIFIC ABILITIES

The appeal of the specific ability approach to cognition is that it is readily grasped and appreciated both by those who use it and by consumers of educational service, i.e., pupils and their parents. The notion that one's child may have a specific disability that causes learning problems has great appeal. Parents prefer to hear that visual-perceptual disabilities cause a child's poor schoolwork rather than that the problems are a matter of low intelligence.

Another reason for the appeal of the specific ability movement is that it offered great hope to parents and teachers when it first became popular (in the modern era) during the early 1960s. Many people believed that the specific ability approach could overcome many learning problems that were not being helped through traditional academic or remedial means. It seemed possible to diagnose various abilities and their disabilities through observations, surveys, scales, and tests and to provide training that would assist specific abilities to mature, to correct their uneven development, or to remediate their deficient ones, or to help weak abilities through the use of strong abilities. Many intervention and remediation programs were developed along these lines. They are usually known as *process training approaches*. Most specific ability theorists developed training programs based on this theory. Handbooks to assist in specific ability (process) remediation have also been created (Mann & Suiter, 1974).

Is the specific ability approach valid? The answers are not simple. Surely it is a matter of commonsense observation that there are specific differences in human behavior, and since this is true, doesn't it seem likely that these specificities are caused by specific abilities? Can we doubt the importance of auditory perception when we observe the difficulties that the deaf have with language concepts? Do we doubt the importance of visual perception when we observe the restricted conceptions that individuals born blind have of physical space? Surely touch and kinesthesis provide information essential to the development of proper bodily movements and hence to writing and other academic skills. There seems no doubt on such issues.

Yet efforts to differentiate specific abilities as distinct and separate stable components of cognition that can be easily and accurately assessed have been severely criticized. Efforts to train specific abilities have come under stronger attack (Newcomer & Hammill, 1976). There is no substantial support for the effectiveness of process training in terms of helping either handicapped pupils or those suffering from academic difficulties. Specific cognitive abilities are legitimate hypothetical constructs from the standpoint of neurology, from psychometric studies, on the basis of tests of specific ability, from the standpoint of the occasional successes of process (specific ability) training approaches, and on the basis of commonsense observations.

We face many problems, however, when we try to work with specific abilities. For example, we are not always sure that the specific ability tests actually measure the phenomena corresponding to their names (Mann, 1979). Specific ability tests suffer from unreliability that makes effective diagnosis for any given individual extremely difficult (Salvia & Ysselydke, 1981). Many of these tasks or tests designed to assess particular specific abilities may be solved through the use of other ones. For example, given an oral mathematics problem (using the auditory modality), a pupil may translate it into visual images and solve it effectively through visual processing, if weak in auditory processing abilities. We cannot know when one type of ability switches in or out on the basis of our tests. We do not have any paper-and-pencil tests sensitive enough to detect switching processes. Furthermore, different types of specific abilities appear to be required at different stages of learning. Again our tests do not help us to understand when a particular ability is important for learning.

Finally, when learning or dealing with problems, we tend to use all of our abilities together, so any given cognitive ability may not of itself make an important difference in what we do. That is why *g* predicts so well.

Let us look at this issue further from the viewpoint in Chapter 1. One reason that specific abilities approaches have not been particularly effective either in predicting school outcomes or in directing courses of remediation can be provided by the perspective on cognition provided by hierarchical theories of intelligence. From a hierarchical perspective, general ability factors account for most cognitive activity. And the more specific a cognitive ability is, the less it is significantly involved in any particular cognitive activity, the less it predicts achievement, and the less important it probably is to train or remediate or to adjust curriculum for. Thus general perceptual ability generally accounts for a slight amount of the success in overall school achievement at higher age levels (more at lower ones), and specific perceptual abilities account for even less—perhaps to a degree where they aren't worth assessing for purposes of remediation, though some researchers certainly disagree, e.g., Kavale (1984).

Beyond all this, assuming that specific abilities should be trained, why should we carry out this training separately and apart from other types of instruction in school, recreation, and work-oriented areas? Playing a game of ball certainly engages, and even trains, many of the motor and perceptual motor abilities that the proponents of such specific abilities believe important. Certainly reading and writing involve and train auditory visual abilities and kinesthetic abilities, while mathematics teaches us to use logical abilities. Most school activities compel our pupils to develop and use attention, imagery, memory abilities, and so on.

Why then should we try to remediate or train such types of specific abilities directly? One reason that has been suggested is that by isolating a defective ability for special treatment, we can perhaps do a more effective job of training or remediating it.

Sabatino (Sabatino, Miller, & Schmidt, 1981) thus believes that the effort to train specific cognitive abilities should be renewed. Mann (1979) on the other hand believes that while the idea of retraining or remediating specific abilities is too appealing ever to be discarded entirely, it isn't as a rule the best way to proceed. He advises that the jury is still out insofar as the value of specific ability (process) approaches to training and remediation is concerned, and he suggests that we should not enthusiastically embrace specific ability approaches when they have failed us so badly. He believes that it is up to the proponents of specific ability assessment and training to show clearly where and when their techniques are genuinely useful.

Both Sabatino and Mann believe that it is worthwhile to assess specific abilities, whether or not one believes that they should be trained, if for no other reason than to provide teachers with additional clues as to their pupils' learning characteristics. Also, though research has by and large shown negative results in respect to ability training, some positive results have been found. In any case, negative results mean *not proven* rather than *wrong*—insofar as scientific hypotheses are concerned. We shouldn't close our minds altogether to the possibilities that specific ability approaches may prove useful.

Chapter 6

Piaget and Developmental Cognition

There was a time, not long ago, whenever cognition was mentioned in psychological or educational circles, Piaget's name was likely to come to mind immediately. Many prominent psychologists and educators were convinced that his research and theories would revolutionize educational practice; among these were Bruner (1961), Maccoby and Zellner (1970), Weikart (1971), and Elkind (1976). It is safe to say that almost every teacher, some years ago, was exposed to the Piagetian ''revolution'' in one form or another. Some of the theories and approaches reviewed in Chapter 4 reveal Piaget's influences.

Piaget's influence on psychology and education has been considerably diminished. Partly this is due to changing fashions. It is also due to the fact that Piagetian concepts are not as easy to apply in everyday classroom teaching and remediation as once thought possible. It is further due, in special education at least, to the popularity of behavioral methods. Currently Piaget's influences are strongest at early childhood and preschool levels, e.g., Kamii (Kamii & DeVries, 1978) and Lavatelli (1970). This is perhaps as it should be since the great Swiss psychologist invested so greatly in research with young children.

It is essential that any book concerned with the modern scope of cognitive research and theory examine Piaget's work. Beyond this, an appreciation of Piaget's ideas is enriching for anyone concerned with remediation and special education. Although special educators were relatively late in responding to Piaget's ideas (Robinson & Robinson, 1976), many were to embrace them with enthusiasm, particularly after Inhelder's book *The Diagnosis of Reasoning in the Mentally Retarded* (1968) showed that Piaget's conceptualizations could be readily applied to handicapped populations. Interest in Piaget was less pronounced in learning disability and remedial education circles probably because his findings and ideas did not readily lend themselves to specific remedial activities. This is not to say that there was no interest in these circles. Kephart, whose theories were reviewed in Chapter 5, was admittedly influenced by Piaget. More recently Reid (1978) and Reid and Hresko (1981) have published books that apply to learning problems.

Murray (1978) in his chapter ''Some Cautions of the Implications of Piaget's Theory for Education of the Handicapped,'' observed that Piaget's theory was not an educational one and that ''Piaget has said virtually nothing practical about education and still less about the nature and education of the abnormal child'' (p. 283). Nor was Piaget particularly interested in remediation. This does not mean, however, that Piaget cannot help us understand learning problems. The example in Chapter 1, contrasting behavioral and cognitive approaches to time, is but one demonstration of the insights that he provides educators. Additionally, many remedial and special educators still believe that Piaget's theory can play an important role in remediation and the education of exceptional children (Bricker, Macke, Levin, & Campbell, 1981; Reid & Hresko, 1981).

Piaget was not the clearest of writers. Additionally he was constantly reformulating his ideas. Finally, he wrote in French, which means that most Americans encounter his ideas in translations, not all of which have been well done. Many other writers have attempted to interpret his research and theories to make them more understandable to the average reader. We have chosen to use several of them as guides in preparing this chapter, since by so doing we can best give the readers a view of how Piaget's work is interpreted in the United States. They are Ginsburg and Opper (1979), Phillips (1981) and Wadsworth (1978, 1979). We recommend the study of these writers to those interested in studying Piaget's ideas in greater depth before they proceed to read Piaget himself. Because Piaget's concepts are very complicated and because he was constantly revising them, our chapter oversimplifies his work.

PIAGET'S BACKGROUND

It is not possible to understand the nature of Piaget's cognitive theories without understanding something of the many influences that shaped his conceptions of cognition. Thus, we find that Piaget carried out his doctoral work in the natural sciences, rather than in psychology or education, and that biological studies strongly affected his views of cognitive development. He intensively studied mollusks and was intrigued by the ways that successive generations of this primitive animal alter their physical structures to adapt to changing physical environments. When he later studied children's cognitive development, he decided that human development, too, was a matter of biological processes being shaped by adaptive needs.

Piaget's ideas were strongly influenced by his exposure to those of Binet and Binet's tests, as he freely admits in the preface he wrote to Binet's *Les ideés modernes sur les enfants* (1973). He also worked on tests when serving in the psychological laboratories that Binet had inaugurated. And it was working with Binet-type test items that he first became intrigued with children's "wrong answers" to test questions. In time Piaget became convinced that their wrong answers, more than their right ones, could provide keys to an understanding of their mental processes. It was, in fact, due to his analysis of "wrong" test answers that Piaget concluded that children's cognitive processes are qualitatively different at different developmental stages (Ginsburg & Opper, 1979).

Beyond biology, and beyond psychology, Piaget was strongly influenced by the writings of the great philosophers, to whose work he had been exposed as a student. Some of them, for example, the great German philosopher Immanuel Kant (1724–1804), conceived of the mind as being innately structured to think in certain ways. Others, including the French philosopher-psychologist-educator Jean Jacques Rousseau (1712–1778), believed that mental development proceeds through a number of distinct stages from infancy to adulthood. These philosophical ideas—a mind naturally structured to think in certain ways and developing through different stages—were to become cornerstones of Piaget's cognitive theories.

PIAGET'S METHODS

American psychologists are used to studying their subjects under controlled experimental conditions and doing so in an objective fashion. In contrast, Piaget studied children under everyday conditions using what can be called *clinical-descriptive* and *clinical-inquiry* methods. His approach typically consisted of the following components: posing problems for children to solve, observing their efforts, and asking them questions (actually interviewing them) as to the reasons for their solutions. He posed the same questions to children of different ages (and at different stages of cognitive development) in order to determine how thought processes change with age.

Piaget has been criticized as being unsystematic and subjective in his research. He has also been criticized for having worked only with small numbers of children and for not using statistics (Travers, 1977). It is true that behaviorists also work with small numbers of children and that they do not employ traditional statistics. Behaviorists, however, carry out more carefully controlled and regulated types of research than did Piaget.

Piaget justified his methods on the grounds that they, rather than vigorously controlled experiments, were the best ways through which a researcher could understand children's thought processes. Additionally, he carried out exceedingly long, thorough, and detailed studies of his subjects, with some of whom he worked for many years. This is in sharp contrast to the usual in-out research carried out by psychological and educational researchers.

AN OVERVIEW OF PIAGET'S CONCEPTION OF THE MIND

Binet's work influenced the ways that Piaget conceived of and studied cognition (Ginsburg & Opper, 1979, Piaget, 1973). Piaget more or less equated cognition (the mind) with intelligence; it may be said that "the major aim of Piaget's research was to discover what actually constitutes intelligence" (Ginsburg & Opper, 1979, p. 12). Piaget, however, did not conceive of intelligence in psychometric (intelligence tests) terms, for example, as a particular mental capacity to be assessed quantitatively and be used to predict success in school. He rather thought of it in dynamic terms as a "system of living and acting operations" (1950, p. 7) and a "particular instance of biological adaptation" (1952, pp. 3–4).

Piaget believed that a mature person's intelligence operates in logical mathematical terms as a matter of biological necessity (Travers, 1977). The universe, Piaget pointed out, is a logical mathematical system, i.e., governed by logic-mathematical laws (Phillips, 1982). We as humans are at a physical disadvantage in the world when compared to many other animal species, i.e., in strength, speed, predatory tools, even in our protective coverings. In order for us to compete with other species, our brains have had to develop in ways that permit us to utilize the world's logicomathematical rules to develop tools and technologies. Piaget's research sought to determine how children develop cognitively to levels where they eventually are able to think in truly logical ways. This is a major reason why so many of his experiments require mathematical or other types of logical solutions.

Through his research Piaget found out that older children are not only more accurate than younger children in their solutions but that the reasons for their solutions (the logic behind them) are quite different. One way that he demonstrated this was by asking children of different ages the question "What weighs more, a pound of feathers or a pound of lead?"

This is an old question, indeed, but Piaget made superb use of it to make his points. He found that a four-year-old child doesn't understand the question at all. A six- or seven-year-old child will say that the lead weighs more because it is heavier, which is a wrong answer though a logical one in the sense that it is a deduction from the premise that lead is a heavier material than feathers. A normal nine-year-old child can solve the problem easily because the child knows that a pound of anything is still a pound. Thus Piaget found four-year-olds unable to understand the question, while nine-year-olds both understood and answered it correctly. The explanation for the difference in answers is that children of different ages are also at different stages of logical (cognitive) development.

We can thus understand why, though he is usually considered a psychologist, Piaget has described himself as a *genetic epistomologist* and his studies as being those of *genetic epistomology*. Genetics is a branch of science concerned with development, while epistomology is a branch of philosophy that inquires into the nature of knowledge. Piaget was concerned with the development of knowledge.

Other names have been used to describe Piaget and his work. Because he conceived of human cognition (intelligence) as a biological system that develops through constant interactions with the environment, he and his theories have been called *interactionist*; the implications of this become clearer later.

Piaget and his theories have also been labeled *constructivist*. This is because he believed that the world around us can be understood only in terms of our interpretations of it. We can never "know" the real world directly, i.e., in terms of its actual physical characteristics. Rather we construct it—its *reality*—in our minds, in accordance with our mind's characteristics and capabilities, and our "constructions of reality" differ according to our level of cognitive development. A young child's construction of reality is far different from that of an adult, and a retarded pupil's constructions differ from those of a gifted pupil. At the highest levels of cognitive achievement, individuals are able to construct realities that go far beyond physical appearances. Newton and Einstein are examples of individuals who did this. So are Shakespeare and Freud. And so is Piaget.

BASIC PIAGETIAN CONCEPTS

Intelligence

We begin by again examining Piaget's conception of intelligence. We must do so since, as explained earlier, Piaget essentially equated cognition with intelligence, and the study of cognitive development to be the study of how children develop their intelligence to the level of logical mathematical thinking (Travers, 1977).

Piaget was interested in the general rather than the individual aspects of intelligence; he was not interested in finding out how or why individuals differed from each other in intellectual ability (Modgil & Modgil, 1982). As Ginsburg and Opper (1979) put it, he sought to study intelligence from the standpoint of "the individual's optimum level of functioning at his current developmental stage" (p. 14). Piaget was not particularly concerned with the everyday practical implications of intelligence, i.e., how intelligence affects a pupil's school performance. Nor was he particularly concerned with children's cognitive deficits (Fincham, 1982).

Furthermore, Piaget downplayed the role of language in the development of intelligence (Siegel & Hodkin, 1982; Elliott & Donaldson, 1978b). This is not to say that he did not recognize the importance of language to thought, but he did not regard it as being essential to cognitive development in the way that many psychologists would consider it, e.g., Fodor (1975), Luria (1966), and Vigotsky (1962). Also, Piaget was not interested in studying emotional or motivational processes apart from cognition (Ginsburg & Opper, 1979).

Piaget was interested in the biological aspects of intelligence (Travers, 1977). He emphasized that intelligence is not static ability or a set of abilities that can be identified by some fixed number like an IQ. It is rather, he wrote, to be understood as an ongoing process developing from the child's continuing interaction with its environment.

Distinction between Cognitive Development and Learning

Piaget made a distinction between learning and cognitive development. While learning is important, it is subordinated to cognitive development and is only a particular aspect of it. Learning is a matter of acquiring specific types of information or skills; it increases the child's cognition only in limited narrow ways. Cognitive development is a matter of the child transforming the mind on the basis of its active experiences (Voneche & Bovet, 1982). Siegel and Hodkin (1982a, 1982b) have objected to this point of view on the basis that it makes learning to be a mechanistic process—which they insist it is not. In this chapter, we do not make distinctions between learning and cognitive development since this is too fine a point for an introductory text.

Equilibrium

Organisms constantly seek to establish an equilibrium with their environments. All of their physical interactions, i.e., with other organisms, objects, situations, changes in temperature, represent efforts to achieve equilibrium. A child's cognitive interactions, too, are efforts to achieve equilibrium. And what does *equilibrium* mean? While Piaget used it to characterize biological (physical and cognitive) processes, he borrowed the term from physics. It indicates a balance between two or more factors. As it pertains to a child's intelligence (cognition), it means the establishment both of a harmonious balance between a child's cognitive structures on one hand and the environment on the other and of a balance among the child's cognitive processes.

Piaget interpreted intelligence in two ways from the standpoint of equilibrium. It is first a cognitive goal that the organism tries to achieve by establishing an equilibrium with its environment; Piaget (1950) called intelligence a "form of equilibrium" (p. 6). It is also the instrument that the organism uses to achieve equilibrium.

Organisms never achieve a final stage of equilibrium. The nature of living is that it continually destabilizes previously established states of equilibrium and requires new efforts to reestablish them. A child's cognitive state of equilibrium is, at any given time, a temporary achievement. New cognitive demands made on the child destabilize earlier equilibriums and activate efforts to establish new ones. When a child reaches a particular state of equilibrium, the very cognitive achievements made possible by this achievement destabilize this state and activate new equilibration efforts. Piaget's life's work can perhaps be epitomized as being devoted to the study of the ways children use their intelligence to achieve equilibrium with their environments and how they develop their intelligence by so doing. We reexamine those constructs later in this chapter.

NATURE OF INTELLIGENCE

Piaget conceived of intelligence in terms of structures, functions, and contents. We need not concern ourselves to any great degree with the content side of intelligence in this chapter, i.e., what it is an individual is thinking about. The contents of a person's mind (intelligence) change vastly from the beginning years of life, when they are largely of a sensorimotor or perceptual motor nature, to later mature years, when they are likely to be of an abstract and logical nature. But Piaget was not overly concerned with the contents of intelligence—in what children are thinking about. He wanted to understand the whys and hows of intelligence, its structures and functions rather than its whats (its contents).

COGNITIVE FUNCTIONS

Piaget did not particularly concern himself with the physical side of cognition; as far as he was concerned, heredity preprogrammed the nervous system in broad general ways that enabled it to support cognitive functions. All species according to Piaget have two basic, in- herited tendencies. He called these *invariant functions* because they determine the course of biological (physical and cognitive) functioning throughout an organism's lifetime.

These invariant functions are organization and adaption. They are functional counter- parts, going on simultaneously, each essential to the other. The organism, in order to adapt cognitively to the environment, must constantly keep reorganizing its cognitive structures.

Organization

Let us examine the invariant functions in greater detail. We begin with organization. There is a tendency on the part of all species to organize their physical (bodily) and psychological (cognitive and intelligence) processes into coherent systems (Ginsburg & Opper, 1979). It is not enough for a body to possess the physical structures of digestion, e.g., a mouth, teeth, salivary glands, stomach, for digestion (a type of adaptation) to take place. The body's digestive components must be organized—systemized to work interac- tively—for digestion to proceed properly.

Because of the qualitative organization (really reorganization) of cognitive structures, as humans mature, they develop from a mental level where their cognitive structures can cope only with problems of simple perceptual or motoric nature to one where they can deal with them symbolically and logically.

Adaptation

The invariant function of cognitive organization is a hypothetical construct inferred from the behavior of particular organisms. It is used to explain how organisms are capable of cog- nitive adaptation, i.e., problem solving in various forms. The invariant function of adapta- tion is also a construct, but it is one that is clearly expressed in behavior. We can observe it when a handicapped child tries to put pegs in a board or when a poor reader struggles with a book passage. Piaget developed his theories from his observations of children's adapta- tions.

An easy physical example of assimilation and accommodation is provided by eating. When we eat something, we assimilate the food by putting it in our mouths. But in order to do this, we must adjust, i.e., accommodate our mouths to the particular food we are eating. Our mouth, its structures, and their functions change to accommodate various foods in various ways. We open, shape our lips, and use our teeth and tongue in different ways and degrees depending on whether we are simply tasting a particular food or are really hungry to eat it, whether it is hot or cold, whether it is liquid or solid, tart or sweet. Our saliva is secreted in different amounts for different foods.

Let us provide another physical example of assimilation and accommodation at work. When we digest food, there is an interaction between the digestive system and the food. The digestive system attempts to assimilate the food for nourishment. But in order to do this, it must accommodate to it. Thus the stomach expands, certain organs release digestive fluids, the supply of blood to the stomach is altered.

In both of our physical examples we have shown that assimilation and accommodation work together. The body's physical structures seek to take in (assimilate) elements of the external world. In order to do this effectively, they must adjust (accommodate) to the (external) demands placed on them.

Intellectual adaptation proceeds in a similar fashion. We assimilate information from the environment. This expands, enriches, and sometimes changes our cognitive structures. But our cognitive structures must accommodate, i.e., adjust themselves in varying degrees, to that information to make its assimilation possible. While it is true that at any given time and in any given cognitive activity, either assimilative or accommodative processes may dominate, both go on simultaneously at all times, and each is essential to the other. A baby wants to pick up a toy—to assimilate it to the baby's ways of playing. In order to do this, however, the baby must accommodate to the toy, by adjusting eyes so that they focus on the toy, arms so that they can reach it, hands so that they can hold it. A pupil wants to assimilate new information about a topic in science. The pupil must accommodate to the information as it is presented in various forms, e.g., in textbooks, encyclopedia, on a computer terminal. A pupil will try to assimilate social studies information to pass a future test and accommodate ways of studying differently, depending on whether an essay or a multiple-choice test is expected.

Let us recapitulate what we have learned to this point. Piaget conceived of cognition in dynamic and active terms. Intelligence doesn't just develop because of physical maturation, through an increase of S-R or behavioral units. It is created and developed—more properly it creates and develops itself—through interactions with the environment. These involve the functional invariants of organization and adaptation. Organization makes adaptation possible. Adaptation creates organization. Adaptation involves the complementary processes of assimilation and accommodation. Through the latter the organism seeks to achieve equilibrium between itself and its environment. Cognitive development proceeds as a result of efforts to achieve equilibrium.

Equilibrium

We have discussed equilibrium to this point in terms of relationship between the organism and the outer world. We must study it from the standpoint of internal cognitive operations, for equilibrium is also to be interpreted as a proper balance between assimilation and accommodation.

Equilibration is a self-regulatory biological process that is continually activated within the organism in its efforts to achieve equilibrium. It seeks to reconcile all of the factors that are involved in cognitive functioning (Wadsworth, 1979). Its goal is to achieve ever more stable and coherent states of cognitive equilibrium.

Equilibration is also the mechanism that works during an individual's period of cognitive development to help achieve higher levels of cognitive development since it forces cognitive structures to mature (Ginsburg & Opper, 1979). Piaget conceived of learning as a process of equilibration.

The importance of this inner cognitive balance is easily understood. If a child only assimilated information and never accommodated to it, everything would seem the same, for the child would not be able to differentiate one type of information from another. The child would react to all things similarly because the child couldn't distinguish among them. On the other hand, if the child always accommodated to information but never assimilated, the child would be aware of and responsive to many specific items of information but could never see similarities among them. Everything would be a new experience (Wadsworth). Such extremes are impossible in living things. But overassimilation and overaccommodation may explain some learning problems.

The concept of equilibrium is an essential one for educators interested in translating Piaget's ideas into instruction. A schoolchild, like all other organisms, constantly seeks to establish equilibrium between assimilation and accommodation through the self-regulatory processes of equilibration, which attempts to reconcile all the factors of cognitive functioning. When the child experiences a state of cognitive disequilibrium, efforts are renewed to establish a new state of equilibrium, i.e., through further assimilations and accommodations. The goal of all efforts to achieve states of cognitive equilibrium is that of assimilating more information effectively; but obviously some type and degree of accommodation are always necessary to accomplish this.

During the period of cognitive development, the child's cognitive structures change qualitatively as a result of accommodation. These qualitative changes constitute cognitive development. Assimilation, on the other hand, quantitatively changes children's cognitive structures; so in a sense it is less important than accommodation to cognitive development. Nevertheless it must be remembered that the purposes of accommodation are to make further assimilation possible. Thus we cannot really separate it from assimilation.

COGNITIVE STRUCTURES (SCHEMATA)

Our discussion of functions before structures may have struck some readers as putting the cart before the horse. We proceeded in this manner because an understanding of Piaget's views on cognitive functions helps us to understand better the nature of cognitive structures (as he conceived them to be) since cognitive structures are formed through the interactions of cognitive functions.

We organize our behaviors and our cognitive activities in order to adapt to the environment. The interplay of adaptation and organization creates generalizable cognitive structures and then causes them to expand, develop, mature, and change. These cognitive structures control thought and behavior. Piaget called them *schemata* because he wished to call attention to their organizing qualities.

Humans progress through a series of distinct stages cognitively as they move from infancy to maturity. Each of these stages is characterized by distinct types of schemata. Early in life these structures are innately determined reflex behavioral ones—controlling specific behaviors, e.g., sucking, the flailing of arms. Nevertheless they rapidly develop through experience into truly cognitive structures. Throughout the period of a child's cognitive development, the cognitive schemata are constantly changing in order to manage more and increasingly complex and demanding varieties of behavioral and cognitive activities. They change quantitatively by assimilating more information. They change qualitatively, i.e., are restructured, because of the need to accommodate new information cognitively. Schemata not only change qualitatively in the process of accommodation. They also become components, together with other schemata, of broader, more encompassing, higher-order schemata as the organism matures. Thus the original simple schema that controlled thumb sucking in an infant is later combined with simple reflexive arm and hand movement schemata to create a higher order and (relatively) complex thumb-sucking "habit" (schemata).

The hypothetical construct of schemata constitutes still another key component of Piaget's theories. Schemata are generalizable cognitive structures that organize and control cognitive and behavioral activities. They are the basis of a child's construction of reality. That is, the ways that a child interprets, understands, and responds to the world at any given time are dependent on the number and types and sophistication of the available cognitive schemata.

Characteristics of Schemata

Schemata are organized and coherent; imply inner activity on the part of the child (or adult); are the basic structures that underlie, organize, control, and direct behavior and cognition; create generalizable cores of human activity (Ginsburg & Opper, 1979); and imply regularity (as opposed to random unsystematic and disconnected and unregulated activity).

Development of Schemata

A child's earliest schemata, as observed earlier, are sensorimotor reflexes. Subsequent ones develop through the operation of the functional invariants as the child interacts with its environment. True learning—which results in knowledge and affects schemata—is an active process and is achieved by the child acting on the world. That is, cognitive schemata develop through child's physical and cognitive manipulations of the environment. They also result because of inner activity, i.e., within the child, the cognitive equilibration activities that constantly reorganize schemata. All schemata are founded on the child's sensorimotor behaviors. The earliest cognitive schemata are completely physical in nature. They develop from and are expressed in physical activities. The most advanced and mature schemata, even though they are expressed in abstract and symbolic thinking, still show physical, i.e., sensorimotor, traces.

Schemata develop through the interplay of the invariant functions of organization and adaptation, the goals of which are to enable the child to achieve higher, more coherent, and more stable states of equilibrium. On the adaptive side the child is constantly assimilating new behaviors and cognitive activities within existing schemata. At the same time the child is accommodating (and therefore changing) schemata to accommodate them to novel or problematic types of information and new behavioral demands. And just as the invariant functions control the development of schemata, the formation of new schemata constantly reshapes the ways in which the invariant functions express themselves.

Cognition's invariant functions remain the same through an individual's lifetime. Cognitive structures (schemata), in contrast, change in a systematic, regular sequence as the child develops. That is, they proceed through stages of development, each of which is characterized by different types of schemata. Let us restate this important distinction between invariant functions and schemata. Organisms are constantly required to adapt to the environment and always use the same invariant functions to organize their responses (behavioral and cognitive) for this purpose. The cognitive structures that make this adaptation and organization possible, however, change from one cognitive developmental stage to another.

Development of Cognitive Structures

Cognitive schemata begin as innate reflexes. These reflexes rapidly assimilate new information and accommodate to new demands so that more complex and advanced schemata soon emerge. Thus while the initial schemata are best described as behavioral, subsequent ones (created from these reflexes) are cognitive.

Schemata expand through assimilation but change through accommodation. Some accommodations incorporate and integrate earlier separate schemata into broader more complex ones.

As the child matures, new schemata develop. They are drastically different from and advanced over the predecessors. This is why Piaget discussed cognitive development as proceeding in stages. It is important to observe, however, that new schemata develop on the foundation of earlier more primitive and immature ones and incorporate and reorganize the latter within them. Thus, no matter how abstract thought may be, it still shows its sensorimotor origins in some fashion.

Cognitive development is inherent in the child's nature. While the child also "learns" through reinforced associations, such learning is peripheral to true cognitive development. Reinforcements develop narrow splinter skills. They may influence the ways that cognitive schemata control behavior. But they cannot create schemata.

It is clear that Piaget was scornful of behaviorism. He even minimized the value of reinforcements (rewards) in encouraging, i.e., motivating, learning. He attributed most motivation to the processes set in motion by disequilibrium. That is, motivation to learn is created when a child's existing schemata cannot manage experiences. This creates a conflict that activates the processes of assimilation and accommodation. The first of these adds (quantitatively) to the breadth of knowledge; it expands schemata, which is sometimes sufficient to reestablish a state of equilibrium. The second of these is required when existing schemata cannot assimilate information and must (quantitatively) change, so that assimilation can proceed. In the case of either quantitative or qualitative changes in schemata, it is disequilibrium that motivates change and creates learning.

Schemata generalize and expand their applications through assimilation; this enables them to control ever broader ranges of thinking and behavior. An example of this is found when a child first identifies a dog as a "doggy," and then begins to call all four-legged animals a dog. In so doing, the child is demonstrating that the doggy schema has expanded to include and to manage data not originally associated with it. While we don't usually think of such thinking as reflecting cognitive development, it indeed does so.

More in keeping with our ideas of cognitive development are schemata's accommodative changes. Our doggy schema again provides an example of this. When the child finally learns to identify cows as cows and cats as cats, while still calling the dog doggy, and identifies all of them as animals, the original gross and overassimilative doggy schema has obviously been replaced by more sophisticated cognitive structures. And it is this sort of cognitive development that we usually describe as cognitive growth. Along these lines Wadsworth (1979) observes that Piaget's general "hypothesis is simply that cognitive development is a coherent process of successive qualitative changes of cognitive structures," each of which derives "logically and inevitably from its predecessor" (p. 28) "[which it] incorporates . . . in a newly organized form." Advanced schemata build on the foundations of older ones and "complete, correct or combine with them" (p. 32).

STAGES OF COGNITIVE DEVELOPMENT

Until Piaget most certainly recognized (indeed identified) continuities in cognitive development, he also believed that it proceeds in distinct stages, each separate and different from the one that precedes and succeeds it in important ways. There has been considerable debate as to whether Piaget originally intended that each stage be conceived of as beginning and ending abruptly as it supplants or is supplanted by other stages. It is the general consensus that the various stages blend or merge into each other and that the close of one stage has components of and resembles the beginnings of the stage that succeeds it. It is for this reason that most Piagetians now prefer to identify the major stages as *periods*, since this sounds less abrupt or distinct than the term *stages*. And others have downplayed the stage notion altogether (Phillips, 1981). It is interesting, in light of such efforts, to note that Piaget, in an article written in his final years, continued to call *stages* what others insist on calling *periods* (Piaget, 1972).

In any case, Piaget conceived of clearly delineated periods of cognitive development, each characterized by different types of cognition. And he believed that at different points during development there are marked and dramatic improvements in the way normal children think.

Recently Piagetians have somewhat deemphasized the importance of stage theory (Voneche & Bovet, 1982). The latter, however, is still influential enough in education to justify extensive discussion.

Assumptions of Piaget's Stage Theory

Piaget conceived cognitive development to be divided into four broad periods (stages), each which in turn is divided into subperiods. Each stage and substage is characterized by the dominance of a particular type of cognitive functioning. Table 6–1 presents a brief review of these stages.

A key tenet of Piaget's stage theory is that all children must pass through the same stages or periods of cognitive development in exactly the same order. Not all children fully proceed through all of the stages; i.e., the severely and profoundly handicapped don't usually progress beyond the period of sensorimotor development. Some children pass more quickly through them than do others; a bright child develops faster cognitively than does a slow learner. But the sequence of development is invariant. It does not change. There is no skipping of any stage or period. Since each development stage (period) is characterized by a particular type of "intelligence," all of the child's cognitive activities and behavior at that stage have similar characteristics. While there may be specific areas of cognition or behavior in which the child is accelerated or lags (shows décalages), there is still an overall uniformity to the ways the child thinks and behaves.

Table 6–1 Summary of the Periods of Cognitive Development

Stage	Characteristics of the Stage	Major Change of the Stage
Sensori-motor (0–2 years)		Development proceeds from reflex activity to representation and sensori-motor solutions to problems. Primitive likes and dislikes emerge. Affect invested in the "self"
Period 1 (0–1 months)	Reflex activity only; no differentiation	
Period 2 (1–4 months)	Hand-mouth coordination; differentiation via sucking reflex	
Period 3 (4–8 months)	Hand-eye coordination; repeats unusual events	
Period 4 (8–12 months)	Coordination of two schemata; object permanence attained	
Period 5 (12–18 months)	New means through experimentation—follows sequential displacements	
Period 6 (18–24 months)	Internal representation; new means through mental combinations	
Preoperational (2–7 years)	Problems solved through representation—language development (2–4 years). Thought and language both egocentric. Cannot solve conservation problems	Development proceeds from sensorimotor representation to prelogical thought and solutions to problems. True social behavior begins. Intentionality absent in moral reasoning.
Concrete operations (7–11 years)	Reversability attained. Can solve conservation problems—logical operations developed and applied to concrete problems. Cannot solve complex verbal problems and hypothetical problems	Development proceeds from prelogical thought to logical solutions to concrete problems. Development of the will and beginnings of autonomy appear. Intentionality is constructed
Formal operations (11–15 years)	Logically solves all types of problems—thinks scientifically. Solves complex verbal and hypothetical problems. Cognitive structures mature	Development proceeds from logical solving of concrete problems to logical solving of all classes of problems. Emergence of idealistic feelings and personality formation. Adaptation to adult world begins

Source: From *Piaget's Theory of Cognitive and Affective Development*, third edition, by Barry J. Wadsworth. Copyright © 1971, 1979, and 1984 by Longman Inc. Reprinted by permission of Longman Inc., New York.

FACTORS INFLUENCING PASSAGE THROUGH COGNITIVE STAGES

Four broad factors have been suggested by Piaget as influencing cognitive development. None affects cognition independently. All are interactive. Together they determine the degree and rate of cognitive development through each stage and from one stage to another. The four factors are (1) maturation, (2) physical experiences, (3) social interaction, and (4) the process of equilibration.

Maturation

Maturation clearly affects a child's neurological and endocrinal, motor, etc., development—the physical side of cognitive development. Nevertheless Piaget downplayed the importance of physical factors. He and his associate Inhelder stated that the nervous system can do no more than determine the totality of possibilities and impossibilities at any given stage of cognitive development.

Physical Experiences

We have already discussed Piaget's insistence that the environment by itself doesn't modify cognition. A child develops cognitive schemata, i.e., develops cognitively, through activities. These activities may be visible ones, e.g., displayed in the child's manipulation of things. There may also be invisible ones, i.e., proceeding in the child's mind. But in both types of activities the child is acting on and interacting with objects, people, situations, events, etc. In the early years the interactions are physical. In later years much of it proceeds on a mental basis.

Social Interactions

Children's relationships with other children and adults are of great importance to cognitive development. Many schemata have a purely physical core; e.g., mathematical schemata emerge out of the physical acts of counting, seriation, and other quantitative physical activities. But other schemata are essentially social in nature and can develop only through interactions with people, for example, schemata concerned with such ideas as honesty, justice, liberty. Beyond this, social interactions expand and correct a child's thought even on purely physical issues. Even those schemata that mediate mathematics and science are altered because of social influences.

Equilibration

Schemata develop through equilibration. Disequilibration results whenever existing schemata cannot cope with events. It activates the process of equilibration, i.e., of new assimilations and accommodations that continue until schemata are altered either quantitatively or qualitatively so as to be able to establish a new equilibrium. That is the nature of true learning. That is the way of true cognitive development.

We are ready to examine Piaget's stages (periods). During our review, we introduce a number of new and important Piagetian constructs.

Sensorimotor Stage (0–2 Years)

Piaget made the point that cognitive development begins at birth. While thinking as a true sense does not begin at that time, an infant's primitive reflexes create the foundations for all later cognitive development. It has even been said that the infant's behavior shows some degree of abstract cognition, e.g., reflective abstract (Reid & Hresko, 1981).

Cognitive growth begins during the early months. At the beginning of the sensorimotor stage the baby is capable only of reflex behaviors but will be able to solve a variety of problems at the close—as any proud parent can tell you. At the beginning infants deal with everything in terms of their own bodies. At the close of the period, the baby "is able to recognize himself as . . . one element in the universe, and the universe is now experienced as external to himself" (Wadsworth, 1979, p. 39). That is, there is true thought.

Piaget divided the sensorimotor period into separate and distinct stages (see Table 6–1). Each represents an advance over its predecessor. Each shows the child cognitively and behaviorally active in new ways.

Substage 1 (0–1 Month): Random and Reflex Reactions

The baby is born with sucking, crying, grasping, and other reflexes. These are the beginning schemata. They are more behavioral than cognitive, but they represent the beginnings of cognition.

The processes of assimilation and accommodation are in evidence from birth on, as the baby seeks to adapt to the environment. These processes rapidly organize the early primitive reflex schemata into higher level structures. There are ready examples of this everywhere in the baby's behavior. The baby's initial behavior is largely assimilative. The baby sucks anything close to the mouth, it grasps anything the hand closes on. But in a few weeks there is also evidence of accommodation. The baby now searches for a nipple when hungry. The baby sucks that nipple in different ways depending on the type of nipple and its placement for feeding. Behavior is now adapted and reflects inner cognitive organization and it also represents meaningful learning, for the baby's original sucking schema has developed into a relatively complex cognitive structure that incorporates the original sucking reflex and information from the infant's earlier sucking experiences. The child's new schemata can coordinate a variety of behaviors. The baby, however, at this substage has no true conscious awareness of what is being achieved.

Substage 2 (1–4 Months): Primary Circular Reactions

During the second substage of sensorimotor development the basically reflexive behaviors of the earlier stage are modified considerably. The baby develops habits that indicate the development and operation of more complex schemata. These new schemata are created through what Piaget called *primary circular reactions*.

A primary circular reaction develops through the process of trial and error. The infant tries to repeat behaviors discovered by chance to be gratifying. Thumb sucking is an example. The child pops a thumb into the mouth by accident, finds it a pleasurable experience, and then purposely tries to repeat the action. In so doing the baby coordinates schemata that were previously distinct—schemata governing eye movements, finger movements, and sucking movements—into complex cognitive and behavioral schemata. This is a result of the infant's actions on and interactions with the environment. From these actions the infant has learned to move arms and hands in certain ways in order to suck the thumb, to push away covers or other obstacles, and to put the thumb into the mouth with a smooth coordinated movement. Behavior patterns of this sort are called *circular* because the satisfaction created by sucking stimulates efforts to repeat certain activities and sets a circle of events into action.

The infant develops a number of other primary circular reaction schemata during the second substage of the sensorimotor period. For example, the baby follows visual objects with eyes and orients to sound.

Something else is going on cognitively during this initial substage. The baby is beginning to anticipate events and is showing signs of curiosity and imitation. The infant is also developing (creating) a notion of the surrounding physical world.

Substage 3 (4–8 Months): Secondary Circular Reactions

During this substage of the sensorimotor period the infant becomes increasingly aware of and oriented toward things and events apart from the self and the infant's own activities. The baby begins to crawl and manipulate things extensively. Sensorimotor development is proceeding rapidly, though the infant cannot yet fully integrate eye and hand movements.

The primary circular reactions of Substage 2 were characterized by the child reproducing pleasurable events involving the body. During Substage 3 the baby is also able to engage in secondary circular reactions. This means that the baby develops ways of reproducing satisfying events accidentally discovered in the environment. The baby picks up a rattle by chance, finds it fun to shake, and tries to shake it again. A secondary circular reaction is in progress.

The baby also incorporates new sights and sounds and muscular reactions into existing schemata through what is called *imitative assimilation*. The baby begins to develop an understanding of objects through the manipulations. The infant seems to know that things exist apart from the self; for example, if something disappears from view, the baby appears to make an effort to search for it.

A significant cognitive accomplishment during this period is the beginning notion of object permanency in the baby's mind. This develops as a result of the baby's active manipulation of things. Object permanency is an appreciation of the fact that objects exist in their own right and remain the same even though they may look different from different positions.

During the previous substage an object that was hidden from sight no longer existed from the baby's standpoint. The idea of the object did not persist in the baby's mind. It was gone forever. This was indicated by the fact that the baby didn't search for an object once hidden. During Substage 3, if an object is hidden, the baby will search for it. This indicates that the baby knows the object is there even when unable to see it. The baby now has schemata that support the idea that the object has an existence of its own, i.e., a permanence. Such new schemata, however, are tentative and limited.

Substage 4 (8–12 Months): Coordination of Secondary Schemata

The fourth substage, characterized by more sophisticated and elaborative schemata, marks the onset of what Piaget called *intentional behavior*. That is, the baby is able to apply older patterns of behavior to new problems. In Substage 3 the infant engaged in secondary circular reactions after accidentally discovering what they accomplished. In Substage 4 the infant "knows" what is wanted before doing it, and the baby coordinates, i.e., combines two or more schemata, to accomplish its purposes. The baby thus engages in intentional behavior for the first time. In Substage 4, when seeing a toy, the baby deliberately reaches for it.

During Substage 4 the baby also begins to understand physical relationships. For example, the baby starts to recognize that things are in front of or behind other things, and that one object may have to be removed to reach another.

The baby is also learning to respond to signifiers, an indication of being able to use symbols in a rudimentary fashion. When mother puts a spoon in front of baby's mouth, the baby opens the mouth if anticipating some liked food and closes it when anticipating not liking the food. If a mother gets up, the baby may cry, expecting her to leave the room. Such actions indicate responses to signifiers.

During Substage 4 the baby also begins to develop a true appreciation of causality. That is, it begins to understand that persons and objects apart from the self can make things happen.

Substage 5 (12–18 Months): Tertiary Circular Reactions

In the previous substage the baby engaged in intentional behaviors by coordinating and using familiar schemata to solve new problems. In Substage 5 the baby becomes able to create new schemata to solve problems when existing schemata are not adequate. The baby uses trial and error to solve problems rather than relying on previously formed habitual schemata (Wadsworth, 1979).

The baby also tries to find out things for their own sake—to satisfy curiosity (rather than just to satisfy self). This is a time when babies play with nesting blocks, pull things apart, let things drop out of their hands (to find out what will happen), make water splash; they are trying to learn more about their environments and how things work. Piaget called these sorts of behaviors *tertiary circular reactions* because they involve doing things for their own sake rather than from a desire for personal pleasure. In primary and secondary circular reactions babies were involved with their own actions and their own gratification. In tertiary reactions their interest is "externalized."

The schemata making tertiary circular reactions possible develop as a consequence of the baby's growing understanding that objects exist and have qualities altogether apart from self and personal needs. In order to learn more about these objects, the baby makes accommodations. These create complex and sophisticated schemata capable of assimilating wider and more diverse types of information.

The baby's growing understanding of object constancy during this substage, i.e., that objects exist apart from oneself, is shown by the newly developed ability to deal with the serial displacement of objects. Before Substage 4 the baby wouldn't look for objects if they were hidden from view. During Substage 4 the baby searched for the object but not always in the place where it was hidden, i.e., was unable to handle sequential displacement of objects. That is, if an object usually hidden in Place A were later hidden in Place B, the baby would persist in searching for it in Place A. In Substage 5, however, the baby is able to attend to the demands of new experiences. If an object is hidden in Place A, the baby searches in Place A; if in Place B, the baby searches in Place B. The baby can, however, understand only visible displacements but cannot follow invisible ones. Thus if the object is hidden at a certain spot and then moved about after being hidden, the baby will keep searching for the object only at the spot where it disappeared from view. This is because the baby is not capable of creating mental representations of objects and cannot keep an image of an object in mind once that object has disappeared from view.

The baby continues to increase an understanding of causality during Substage 5. It is increasingly aware that things often happen because of events beyond one's own personal control. While earlier understanding events only after they occurred, the baby now has prevision, i.e., is able to understand that something may happen before it actually does.

Substage 6 (18 Months–2 Years): Invention of New Means through Mental Combinations

Substage 6, the last of the sensorimotor subperiods, is a transition stage leading to the next major period of cognitive development. During this substage the baby actually becomes capable of true thought and is able to represent mentally things and events in the mind using images, symbols, and language. The baby is able to think about things without those things actually being present.

Substage 6 is identified with the concept of invention of new means through mental combinations. The baby is capable of mental representation, is able to solve problems by thinking, as well as through physical actions. In Substage 5 the baby experimented by manipulating things physically but now "experiments" by representing objects and carries out actions with them within the thought processes. No longer controlled by the events of the external world, the baby is able (for the first time) to deal with possibilities, that is, is able to think through , i.e., try things out mentally, without actually engaging in behavior. The baby's problem-solving activities have become internalized.

This new power and mental representation is demonstrated by the phenomenon of object constancy. Since now able to manipulate images of objects in its mind, the baby can mentally picture the possibilities of an object being moved after it is hidden and can now for the first time deal with invisible displacements. Thus when one of the baby's toys is hidden under a blanket and then moved (away from its point of disappearance), the baby will search for it in different places.

The two-year-old baby's new powers of mental representation also improve the ability to deal with causality. The baby doesn't have to see things happening to understand that one object may affect another or that one event may result in another.

Summation of the Sensorimotor Period

The invariant functions are at work throughout each of the substages of the sensorimotor period, both quantitatively and qualitatively changing the infant's cognitive schemata. During each of the sensorimotor substages distinctly new and superior generations of schemata are developed, each succeeding generation of schemata incorporating within itself the earlier, simpler schemata of the previous stages. During each substage all cognitive schemata develop concurrently and are interdependent. And the development of one schema is dependent on the development of other schemata. Thus the development of object constancy requires that the baby be capable of cognitively appreciating both shapes and space. Similarly the baby must be able to coordinate hand-eye actions to carry out intentional behavior.

Piaget has provided an interesting example showing the surprising maturity of thought of a child completing the sensorimotor stage. Piaget blocked the gate to his garden with a chair that could not be seen from the other side. Piaget's son (at   Substage 6 of sensorimotor development) tried to push the gate open but could not. He suddenly understood the problem and went around the garden wall to the other side of the gate and removed the chair—which made it possible to open the gate. The child was capable of this solution because he was able to picture or represent the cause of the obstruction in his mind and to understand the cause-and-effect relationship of chair to the blocking of the gate. He solved the problem through the invention of new means through mental combination (Ginsburg & Opper, 1979).

At the close of Substage 6 the sensorimotor period is completed (about two years of age in a normal child). By its close the child has reached the level where cognitive functioning can proceed on a conceptual-symbolic basis. This does not mean that the child will no longer rely on physical sensorimotor schemata to guide thinking; they will continue to play a significant role in thinking. They are, however, gradually becoming subordinated to truly mental schemata.

Preoperational Period (2–7 Years)

The preoperational child achieves a cognitive level, with the ability to *think*, i.e., conceive of things and situations mentally, and to solve problems mentally. The child, however, is still very much dependent on the physical environment for what is thought. Thoughts are determined by what the child actually can see, hear, touch, and otherwise experience. For a variety of reasons, including this continued dependence on physical experiences, the preoperational child is still unable to think logically (until the close of the period). Since it is logical thought that defines operational thinking, the child is preoperational.

The preoperational stage is actually divided into two substages. The first is the preconceptual period (two to four years of age). The second is the perceptual or intuitive thought period (ages four to seven). In the preconceptual period the child uses language and mental images in thinking. In the period of intuitive thought the child solves problems on the basis of personal intuitions (hunches).

Characteristics of Preoperational Thought

The child's thinking throughout the preoperational period—except toward the close, when it blends into the operational period—is still illogical. It is characterized by transductive rather than inductive or deductive (logical) reasoning. *Transductive reasoning* is reasoning from one idea to another without logically relating the ideas. Thus the child may interpret the things seen in some physical relationships as belonging together by some necessity. The child also thinks that things happening together have a cause-and-effect relationship to each other, even when they are completely unrelated.

Syncretic thinking is a form of transductive reasoning in which the child draws conclusions on the basis of features that are conceptually irrelevant. One of Piaget's daughters at the preoperational stage wished to eat an orange. She was told that she couldn't do so because the oranges were still green. After drinking a cup of tea and observing that it was yellow, she decided that since the tea was yellow, the orange had to be yellow too and she should have one to eat (Ginsburg & Opper, 1976).

Juxtapositional reasoning is another type of transductive thought. Here the child draws conclusions based on the basis of details, while overlooking the main point of things. Because of these tendencies the child cannot adequately classify objects. Asked to put together a group of toy objects on the basis of their similarity, a child will assemble a church, tree, motorcycle, and bench because once these objects were seen together. Asked to tell the examiner why different objects float, the child explains the floating of the objects on the basis of different, unrelated, and usually irrelevant details. Thus a big sailboat floats because it is big, a little one because it is flat. The preoperational child cannot develop logical generalizations (to explain floating and other phenomena) since the mind is fixed on obvious but irrelevant features. The reasons for the child's preoperational deficiencies in logical thinking become apparent as we discuss preoperational thought processes in further detail. Our discussion of the preoperation period describes what the child can and cannot do. The "cannot do" aspects of the preoperational period clarify what is meant by operational thought, the type of thinking that characterizes the subsequent stage of cognitive development.

Advances That Characterize Preoperational Thought

Let us begin by examining the preoperational child's cognitive achievements. They are impressive. As we know, a child at the end of the sensorimotor period is able to function in a representational (and therefore conceptual) fashion. The child is increasingly able to deal with problems internally and has come to depend less on actual physical solutions to its problems. Representation, i.e., conceptual cognitive functioning, characterizes the preoperational period. The preoperational child also shows the ability to think over time, something that the sensorimotor child was incapable of. Piaget once compared sensorimotor intelligence to a motion picture film taken at very slow speed, so that its pictures are seen in succession one at a time. In other words sensorimotor thinking lacks a sense of continuity, and can deal only with immediate experiences. The preoperational child clearly moves beyond such limitations. That child can think in terms of the past and future as well as the immediate present and is no longer restricted to the here and now. The child can also review in the mind what went on before and what might happen in the future and integrate both with the events of the present. The preoperational child can also span time rapidly in thinking so that thought is more sustained, coherent, and organized (and more relevant) than that of a sensorimotor child.

A most important advance of the preoperational stage is the development of schemata that support semiotic functions. That is, the preoperational child is able to use symbols to represent things that are not actually present. The child can use small toys, pictures, or even words to represent real objects; a toy tricycle, the picture of a cycle, or even the word tricycle can substitute for an actual tricycle in thinking. This ability to use symbols liberates the child's thought processes. The child's new freedom of thought is expressed in play, within which the child engages in what Piaget called *internal imitation*; i.e., the child imitates or duplicates real-life situations and events through the symbolic vehicles of play. This newly developed symbolic ability represents a considerable advance over the sensorimotor child's ability to use signifiers. Signifiers suggest the existence of things while symbols actually represent them in the child's mind and can be manipulated mentally.

The child's language develops significantly during the preoperational period and aids cognitive development in a variety of ways. It does so by expanding the child's communications with others that have a maturing influence on its thinking. It also adds to the symbols that the child can use, accelerating and sophisticating the internalization of actions. As a consequence of language, the speed and power of the preoperational child's thinking processes are increased. Without language, cognitive development is necessarily slowed down and diminished. Piaget, however, insisted that language should not be confused with thought. The two, he insisted, are different, though both have origins in the same sensorimotor schemata. Deaf children are generally able to develop   normal cognition, despite their language deficits, if they share sensorimotor experiences in common with normal children.

Socialization experiences play a significant role in shaping thinking during the preoperational period. One of the reasons that language is important to cognitive development is because it is a major means through which children can be influenced, i.e., socialized by other children and adults. Socialization opportunities increasingly provide preoperational children with new ways of understanding themselves and the world around them and also provide models of thought and behavior to imitate. Social experiences play a major role in helping the preoperational child to become operational; they help to correct and redirect its thinking.

Limitations in Preoperational Thinking

We are ready to consider some of the preoperational child's limitations in cognition. They represent obstacles to the development of truly logical thought: the ultimate goal of cognitive development.

Concreteness

The first of the preoperational child's cognitive weaknesses that we examine is cognitive *concreteness*. Though able to manipulate symbols effectively, the child is still very concrete in thinking. For even though capable of thinking in terms of symbols, the child can use only symbols that refer to actual physical experiences. When thinking, the child still thinks as if actually participating in the situations that the symbols represent. The child's thought processes are thus dominated by perceptions and images (of actual things and events); the influence of sensorimotor events is still quite powerful.

Egocentrism

The term *egocentrism* has been used by social and behavioral scientists in a number of ways. In popular terms it has come to mean that someone is self-centered, concerned only with the ways oneself thinks and feels about things.

Piaget's use of the term *egocentrism* has some aspects in common with this popular interpretation. But it also indicates a particular cognitive state. *Egocentrism* means that the individual believes that only what the self believes can be true. It is a special limitation in cognition for the preoperational child.

When Piaget described the preoperational child's thinking and behavior as being *egocentric*, he meant that the child is convinced that what the self believes or does or feels at any time is the only correct way possible. No one else's opinions can be right—unless they agree with one's own. Others must believe what the preoperational child says because of saying it. The preoperational child never questions the validity of one's own views. When shown contradictory evidence, the evidence must be wrong. Egocentricity is a major reason why preoperational children become so frustrated when they are corrected by adults.

The preoperational period is a long one. Throughout it the processes of cognitive development and social pressures keep working so that as the period progresses, the child does finally begin to question one's own thoughts and opinions, to appreciate others' points of view, to modify thinking in the direction of social consensus, and to diminish in egocentricity.

While calling particular attention to egocentrism at the preoperation stage, Piaget made it clear that it is found at all levels of development. The sensorimotor child, for example, is completely egocentric. And after the preoperational period, egocentrism is likely to appear any time new schemata are developed. Such occasions arouse attitudes of cognitive defensiveness on a child's part. Thus during adolescence, when the capabilities for fully logical thought finally emerge, there is likely to be a flare-up in egocentrism. As everyone knows, adolescents often believe that only their points of view are accurate. This accounts for much of their self-righteousness and their so-called defiance of authority.

During the preoperational period the child's egocentrism prevents the development of logical thinking by maintaining the child's cognitive status quo. The preoperational child resists accommodating schemata to facts.

Centration

Centration, too, is an important characteristic of preoperational thinking. It is another side to the child's concrete and egocentric thought processes. Centration refers to the tendency to focus on certain narrow aspects of perceptual experiences at the expense of the other parts or the totality of those experiences. In centered thinking the child attends only to a single or few details in a problem—often irrelevant ones—while entirely overlooking others. In observing something happening, the child attends to the beginning and end of the event but overlooks what goes on in between.

Centration is a major obstacle to the development of logical thinking. Logical thinking requires that one take all significant factors into consideration. In order to think logically, an individual must be able to decenter thinking. Since *centration* causes the preoperational child's thinking to be dominated by a situation's most obvious perceptual characteristics, the child cannot think in a truly logical way.

Inability To Attend to Transformations

Another limiting cognitive characteristic of the preoperational child is the inability to observe transformations. When watching a succession of events, or a sequence of changes, the child focuses on their separate elements, one at a time, rather than on their transformation from one stage to another. This is a natural consequence of the child's failure to decenter.

A frequent example of the preoperational child's inability to deal with transformations is provided by a pencil experiment. A pencil is held vertically and then allowed to fall. The beginning state is an upright, vertical one. The final state (after the pencil has fallen) is a horizontal one. The pencil passes through a number of successive (positional) states between the initial and final ones, but the preoperational child is unable to follow these transformations, i.e., the sequence of steps the pencil goes through in falling. This is because the child is unable to decenter thinking from the first and final stages—from the pencil's initial (upright) state and its last (fallen) position. The child thus misses what has gone on in between (see Figure 6–1).

The preoperational child's inability to follow transformations is another major barrier to its thinking in a logical coherent fashion. Unable to understand the flow of events, natural sequences, and the relations of the various steps in a process to others and unable to create a coherent whole from the "pieces" of experiences, the child is also unable to think in a truly logical way.

Figure 6–1 The Pencil Experiment

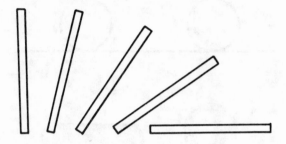

Source: Reprinted from *Piaget's Theory: A Primer* by John L. Phillips, Jr., with permission of W.H. Freeman and Company, © 1981.

Reversible Operations

Reversible operations (in action and thinking) imply that they can be turned around. Cognitively, it means that one can add something to a group of things and take it away in the mind, or one can mentally increase the quantity of something and then diminish it. *Reversibility* means that changes can take place in a closed system in which a change in one part requires a compensating change in another part of the system. It is an essential condition for logical-mathematical operations (Phillips, 1981). It is the other side of conservation. The following are examples of reversibility:

$$4 + 5 = 9; 9 - 5 = 4$$

boys and girls = all children; all children − boys = girls

In both instances, one observes "thought going from one condition to another and returned to the starting point" (Phillips, 1981, p. 85).

Piaget demonstrated the irreversibility of the preoperational child's thought processes in a number of fascinating experiments. For example, a child is shown two plasticine balls of equal size (see Figure 6–2) and is asked whether the balls have the same amount of plasticine. If the child agrees that they do, one of the balls is rolled in a sausage shape, and the child may be asked whether both balls have the same amount of plasticine and are of the same size. Piaget found that preoperational children usually say that one or the other has more plasticine and is bigger (usually the sausage-shaped one), even though the child is aware that both originally looked exactly alike and that one was merely changed in shape.

Piaget attributed the child's faulty conclusions to a failure of conservation, i.e., to an inability to reverse thinking to its operational point of origin. Because of this inability, the child is incapable of understanding that nothing was either added or removed from the original plasticine ball when it was turned into a sausage shape or that it could be remolded into a ball the same size as the other. Nor can the child understand that the additional length of the sausage (which usually makes it look larger or as having more plasticine than the other

Figure 6–2 Piaget's Ball Experiment

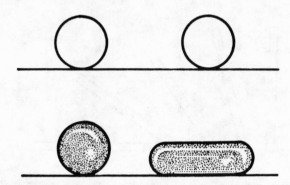

Source: Reprinted from *Piaget's Theory: A Primer* by John L. Phillips, Jr., with permission of W.H. Freeman and Company, © 1981.

---

shape) has been compensated for by a loss in breadth. In short the child cannot understand that the original amount of plasticine in the ball has not been changed at all through its transformation into a sausage shape. The domination of the child's thinking by perceptual irrelevancies prevents reversible thinking.

The preoperational child's irreversibility of thought and failure to conserve have been demonstrated in numerous other experiments. In one of them the child is shown piles of beads that are exactly alike in size and shape. When asked to put equal numbers of beads into two separate containers of different shapes, the child will then say that one or the other (usually the taller) of the containers has more beads than the other because that container looks bigger (see Figure 6–3). Once again we have an example of "illogical" thinking because the child is deceived by perceptual irrelevancies. The factors responsible for the preoperational child's inability to reverse thinking are the same ones responsible for the child's failure to conserve.

Conservation

Piaget identified conservation as an essential operation in logical thinking. The child advancing into the operational stage becomes able to deal with conservations because of advances in logical thinking. At the same time, ability to deal with conservation is required for genuinely logical thinking to take place. *Conservation* is a thinking process that takes into account the fact that the quantity or quality of things can remain the same despite changes in physical appearances.

Preoperational children are concrete and egocentric in their thinking and unable to decenter or follow transformations. They typically attend to things, objects, situations, and events on the basis of appearances and tend to respond to irrelevancies they cannot reverse. Because of these and other reciprocal limitations, the child cannot conserve.

To a preoperational child a balloon that is empty at first but then filled with air is not the same balloon under different conditions but rather two distinct balloons. Attending to irrelevant physical dimensions when deciding how many balloons there are, the child has failed to conserve.

Figure 6–3 The Bead Experiment

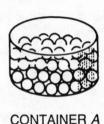 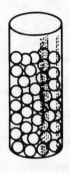

CONTAINER *A*   CONTAINER *B*

Source: Reprinted from *Piaget's Theory: A Primer* by John L. Phillips, Jr., with permission of W.H. Freeman and Company, © 1981.

Summation of the Preoperational Stage

The preoperational child is no longer restricted to thinking through actions. The child is capable of representational thought and of manipulation of symbols, can solve problems mentally, and has a sense of time.

The preoperational child's increasingly mature language facilitates cognitive development by providing the child with additional symbols to manipulate and by otherwise accelerating the pace of thinking. The growth of language accentuates the influence of socialization experiences on the child's thinking processes. These socialization experiences play an important role in maturing the child's thought.

The preoperational child, however, is still dominated by perceptual events in thinking. The child cannot yet engage in true logical thinking. The thought processes are characterized by egocentrism, concreteness, inability to decenter, transform, perform reversible operations, or conserve. There is continual improvement in these areas as the preoperational period progresses. The preoperational child's thinking starts to become operational toward the period's close.

Stage of Concrete Operations (7–11 Years)

During the period of concrete operations, a child's cognitive schemata develop to a level where they are able to support concrete operations. The child becomes operational.

Definition of Operations

Piaget has defined an *operation* as an action that is mental and has reversible aspects; i.e., it can return to its starting point. More specifically an operation can be defined in terms of four characteristics: (1) It is internalized, i.e., carried out in thought, in terms of images and symbols, that is, on a truly cognitive level; (2) an operation is reversible; (3) an operation always implies conservation; i.e., it always has an invariant, some unchanging characteristic; and (4) an operation never exists alone; it is always related to other operations and thus is part of a system.

When finally operational, the child is no longer dominated by its perceptual experiences but can decenter. The child is able to follow transformations, can reverse thinking, can conserve, and is considerably less egocentric than the preoperational child. The operational child is better able to communicate and participate with others on a genuinely cooperative, give-and-take basis. And an operational child is capable of truly logical reasoning, can seriate, understand equivalences, classify things, and deal with causality.

Seriation Operations. This involves the ability to organize mentally items or units according to increases or decreases in size, length, weight, volume, etc. Children begin to seriate length about the age of 7, weight about the age of 10, volume about 12.

Equivalence Operations. The concrete operational child is capable of a variety of equivalence operations, i.e., $A + B = C$, so $C - B = A$. The child can also deal with length, weight, volume, and other equivalences.

Classification Operations. Unlike a preoperational child, an operational one can flexibly classify objects on the basis of several dimensions. Piaget has provided an example of a classification problem unsolvable at the preoperational level but easily managed by a child functioning at the concrete operational level (Wadsworth, 1978, p. 104).

A preoperational child is shown 40 beads, 20 of which are made of wood, 20 of glass. Eighteen of the wood beads and 18 of the glass beads are white in color. Two of the wood and 2 of the glass beads are brown in color. The child is asked to examine the beads and to sort the white and brown ones into separate containers. The ability to do this indicates that the child is capable of making correct perceptual classifications.

The preoperational child is also able to carry out more demanding classification tasks. This child can also classify and sort out the beads on the basis of color or on the basis of being wood or glass.

Despite these intellectual achievements, the preoperational child is still incapable of concrete operations. This can be demonstrated if the child is shown the beads and asked whether there are more wooden or brown beads. The child will answer brown beads. The correct answer is wood beads.

Reversibility and Conservation

The operational child is capable of fully reversible thinking and thus of conservation. The operational child understands that placing objects close together or spreading them does not change their numbers. The child knows that changing the shape of a piece of plastic doesn't make it bigger and that pouring water from a flat dish into a long cylinder doesn't make it more.

One Piagetian experiment in particular clarifies the reversibility of operational thought. This is shown by the operational child's solution of a problem beyond the capabilities of the preoperational child. If the latter is shown three balls of different colors but of the same size, which are placed into a cylinder in the order red, blue, yellow, the preoperational child will correctly predict the order in which the balls will emerge from the bottom of the cylinder; i.e., red, blue, yellow. But rotate that cylinder so that the balls come out in a different order and the preoperational child will still predict that the balls will come out in a red, blue, yellow order. The child is surprised on seeing them come out in the opposite order. The operational child, able to reverse operations, understands what really happens and why it happens.

Causality

The operational child achieved an understanding of causality in a true sense. The child doesn't make cause-and-effect decisions merely on the basis of appearances. For example, the child is able to understand relationships between rate and speed. A preoperational child observes two toy autos going at different speeds and different distances to the same destination point. This child believes that the faster car must arrive earlier even though it is going a much longer distance, because the child can't understand the relationship between distance and speed (see Figure 6–4). *Faster* automatically means *more*. In contrast, the operational child understands that the car driving the longer distance must proceed at a faster speed in order to arrive at the destination at the same time as the car going the shorter distance. This child is able to adjust one dimension to compensate for another. The child is operational.

Décalage

In conservation as well as seriation and classification, a phenomenon that Piaget calls *horizontal décalage* shows itself. That is, while the problems of conservation are solved by operational children, the ages at which this occurs differ from one type of problem-solving area to another. The concrete operational child develops conservation skills for number problems about 6 to 7 years of age, but conservation skills for area and mass problems develop between 7 and 8 years. Conservation of volume, i.e., the ability to understand the displacement of water when objects are immersed, develops much later, indeed is not achieved by most children until 11 or 12, when they have advanced beyond the operational period; in short not all operations are achieved during the operational period.

Cognitive Limitations of the Concrete Operational Period

As stated, the concrete operational child is no longer perception-bound to the degree and in the ways that the preoperational child is. The operational child can decenter perceptive experiences and attend to transformations. The child achieves reversibility of operations

---

Figure 6–4 A Causality Experiment

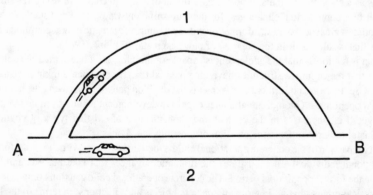

Source: From *Piaget's Theory of Cognitive and Affective Development*, third edition, by Barry J. Wadsworth. Copyright © 1971, 1979, and 1984 by Longman Inc. Reprinted by permission of Longman Inc., New York.

and conservation and can think logically. Nevertheless the concrete operation child is not yet able to function at the highest levels of logical thinking. Operations are still limited to concrete, i.e., physical-observable, tangible situations, objects, problems. The child cannot reason in terms that are divorced from these and thus cannot solve a purely verbal problem or one that involves the application of abstract mathematical formulas (with understanding).

Summation of the Concrete Operational Period

The concrete operational period is a transition stage through which a child must proceed to pass from illogical (preoperational) to fully logical (formal operational) status. A concrete operational child's thinking is no longer dominated by perceptions. The child's thought loses much of its egocentricity. The child becomes able to decenter, observe transformations, carry out reversible operations, and conserve, with transductive thinking giving way to truly logical thought; the child can deal with problems of seriation, classification, time, and speed. Nevertheless the child is not yet capable of abstract reasoning and can reason only in terms of physical, concrete facts of life, things, and situations. At the close of the period of concrete operations the child is ready to move to the final and most advanced stage of cognitive development.

Period of Formal Operational Thought (11–15 Years)

A child capable of concrete operational thought is greatly advanced cognitively over other, subhuman species but is still far short of being able to engage in fully mature thinking. Nevertheless, by the time that the period of formal operational thought is over, the child, now an adolescent, has developed its cognitive capabilities (if normal) to the fullest degree possible. During the formal operational period the child not only becomes an adolescent but also develops schemata to their highest levels; they become qualitatively equal to those of a cognitively competent adult. After completing the period of formal operational development, humans do not develop any new schemata. Cognitive development, qualitatively speaking, comes to an end.

The cognitive structures developed during the formal operational period are sufficient to adjust to and solve any kind of problem. A formal operational person can deal with the forms as well as the contents of problems. Formal operational cognitive structures suffice for all future intellectual challenges, for they are sufficiently advanced and stable so as to assimilate a great deal of new information without requiring dramatic new accommodations (ones that would result in the creation of new schemata) (Phillips, 1981).

That is not to say that the adolescent is capable of thinking as well as a mature adult but rather that the cognitive structures have the potential to carry out such thinking. To say it otherwise, there are no further improvements in cognition potential following the period of formal operations. The individual's later cognitive development results from quantitative changes, i.e., increases in the content and sophistication of existing types of cognitive schemata, rather than from the creation of more advanced ones.

A comparison of the concrete operational child's thought processes with those of a formal operational individual   demonstrates the dramatic advances that take place cognitively during the formal operational period. The concrete operational child can think only in terms of physical things, that is, in terms of concrete objects and situations, in terms of the here and now, and in terms of one operation at a time. In contrast the formal operational adolescent has become entirely free of the concrete, free of the present. The adolescent can think in ways that are entirely divorced from things and can do so in a flexible, combinatory fashion. The formal operational adolescent can "think about thought," "operate on operations," integrate operations. Thinking can go entirely on an abstract or hypothetical level. And it can deal with symbols and symbolisms as symbols and symbolisms rather than as signifiers of other things. An adolescent functioning at a formal operational level is able to understand intellectually philosophical issues and is also capable of scientific thinking. At the close of the formal operational period, logico-operational thought, the highest manifestation of intelligence, is fully established. Thus cognitive development ends.

The new possibilities of thought made possible through the adolescent's development of formal operations temporarily intensify the egocentricity of thought processes. As observed, egocentricity is particularly characteristic of preoperational thinking, but is also a characteristic of cognition any time there are dramatic qualitative changes in schemata. It is therefore not surprising that an adolescent, whose horizons of thinking have enormously expanded because of formal operational capabilities, is initially quite egocentric. This is the basis for much of adolescent willfulness and unwillingness to compromise. At the same time, and in a more positive vein, the initial achievement of formal cognitive operational status often brings with it idealism and moral growth; the adolescent thus is often involved with abstract notions of fairness and justice and with causes.

Summation of Piagetian Periods

Before we proceed to consider the implications that Piaget's work holds for education, it may be helpful to summarize the various periods of development and to call attention to some special features of this development. There are four major stages or periods of development; within each of these are distinct subperiods.

The sensorimotor period (0–2 years of age) is the first of these periods. At its beginning the child functions on the basis of inherited motor schemata. At its close the child has developed increasingly differentiated and integrated sensorimotor schemata that can be used to solve problems with and to "think." During the preoperational period (2–7 years) the child's intellectual development moves to a much higher level. The child is capable of true representational thought. Thinking, however, is entirely egocentric and is unable to conserve or deal with transformations. The child focuses or centers on isolated perceptual aspects of problems. The child cannot engage in logical thinking. The child advancing to the concrete operational period, on the other hand, is fully capable of logical thinking. The child is able to decenter thinking, deal with transformation, reverse, and conserve in thinking. The child, nevertheless, can still think only in concrete, here-and-now terms. By the time the formal operational period (11–15 years of age) is completed, the child, now an adolescent, is capable of mature cognitive functioning. The adolescent is able to deal with abstractions and symbols and to function in a fully logicomathematical way. Cognitive development (of structures) is fully completed at the close of the formal operational period though improvements, i.e., greater knowledge (content) and more sophisticated thinking (functions), will result from further maturity and experiences.

The Stage Concept, Reexamined

According to Piaget a child's cognitive development through each of the four major stages (periods) and their subperiods is invariant. That is, no stage can ever be skipped. The progression through the stages may vary in speed. Some children mature cognitively faster than others. Some children may never progress past a particular stage. Thus severely and profoundly retarded children appear to remain at a sensorimotor or preoperational stage even when they become adults. Furthermore it appears that many normal adults never become completely operational at a formal level. Perhaps no more than half do (Kuhn, 1978). But the sequence of cognitive development is unalterable.

Piaget and his closest followers have insisted that each stage or period builds on the accomplishments of others, that in fact earlier schemata are not lost and do not disappear when new more advanced ones emerge, that in fact advanced schemata are built on and from older less sophisticated ones, incorporating the latter's elements into their own structures. Thus the highest types of scientific thinking still show some evidence of earlier (and primitive) sensorimotor schemata.

Piaget and his followers have also insisted that cognitive development proceeds in a broad, general way. A child's maturing cognitive schemata manifest themselves similarly in a child's reasoning across a variety of situations. They do admit to certain exceptions to this general rule. These exceptions come under the name of *décalages*. A *décalage* is a gap; both vertical and horizontal gaps are found in cognitive development.

In vertical décalage a child functions at one cognitive level in a particular realm of functioning and at another in a second realm. Piaget points out that a child may be able to solve problems with the cognitive maturity of an 11-year-old at a practical plane of action while functioning like a 7-year-old on a plane of verbal thought.

In horizontal décalage the child may show gaps in cognitive functioning within the same realm of cognitive operations. As we have seen, concrete operational children appear to be able to conserve quantities readily at a 6- and 7-year level but cannot deal with conservation of volume until 8 or 9 years of age. Décalages have been some source of difficulty for Piaget's theories. Even though Piaget and his followers believe that they satisfactorily deal with it in their theories, décalage does contradict the idea that cognitive development proceeds in a general fashion. Some décalages in individual children may be considered the equivalents of cognitive deficits.

SOME OBSERVATIONS

This book is not intended to provide detailed analyses of any of the cognitive approaches surveyed. The discussion of Piaget's ideas has been extremely limited, a superficial overview of them. There is always a danger in trying to simplify complicated information. This is particularly true with Piaget because he was constantly altering theories and his thinking was of great complexity. Nevertheless, this review does provide a reasonable basis to understand the implications that his work may have for remedial and special education.

Before proceeding to these topics, however, it should be noted that despite the enormous admiration that his work has received, Piaget's work has also been consistently criticized from a number of different standpoints, some of which have been discussed. The same can be said, of course, for almost any area of cognitive psychology. The constructs of intelligence and special abilities are constantly being attacked. We again call attention here to the criticisms of Piaget's work only because remedial and special educators are more likely to encounter enthusiastic praise of Piaget than they are to read any critical appraisals. Furthermore, many books and articles discussing the implications of Piaget's theories for education seem to proceed as if the writer believes his theories are essentially proven, when in fact they are still theories.

Some major cognitive theorists and researchers indeed believe that his theories are fundamentally incorrect and criticize Piaget's belief that cognition develops in different stages and that more mature cognitive structures build on and merge from earlier ones. Bruner (1972) has complained that Piaget's theory explains only limited aspects of cognition. Philosophers have criticized him on the grounds that he has carried out his research to prove theories rather than developing his theories on the basis of research (Hamlyn, 1971). But Piaget's theories, whatever their limitations, are of value to education.

PIAGET AND EDUCATION

Let us remember that Piaget distinguished between two cognitive types of developmental learning. The first is learning in the narrow sense, that is, learning to acquire specific types of new information or to learn special skills. Such specific learning is important, but it doesn't have generalizable qualities. Learning in the wider sense—cognitive development—means the development of generalizable cognitive structures, i.e., schemata, that control and direct activities in a variety of circumstances. We need not remark what type of learning Piaget was interested in.

For Piaget, becoming educated is not a matter of learning how to do specific kinds of things. It is rather cognitive development, specifically the achievement of the highest (logicomathematical) developmental level of cognition. This is a different view than that of behaviorists who seek to train specific skill sequences. For that matter it is quite different from that of most educators who are concerned with academic skills learning; for Piaget was not concerned that a child learn specific curricula, rather that a child become capable of logicomathematical operations.

Piaget was above all a theorist and a researcher. He sought to discover the principles of general cognitive development and functioning rather than ways of applying them to specific practical problems. He came late to giving any advice to educators. Nor was he particularly interested in the problems of remediation or of the handicapped (Murray, 1978).

There has been a good deal of successful and useful research into the cognitive characteristics of learners, from preschool through adult ages. We mentioned earlier how preschool education has been influenced by Piaget. Nevertheless, it is still difficult to apply Piagetian ideas to educational practices in specific ways. Some critics indeed believe that efforts to apply Piaget to the classroom should be abandoned altogether, while others take a guarded point of view. Thus Sinclair (1976) has observed that Piaget's ideas can serve as a source of general educational principles but that they have "absolutely" no direct implications for the teaching of reading, writing, etc.

As to applications to problem learners and the handicapped, Murray (1978) credits Piaget for having forced educators to conceptualize better the relationships between cognition and perception and to recognize that school learning problems should more likely be attributed to "incomplete structures" than to inadequate or faulty sensory information (p. 283). But like Sinclair, he has made the point that Piaget said "virtually nothing practical . . . either about education or the education of handicapped children" (1978, p. 283).

A number of psychologists and educators have attempted to apply Piaget's principles to instruction. Some have used them to guide curriculum development, particularly in mathematics and science, where ideas such as conservation and causality are clearly important (Kuhn, 1978). Others have suggested that his clinical interviewing techniques can help teachers evaluate their pupils more effectively. Some efforts have been made to create new types of Piagetian intelligence tests based on his concept of cognitive developmental stages. There have been and continue to be efforts to accelerate or even to remediate the cognitive functions that he studied, e.g., to improve conservation, teach decentering, help children to seriate more efficiently (Bricker et al., 1981).

General Piagetian Principles for Educators

A number of the educational principles based on Piaget's work cannot be considered original. Dewey, Montessori, Froebel, and other educational pioneers made similar recommendations at much earlier times. Thus among Piaget's principles we find the following:

- A child learns differently than adults and at different stages of cognitive development.
- Children progress at different paces cognitively so that tasks and lessons should be individualized.
- Sensorimotor learning is essential to cognitive development; concrete activities are needed to assist children to develop cognitively.
- A child needs to learn in an active way, for cognitive development results from the child's own activity.
- Continual opportunities should be provided for a child's current cognitive structures to interact with new environmental experiences.
- Self-regulation is essential for genuine learning and the child should progress at an individual pace—teachers should not force learning.
- Social interaction fosters learning (Ginsburg & Opper, 1979).

DIRECT APPLICATIONS OF PIAGETIAN THEORY

Stage-Based Curricula

Early efforts to apply stage theory to education were made in the country at the preschool level by Lavatelli (1970) and Weikart (1971) and others. Working with preoperational children these investigators sought to promote children's acquisitions of concrete operational concepts. Initially there was enormous enthusiasm about such efforts. They did not, however, progress beyond their experimental beginnings, and it is not clear how useful their efforts were, despite early enthusiastic reports. As Kuhn (1978) points out, almost all normal children acquire concrete operations, whether or not they attend a Piagetian preschool. Even if these programs did help children achieve concrete operational status, it was not much of an achievement.

Since 1970 there has been more curricular emphasis at the formal level of operations, particularly in mathematical and scientific areas, to which Piaget's theories are oriented. There is Karplus's (1974) Science Curriculum Improvement Study (SIS) for elementary grades and later expansions of this approach to junior and senior high school levels. For the older children these curricula attempted to foster formal operational thinking, as well as to teach science concepts. In this vein, Lawson and Wollman (1975) developed a science curriculum to help pupils who are able to deal with science concepts only at concrete operational levels to accelerate their development to a formal operational status. This requires that students first physically manipulate materials and observe the results of their activities. They then are to learn useful symbols, words and phrases, and ways of applying these to the more concrete aspects of their studies. Finally they are expected to apply the concepts they learn within increasingly abstract contexts (Kuhn, 1978).

Such formal operational curricula raise questions. How different are they from any other curricula that seek to teach science effectively? Nothing truly new seems to be involved, except the *goal* of achieving formal operations. Can such Piagetian programs achieve the goal, i.e., move students from concrete to formal operations? It is not at all clear that they succeed in doing so.

Piaget's curricular efforts have also been devoted to programming that may provide assistance to improve specific cognitive mechanisms rather than to accelerate general progress through the cognitive stages (Kuhn, 1978). The Kamii and DeVries (1978) program proceeds on the basis of Piaget's belief that knowledge results from the child's own constructive activities, self-reflection, etc. Their program encourages children to become active, curious, and independent, to pursue their own interests, to have confidence in their ability to figure things out, to speak their minds openly (Kuhn, 1978). Again it is difficult to see what is new or original or specifically Piagetian in such an approach or in Furth and Wachs' (1977) program to help children achieve habits of creative independent thinking through special thinking games.

Educational Emphasis on Piagetian Processes

Piaget has elucidated numerous cognitive processes or combinations, the targets of educational programs and intervention efforts. Thus numerous attempts have been made to accelerate or train conservation processes (though Piaget advised against the practice), seriation, transformation, decentering, etc. Some specific types of intervention, though, focusing on specific processes have attempted to encourage overall cognitive development. One particularly interesting approach that would appear to have implications for remedial and special education is based on the idea of an optimal mismatch.

Remember that cognitive development results from a continuing effort to achieve equilibrium and that disequilibrium, by setting processes of assimilation and accommodation into action (to restore equilibrium), forces cognitive development. Why not create a special type of cognitive conflict that will set off equilibration efforts? Why not diagnose a child's level of cognitive development in a particular area of functioning and then provide activities that optimally challenge the child's schemata? Such is the idea behind optimal mismatch—to create a state of cognitive disequilibrium of just the right proportions so as to urge cognitive development along.

Furth and Wachs (1977) thus state that the teacher should provide activities that "are developmentally appropriate to challenge the child's thinking, but not too difficult as to invite failure" (p. 45). These activities should create just enough disequilibrium to stimulate cognitive growth.

APPLICATIONS OF PIAGETIAN PRINCIPLES TO REMEDIAL AND SPECIAL EDUCATION

As observed earlier, Piaget was not particularly interested in direct types of intervention and remediation. Inhelder (1982), one of his students, however, encouraged intervention with the cognitively handicapped. And a number of special educators have since attempted to accelerate the progress of handicapped learners through one or the other of the developmental stages or to teach them to engage more effectively in such cognitive processes as decentration and conservation. Despite waxing and waning of efforts from one time to another, a considerable amount of effort has thus been devoted to applying Piagetian principles to remedial, handicapped, and other populations (Bricker, Macke, Levin, & Campbell, 1981; Gallagher, 1979).

We initially review the application of Piagetian principles by Ingred Shiiebeeks to the instruction of children with learning problems, ages 8 to 14. Our review is based on an article by Nelson Moses (1981). The statements made represent quotes or paraphrases of statements from this article.

- Principle 1. Learning depends on children's efforts to control and understand problematic transformations.
- Principle 2. Having goals to work toward while experiencing transformations helps children regulate transformations.
- Principle 3. Experiencing transformations helps children control and understand transformations.
- Principle 4. Creating problem-solving strategies facilitates the growth of knowledge.
- Principle 5. Effective learning occurs when children anticipate the results of their actions, observe the results, and compare predictions with outcomes to verify success or failure.
- Principle 6. The ability to control and understand transformations develops as the result of reflexive abstraction.
- Principle 7. Telling children that their actions are good or bad, right or wrong reinforces dependence on a controlling environment. Responding to children by fashioning further interactions that stimulate curiosity, creativity, and reasoning strengthens internal regulation.

These principles are some of the ways that Piagetian ideas are being applied to the education of the children with learning problems. Their very generality may provide useful ideas to all educators. At the same time they do not appear to have specific implications for either remedial or special education.

Piaget and Exceptional Children

As with the learning disabled there have been efforts to assess, instruct, and otherwise help handicapped children using Piagetian principles or methods derived from his experiments. In the area of assessment, studies of sensorimotor development in young retarded children are based on the sequence of cognitive development steps that are expected on the basis of Piagetian theory. Some studies of the mentally retarded institutionalized adults indicate that most remain at sensorimotor levels of development. Others find décalage across and through stages. Thus while Dunst found that the predicted relationship of language to stage development in the profoundly retarded was not on schedule, lags in profoundly retarded pupils' psychosocial development have been compared to their cognitive development (Baumeister & Brooks, 1981). Such findings are contrary to the Piagetian concept of general developmental advances.

In respect to intervention, numerous attempts have been made to teach specific Piagetian tasks to the mentally retarded. Lavatelli, whose curriculum work we discussed, created a special training kit to teach special education pupils conservation, seriation, etc. Cowan has been more ingenious. He has suggested different techniques to correct overassimilation in the mentally retarded and to encourage overassimilation in the direction of more cognitive accommodation. This is through certain types of play therapy and games and activity that emphasize accommodation.

Robinson and Robinson (1976) have suggested that almost all of the sensorimotor behavior described by Piaget is definable in behavioral terms and modifiable through behavioral methods. Along these lines, William A. Bricker, whom we can perhaps call a behaviorist/Piagetian although a contradiction in terms, supports this kind of approach, taking what can be described as a task analytic instructional view on Piagetian training.

Bricker, Macke, Levin, and Campbell (1981) observe that "emerging evidence indicates that even the most severely handicapped student can acquire the correct underlying concept (in sensorimotor and concrete operational domains), and apply that rule in such a way that responses are accurate in a variety of situations" (p. 161).

Bricker believes that it is possible to teach mentally retarded learners specific items of sensorimotor and concrete operational behavior that will help them develop generalized cognitive schemata from their experiences. He points out, however, that mentally retarded children, unlike the normal ones that Piaget studied, cannot be expected to develop cognitively through their own efforts. Thus, it is incumbent on the trained instructor to use Piaget's theory of intelligence as   the basis for determining the necessary and sufficient concepts that must be taught to exceptional children, and then to go ahead and train them.

CONCLUSIONS

Despite recent advances in Piagetian theory and new applications to education, Piaget will never have more than a limited impact on remedial and special education. Piaget's ideas can provide general guides to the assessment and management of learning problems and handicapping conditions, but they are not directly applicable to academic remediation or the education of the handicapped.

These statements are not intended to denigrate Piaget's great achievements. It is true he gave advice to teachers but that is almost obligatory for any important psychologist. He was interested above all in the general cognitive development of cognitively sound children rather than in specific types of academic achievement. He was certainly not interested in remediation. There is no reason, then, why special and remedial educators should expect his theories to have precise applications to remedial and special education. And indeed it is difficult to demonstrate that they have many direct implications for general education. His theories, however, provide a storehouse of good ideas for all areas of education.

Piaget has much to offer to remedial and special educators—in a broad sense. His theories provide us with specific methods of conceptualizing the ways that children's cognitive abilities develop and help us understand behavior from a cognitive standpoint. His theories also assist us to understand better the children's cognitive functioning at different times of their lives and thus to offer instruction appropriate from a developmental point of view.

Beyond these contributions Piaget's views can help everyone whose lives come in contact with children to understand these children and to create positive climates for their cognitive growth. Remedial and special educators are, however, likely to find the cognitive approaches in later chapters more useful for day-to-day applications.

Chapter 7

Information Processing

Information processing is the most dynamic and exciting area of cognitive study. It is more appropriate to speak and write about it as a paradigm than as a theory. That is, it is a particular scientific approach to the study of cognition. A great number of information-processing theories (and models) have been developed on the basis of this paradigm. They all subscribe to the notion that humans are information processors who actively obtain, transform, store, and apply information and that the study of human cognition is "the investigation of the ways in which humans collect, modify, interpret, and understand, and use environmental or internal information" (Merluzzi, Rudy, and Glass, 1981). This statement identifies the modern information-processing paradigm (IPP).

A HISTORICAL PERSPECTIVE ON THE INFORMATION-PROCESSING PARADIGM

While the idea of information processing has a long history (Mann, 1979), the modern influences that shaped the information-processing paradigm (IPP) emerged during World War II. Our historical perspective dates from that time.

Advances in the Study of Servomechanisms

Servomechanisms are the means by which systems self-regulate. The fact that our bodies maintain stable temperatures is due to biological (homeostatic) feedback mechanisms. Living creatures self-regulate on the basis of feedback from their bodies and their experiences. Mechanical systems regulate themselves by making adjustments based on feedback from their operations.

Knowledge of mechanical servomechanisms greatly advanced during World War II. The Germans, for example, used servomechanical principles to guide the flight of the V1 and V2 rockets that they directed against London in the final months of World War II (Howe, 1980). After the war there were rapid strides in the understanding and application of servomechanical principles. Modern space travel shows how sophisticated it has become. It was inevitable that educational psychologists and educators would begin to think in servomechanical terms. Thus, Miller, Galanter, and Pribam came to suggest in 1960 that human learning is also "servoregulated." That is, pupils constantly readjust their learning activities on the basis of the feedback they receive from those activities.

Human Engineering

Human engineering is another major development that contributed to the information-processing paradigm. It too was more or less born during World War II. It is a field of psychology that seeks to help the human operators of equipment to become efficient, i.e., faster and more accurate, in their work, and it involves an understanding and application of servomechanisms. As military technology became more complex during the war, the field of human engineering became important.

The psychologists who specialized in human engineering found it helpful to conceptualize the human operators of military technology as information transmitters and as components of man-machine systems (Merluzzi et al., 1981). They were particularly interested in human decision making and in human operators' role as information processors interposed between a "machine's signal's and its . . . controls" (Lachman, Lachman, & Butterfield, 1979, p. 58). The operators' cognitive processes were studied under conditions that require critical decisions. A submarine commander must make many such decisions when piloting a submarine through dangerous shoals. So does a bomber tailgate gunner deciding when to fire on an enemy airplane or a radar operator determining whether enemy aircraft are approaching. The military psychologists who studied such operators were able to assess precisely a number of distinct sequential cognitive "stages" such as awareness, attention, perception, and judgment in the operators' decision-making processes. They used the information from their assessments to improve the operators' performances. The success of their studies greatly enhanced the credibility of scientific efforts to study cognitive processes.

Communication Science

Communications engineering and information theory also became important during World War II. C.S. Shannon is perhaps the most honored of early pioneers in this area. He was interested in improving phone and electronic information. But he was also interested in general principles of communication and developed a general mathematical theory that could be applied to information transmission in a variety of areas, including human behavior.

Shannon's model of communication conceptualized a number of important information concepts that have thus been important for both engineers and human learning specialists. Simply speaking, the sort of communication model he worked with suggests the following: There is first an information source that prepares a message. A transmitter then sends this message in the form of signals across a channel to a receiver. The receiver "reconstructs" (codes) these signals to create useful information, i.e., communication. Communication between the sending information source and the receiver is constantly in danger of breaking down, because a channel may be inadequate or overloaded, or because distortions and errors (noise) interfere with the production, transmission, and interpretation of information.

The modern information-processing paradigm indeed owes many of its concepts and principles to communication scientists (Lachman, Lachman, & Butterfield, 1979). Among the most important communication science concepts for the IPP are those just mentioned: coding and channel capacity.

Coding

The concept of coding is perhaps the most important concept of all in the information-processing paradigm because coding affects the transmission, utilization, and storage of information at all information-processing levels. Coding has been defined as "a set of specific rules or transformation where messages, codes, signals, or the state of the world are converted from one representation to another, one medium of energy to another or one physical state to another" (Lachman, Lachman, and Butterfield, 1979, p. 68).

In other words information is constantly being transformed from one state to another, and this transformation creates codes. Examples of coding (information transformation) are all about us. Telephones and televisions, computers, records, and audiovisual tapes all encode and decode information. So do our cognitive systems. When reading, writing, or speaking, a child engages in a multitude of encoding and decoding operations. Learning problems are often decoding problems.

Channel Capacity

Channel capacity in information-processing terms is defined in terms of the number of signals that a particular channel can carry within a fixed time. All information channels including those of electronic or human nature are finite and limited in their capacity to manage information. A telephone cable can carry just so many messages at any time. A radio channel can transmit information just so fast and no faster. A computer cannot process data past a certain speed per second. It is possible to conceptualize human capabilities in channel capacity terms. We have upper limits (channel limitations) to what we can perceive, learn and remember and to our problem-solving capacities. We can attend only to a certain amount of information at any time. We can learn just so much information in any given effort. Overcoming or compensating for channel capacity limitations is a challenge for remedial and special educators.

Psycholinguistics

We briefly touched on the psycholinguists' contributions to cognition in Chapter 2. Psycholinguists posed a successful challenge to behaviorist interpretation of language (Chomsky, 1957, 1968; Lenneberg, 1967, 1974). Among other things, they were able to show that behavioral principles are unable to explain language development and language production. They made a convincing case for cognitive explanations of language (Merluzzi et al., 1981). Although psycholinguistic and IPP theories are not identical, many of their concepts are compatible. For example, psycholinguistic and information-processing theories both reject mechanical S-R interpretations of learning. Both emphasize the importance of rules in the head to explain cognition. Both stress the active, transformational nature of cognition.

The Computer

It is possible that modern IPP could have developed had there been no computers. It is not possible to believe that it would have developed to the current degree or in the same way without the computer and the field of study that we call *computer science*. While the phone, radio, and television provide examples of information processing, they do not provide us with any real insight into the human mind. On the other hand, the workings of a computer suggest some fascinating ideas about how the human mind may work.

The computer and the nervous system in no way resemble each other physically. Nevertheless the two have certain functional similarities. They both function as information processors. They both are symbol (code) manipulators. They both transmit, transform, integrate, store, and apply information.

It thus seems possible to conceptualize the human mind in computer terms. It is also possible to program computers so that their operations simulate human cognition; we can even "teach" them to solve problems in ways similar to those that our pupils use. Some information-processing theorists believe it is just a matter of time until computers will literally be able to "think" independently, to become, as it were, "intelligent" machines. There is talk of artificial intelligence (Newell & Simon, 1972).

The computer has strongly influenced the ways that cognitive psychologists formulate information-processing theories. For example, it has encouraged them to describe cognition in terms of inputs and outputs, system architecture, executive processes, programs and production systems.

Verbal Learning

Verbal learning is a research area that has made important contribution to the IPP. Associationistic (S-R and behaviorist) conceptions once dominated verbal learning research. This was a time when verbal learning researchers typically studied learning and memory as applied to simple language units such as letters (and numbers) (Lachman, Lachman, & Butterfield, 1979). Verbal learning researchers were not particularly concerned with the broader issues of learning such as the retention and recall of phonemes, morphemes, sentences, paragraphs; the learning of facts; or the development of concepts. Nor were they much concerned with the ways in which previously learned information and knowledge of rules affected what people were learning. Thus, while verbal learning researchers carried out a great deal of interesting research, it applied more to the laboratory than to real life; it failed to deal with practical learning problems, such as those of reading.

Then in 1956 George Miller published an influential paper titled *The Magic Number Seven Plus or Minus Two*. In this paper Miller observed that humans have a limited capacity to retain items of information in their minds. They can, however, improve their performance if they use a grouping procedure he calls *chunking*. Thus, while it is difficult to recall the number sequence of 569532167 when these digits are committed to memory one at a time, the task is a relatively easy one if the numbers are grouped 569 532 167. Through grouping, the original nine units are reduced to three chunks. Similarly the number sequence 1792177619181941 is impossible of itself for most of us to recall. But if we think of these numbers in terms of meaningful dates (1792, 1776, 1918, 1941), we may readily repeat the entire sequence.

Research like this appeared to demonstrate that learning, memory, and recall cannot be explained in simple S-R terms and that they require active cognitive processing. It made the point that certain cognitive activities can make information more manageable and to some degree can even overcome basic cognitive limitations.

Following in Miller's footsteps, other verbal learning researchers became interested in human capacity (channel) limitations and in ways that could overcome them. Increasingly they turned to the study of the ways that people code, organize, and reorganize information to make it easier to learn, recall, and use. Instead of viewing learning as a product of accumulated S-R associations, many of them began to treat the human learner as an active participant in the learning process (something that Piaget had long emphasized). Verbal learning researchers are in the forefront of IPP research and theory. The IPP's persistent interest in memory is in large part a legacy of verbal learning researchers' interest in this topic.

Later Steps Leading to the IPP

Research into information-processing systems (IPS) proceeded at rapid pace during the late 1950s and 1960s. It is often said that information-processing psychology began with an article by Broadbent on selective attention. Broadbent's book *Perception and Communication* (1958) was a milestone publication. After Ulric Neisser's book *Cognitive Psychology* in 1967 proposed that cognition be conceptualized in information-processing terms, the "cognitive revolution" conquered in psychology.

DEFINITIONS OF INFORMATION PROCESSING

This brief history of the information-processing paradigm should orient readers to the ways in which the IPP developed. We are ready to examine the way the IPP has been interpreted and defined by various experts in the field.

The classic definition of information processing is one provided by Neisser in his book *Cognitive Psychology* (1967). It is indeed the definition that can be considered to have inaugurated the new age of information processing within psychology and education: Cognition is "the process which sensory input is transferred, reduced, elaborated, stored, recovered, and used" (p. 5).

Other definitions have elaborated on this simple one. Thus, Merluzzi and his colleagues (1981) observe that "From the IPP perspective . . . human cognition . . . [relates to] the ways in which humans collect, store, modify, interpret, understand and use environmental or internal information" (p. 79).

Kausler's and Houston's definitions of information processing are somewhat similar. Kausler (1974) suggests that the "scope of [information processing is] . . . the entire flow of information within the human performer, from its registration by sense organs to its entry (or storage) in, and perhaps, recovery (or retrieval from a permanent . . .) memory" (pp. 20–21). Houston (1976) sees cognition as the "flow of information through the human, beginning with the registration of incoming information by the sense organs, through the encoding and storage of this information" (p. 259).

Erickson and Simon's (1981) definition emphasizes the coding aspects of information processing: "According to the human-processing model . . . [there is] a sequence of internal states successively transformed by a series of information processes" (p. 18). Mayer's (1981) definition calls attention to the active nature of human information processing:

> Humans are processors of information; information comes through our sense organs, we apply a mental operation on it and thus change it, and so on until we have an output ready to store in memory or use to generate some behavior.
>
> [In information processing there are] . . . series of cognitive operators (or processes) that a person uses in a given situation, or to put it another way, the various organization of information as it passes through the [information processing] system. (p. 11)

Turvey (1974) defined information processing in a way that highlights its stage and capacity aspects:

Information processing is a hierarchically organized temporal sequence of events involving stages of storages and transformation occurs at points in the information flow where storage capacity constraints demand recoding of information . . . information processing research seeks methods which will decompose the information flow into discrete and temporally ordered stages. (p. 139)

Such IPP definitions are much more consistent than the definitions of general intelligence reviewed in Chapter 4. There are good reasons for this. Since most IPP theorists and researchers have been trained in recent years and under similar conditions, they usually have a similar heritage of concepts and training in information theory, computer science, and verbal learning. They are thus more likely to be similar in their thinking than are intelligence theorists whose span of work extends over more than a century and whose backgrounds have been much more diverse. It is important also to observe that as the IPP research expands, more and greater differences and disagreements are appearing among its constituents.

We cannot go into great detail about all possible extensions or interpretations of the IPP within this chapter. We instead present some of the more traditional IPP models and concepts. The reader will find that we have accentuated memory in our review. This is a natural consequence of computer and verbal learning influences on the IPP. Both verbal learning and computer scientists are always talking about memory.

STUDY OF HUMAN INFORMATION PROCESSING

A number of different procedures can be used to study human information processing. We will study some of the more basic methods in this section because they will help us to understand the ways that information-processing theories are developed.

Self-Reporting Procedures

One basic IPP research study is through the use of self-reporting procedures and protocol analysis. Pupils may thus be asked to report to the researcher how and what they are thinking when learning a verbal passage, solving a mathematical problem, or remembering a story. They tell the researcher about the ways they attempt to learn their materials, the particular steps they use to reach particular learning goals, the reasons for their decisions and behaviors. They give their reports orally or in written form either during or after their actual work sessions. These reports (protocols) are then analyzed to understand the pupils' cognitive functioning.

Computer Simulation

In computer simulation, researchers program the computer to "think" in various ways using programs that simulate the ways people make decisions, solve problems, or recall information. People's self-reports are often used to guide the development of such programs. And just as the self-reports about human cognitive activities can be used to develop computer programs, so have computer programs provided insights into human cognition and provided suggestions as how to "program" pupils better academically.

Laboratory Research

Still another basic IPP research approach is that of laboratory research, in which subjects are studied under controlled conditions. We review one of these laboratory approaches in some detail here because it is particularly helpful to understanding the IPP. It is the decomposition method.

Decomposition of Mental Processing

One of the major assumptions that guided the development of the paradigm is that cognitive processes are noninstantaneous. That is, they take time. It is also assumed that information-processing sequences can be broken down, i.e., decomposed, into separate and distinct component processes. IPP researchers often use decomposition methods to study the time required by the different types of cognitive processing. These methods owe much to the original subtraction method developed by Donders during the nineteenth century (1868).

Donders proposed that mental processes be measured according to the time they require to operate. He originally used three reaction time tasks for this purpose. In the first (detection) task, the subject responded as quickly as possible to any stimulus shown (by pressing a button or lever). In the second (discrimination) task the subject was shown a number of different stimuli and was asked to respond to only one of them. In the third (choice) task the subject not only had to discriminate among different stimuli but also had to choose from and respond differently to each of the stimuli. Whereas Donders subtracted the time required to achieve Task 1 from the time required to achieve Task 2 in order to estimate the time required for the cognitive processes involved in discrimination, he subtracted the time required for Task 2 from that required for Task 3 so as to estimate the additional time involved in making a choice.

Using improved and elaborated versions of Donders' methods, modern information-processing researchers have successfully studied the time requirements of specific cognitive processes by either adding to or reducing, complicating or simplifying the cognitive demands made on subjects. We study several situations later in this chapter to show how decomposition methods have been used to study learning problems.

Some Comments on IPP Research Methods

All research methods focus on some aspects of a topic and ignore or neglect others. They also proceed on assumptions that may or may not be true.

In the case of IPP research, self-reports, computer simulation, and reaction time studies of cognition make us look at cognition in arbitrary and circumscribed ways. Self-reporting is an incomplete way of explaining how and what we are thinking about when we are doing something. It cannot exactly describe our thought processes. Similarly while a computer program may simulate human thinking, this doesn't mean that our minds truly work like computers. Nor can our mental processes be fully explained in terms of reaction times. Nevertheless such types of IPP research have provided new insights into cognition.

IPP MODELS

Information processing is usually described as processing within a system, an informa-tion-processing system (IPS). Information-processing research is usually guided by graphic

Figure 7–1 Diagram of Principal Components of Perception and Memory System

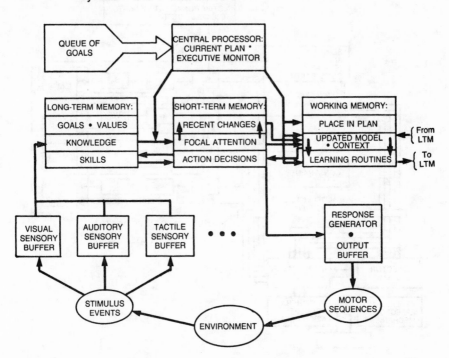

Source: Reprinted from *Handbook of Learning and Cognitive Processes, Vol. 1, Introduction to Concepts and Issues* (p. 37) by Gordon H. Bower, edited by W.K. Estes. Copyright 1975 by Lawrence Erlbaum Associates. Reprinted by permission.

models (see Figure 7–1) that indicate the movement of information through IPSs. These models are abstractions. Our mind doesn't actually consist of series of interconnected boxes or networks, and its processes are far more complex than IPP models suggest. IPS models, however, do help us to conceptualize information processing more readily. They also provide guides to researchers who "try" the models out to determine how effectively they explain various aspects of cognition. IPP investigators test the adequacy and accuracy of their models if they turn out to be inaccurate or inefficient.

Some information-processing models are very broad. Indeed they presume to provide general guidelines to all types of cognition (see Figure 7–1). Others are more specific. Some, for example, deal with reading (see Figure 7–2); others, with the acquisition of particular motor skills (see Figure 7–3).

Traditional information-processing system (IPS) models are presented in a diagram flow-chart form. This is true of those shown in Figures 7–1, 7–2, and 7–3. The blocks in these diagrams (they can be any type of geometric figure) represent the components of the cognitive system being studied or its stages. The various interconnections (interrelationships) among the IPS's components are typically shown by lines or arrows; the latter

Figure 7–2 Reading Model

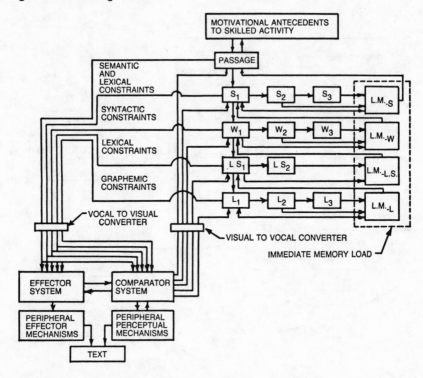

Source: Reprinted from *Development in Human Learning* edited by E.A. Lunzer and G.S. Morris, © 1968.

Figure 7–3 Feedback Model

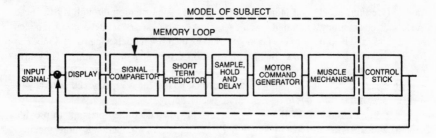

Representation of three classes of constructs: covert oral responses (r_o), covert nonoral responses ($r_{\bar{o}}$), and covert neurophysiological processes (p_n). Complex interactions are represented here with arrows, though the representation of them as neuromuscular circuit components is more realistic.

Source: Reprinted from *The Experimental Psychology Series* (p. 7) by Richard W. Pew (edited by B.H. Kantowitz). Copyright 1974 by Lawrence Erlbaum Associates. Reprinted by permission.

Figure 7–4 Conceptual IPP Model

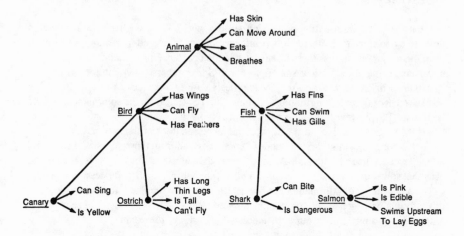

Source: Reprinted from "Retrieval Time from Semantic Memory" by A.M. Collins and M.R. Quillian from *Journal of Verbal Learning and Verbal Behavior,* with permission of Academic Press Inc., © 1969.

indicate the direction in which information processing proceeds and the interaction among the IPS's components. However, not all IPP models of research are of a flow nature. Some that deal with information structures may use "patterns," models that represent the relationships among units of cognitive content, e.g., concepts or the parts of a sentence (see Figure 7–4).

The most familiar type of IPP model, however, is the flow model. And it is the one to which we devote most of our discussion. (See Figure 7–5.)

Figure 7–5 Flow Model

Information Processing Model

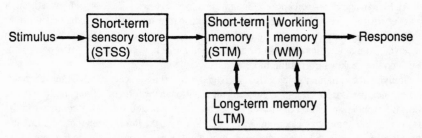

Source: Reprinted from *The Promise of Cognitive Psychology* by R.E. Mayer, p. 25, with permission of W.H. Freeman and Co., © 1981.

GENERAL ASSUMPTIONS ABOUT INFORMATION-PROCESSING SYSTEMS

What makes an information-processing system work? What controls the information flow from one stage to another? How is information coded, stored in memory, or recalled from memory? We discuss these issues later in the chapter. Our immediate concern is to understand some of the basic assumptions that IPS researchers employ in their work.

A human information-processing system deals with two sources of information. One source is that of the external stimulus input into the IPS, i.e., from the environment and the body. An IPS, however, cannot directly process external stimuli. The latter cannot get inside the system. The IPS must deal with the representations of those stimuli.

That is, the IPS works with the "codes" created by and from those stimuli. These codes at one level are neural impulses. At other levels they are sensations, images, memories, etc., that somehow represent external stimuli within our information-processing systems.

The other source of information in a human IPS is its own internal information. Some of this information is genetically programmed into our nervous systems by our genes. Some has been programmed in by our experiences—by teaching, for example.

Structural Limitations to Information-Processing Systems

An information-processing system can manage only so much information at any given time and at any given stage. All IPS components are structurally limited in their information-processing capacities. This is clearly evident from our everyday experiences as well as from the results of IPP experiments. We can attend only to a certain amount of information at any given time. We can store only a finite amount of information in our memory within a certain time. No one can remember everything taught.

Various animal species differ from each other in respect to their cognitive structural capacities. There are also intraspecies variations. Thus while all humans have the same kinds of cognitive structures, some have larger or more efficient ones. Differences in structural capacities may explain what we regard as native differences in intelligence, as well as differences in specific abilities.

Coding at All Levels of Information Processing

The concept of coding, as observed, is at the heart of the IPP. Information processing is a matter of transforming information into codes (Hunt 1975a).

All human activity—perception, thought, memory, behavior, etc.—is achieved through a variety of coding (and recoding) operations. Information always passes from one information processing component or stage to another in the form of codes. At one stage the code received from a previous one may be transformed into a new code that is being passed on. Such coding makes information more usable.

Studying the computer helps us to understand this coding process much better. Computers physically record and manipulate all its information in the form of a binary number code, i.e., different combination of 0s and 1s that are electrically coded by the computer in the form of on-off patterns of electronic switches. However, the information that the computer operator inputs into the computer must go through a number of other coding processes before it is finally coded at this basic level. The ordinary English words or calculations typed into the computer are transformed into a special computer language (code) within the computer. The computer takes this language (code) and transforms it further until it is finally coded in the machine language code the computer actually can work with. Penultimately the computer thinks and remembers and performs in terms of patterns of 0s and 1s. Ultimately it performs with high and low (on-off) electronic states. This is true whether the computer processes simple words or complex documents, single numbers or advanced trigonometry formulas, the recording of beeps or the final bars of a Beethoven symphony.

The computer always and only works with codes. So do human information systems. From the moment our sense organs are stimulated to the moment we carry out some type of behavior, our neurocognitive systems are coding and recoding information, i.e., condensing it, abstracting it, elaborating it, transforming it. We are usually consciously aware of ourselves as thinking and remembering in terms of images, i.e., words and pictures, numbers. The latter, too, are codes—analog ones that resemble but are not the same as the physical stimuli they represent. Most of our thinking, however, proceeds in the form of cognitive codes that are not readily identifiable or understandable by our conscious minds. Ultimately they are physical and electrochemical in nature.

The computer stores an English paragraph or mathematical calculations in its memory in the form of machine codes (electrical on-off states) and then later transforms (recodes) these into   printed English or numeric displays on its screen. We too store information in our memories in the form of unrecognizable (by us) codes but later recode this information in our minds in the form of meaningful images, ideas, thoughts, feelings, or purposeful motor behaviors.

How many different human information codes are there altogether? We don't yet know. Initially there are clearly different ones for the sensory information that develops in our different sense organs, e.g., separate visual information (iconic) codes, auditory (echoic) codes, tactile ones, etc. It is also thought that information is coded differently at various information-processing stages. Thus it seems that verbal information is coded acoustically at a superficial processing level but semantically at a later, "deeper" level.

In a computer, information may be processed at different stages of its operation simultaneously or serially. What happens with the human information-processing system? Initially, at the point of information registration on our sense organs, both kinds of processing appear to go on. Visual perception certainly appears initially to require simultaneous processing. Auditory perception on the other hand appears to rely on serial processing.

Whether both types of processing go on at the same time in the same modality is unclear. What happens at later stages? Some researchers believe that information processing is mainly serial (Newell & Simon, 1972). Others believe that parallel and serial processing both go on throughout the IPS (Paivio, 1975). Still others believe that simultaneous processing may be typical (Hinton & Anderson, 1981). It has been suggested in some quarters that the two brain hemispheres are specialized so that the right hemisphere typically processes and codes information simultaneously while the left hemisphere does so serially. A recently developed intelligence test proceeds on this premise (Kaufman & Kaufman, 1983).

MAKE-UP OF AN INFORMATION-PROCESSING SYSTEM

Computer ideas and terminology have strongly influenced the way that IPP theorists conceptualize the composition and functioning of particular information-processing systems. This is already apparent. It becomes even more evident as we proceed to describe a typical information-processing system (Merluzzi et al., 1981).

Internal Architecture: Hardware

A computer consists of a variety of hardware components, e.g., switches, logic, and memory chips, wiring, fuses. Some computer components respond to information input; others direct the flow through other components, make decisions, execute actions, and check on performance. Some computer components store information temporarily, others store information permanently. The computer's hardware, its internal architecture, is fixed, i.e., unchangeable.

It is easy to compare our cognitive systems to those of the computer. Our brains and other parts of the nervous system can be considered to be the biological hardware or internal architecture of a human IPS. At another level so can our intelligence and special abilities (Merluzzi et al., 1981).

In IPP terms, the hardware of a cognitive information-processing system consists of a number of different components. For example, there are sensory and motor buffers (stores). Sensory buffers receive, temporarily hold, organize, and code the information created by sensory stimulation to prepare it for further transmission; they then send the newly coded information along to other parts of the IPS. The motor buffers store and organize motor commands before their execution. Between the input and output stages represented by sensory and motor buffers are a variety of other structural components. Some, like the central processing unit (CPU), manage, manipulate, and otherwise control information-processing activities. Others like short-term memory and long-term memory store information for varying lengths of time.

External Architecture: System Architecture

The system architecture or external hardware of a computer refers to the format within which its hardware components are laid out, organized, and attached or "wired" to each other; in a human IPS it is assumed that our cognitive capacities are arranged in certain preset ways that determine how information moves in the system. Thus, a human IPS architecture is also of a fixed nature; its arrangements are predetermined by heredity or modified by maturation and experiences.

The IPS can, however, employ its arrangements with a considerable degree of flexibility. An analogy used to explain this point is that of a highway system. This too consists of a prearranged (fixed) network of roads, access lanes, exits, roadside rests, etc. Nevertheless, though the system is fixed, a person may drive through it in a variety of ways. The driver may select one road over another in the system, exit at one point rather than another, go down the highway quickly or slowly, pull over to rest for a while, turn around (Merluzzi et al., 1981).

Control Processes and Programs

A computer's control processes and programs determine how it operates. They "decide" what the computer will do, the information it will record or recall, the problems it will solve, the manner of their solution, and the execution of specific behaviors (such as those of a robot welding machine). To a great degree the computer's hardware and system architecture determine the nature of its control processes. There are, for example, one or more electronic central processing units in a computer. They directly control much of the computer's processing efforts. The computer can also use specially written programs (software) as control processes for its operations. Control processes at all levels, whether created by the computer's hardware or inserted in the form of special programs (software), allow the computer to choose the operation it will carry out. Some can even overcome or make up for some of the computer's physical limitations or deficiencies.

In a similar fashion IPS theorists emphasize that human information-processing systems employ control processes that determine the selection of information to be processed and its recall and use. Still others determine how that information is coded, organized, and enriched. As with the computer, some of an IPS's control processes are built in or pre-programmed into its hardware (its physical nature), i.e., inherent in our nervous systems. Other are programmed into the IPS by our experiences (our equivalents of computer software). As with the computer, special programming may help us to overcome our cognitive system's limitations or deficiencies.

A distinction can be made between voluntary control processes and those of an involuntary nature (Atkinson & Shiffrin, 1968). The former are ones that an organism can volitionally and consciously control. The latter are involuntary or automatic. Involuntary control processes include features as access rate to stored memory information and the speed with which we forget. The distinction between voluntary and involuntary control does not appear to be an either/or phenomenon. Thus we can partly control our attention processes even though much of what we call *attention* operates automatically—indeed without our being aware of its operations.

Executive Processes

Control processes, as we have observed, determine the way an IPS operates. Some of them control other processes or have broad regulatory aspects. Because of this they are often given names of an "executive nature." Some are actually called *executive processes.*

Bower (1975) provides a vivid description of executive processes:

> In a hierarchial program one in which more and more programs or routines direct other sub-routines, the top level routine is called the executive. . . . The executive calls, selects or determines the use of routines [programs] at the next lower level and keeps track of where these sub-routines are to return their results. The executive monitors the number of [achievement of subgoals toward a long term objective] . . . generated in using a particular method [say in a problem solving situation]. It also evaluates (from feedback) how the current plan or program is progressing. The executive may interrupt and switch to another sub-goal if that other one suddenly seems important or if the current method of attacks on a subgoal seems not to be progressing in satisfactory fashion [i.e., in respect to achieving the language goal] . . . [or when] . . . the executive also notices . . . a subgoal has been completed [and its] . . . results may be used in selecting the next steps or next goal to be worked out. The executive is itself just another bit of program and it is quite deterministic in its action. (p. 33)

In the past, talk of such conceptualizations would have been grounds to criticize IPP theorists for talking about supernatural forces and therefore of not being scientific (since a science deals only with physical phenomena). But it is clear now that control processes are no more supernatural than is a house thermostat. A thermostat controls the temperature that the house owner wants in the house. In order to do this it must "remember" a particular temperature setting, to interpret changes of temperature, to make decisions whether the house is too warm or cold, and to execute commands (to the furnace). And it supervises temperature control. So control processes and executive control processes are not mysterious after all.

Cognitive Strategies

The IPS control processes are of great interest to remedial and special educators since they may be particularly susceptible to training and remediation. In particular this appears to be true of a particular type of cognitive processes that are responsible for the fact that "many tasks can be carried out in several different ways [by the IPS]" (Young, 1978, p. 357).

Some cognitive strategies are automatic, switched on or off in a preprogrammed fashion. These are sometimes identified as *production systems* (a computer term) to make it clear that they are not necessarily voluntary or consciously used (Young, 1978). Some cognitive strategies, however, appear to be very much under conscious voluntary control and to be trainable or remediable. Chapter 9 is devoted to the topic of cognitive strategies under voluntary control.

Attention: How the IPP Explains It

Before we proceed to discuss the IPP, it may be helpful to examine how it has been used in the study of one of the most popular and important of modern cognitive constructs, that of attention. Remedial and special educators are frequently concerned with attention, i.e., with problems of inattentiveness, distractibility, lack of concentration, and disinhibition.

What is *attention*? Is it simply a way of describing that someone is "on target," looking at things one is supposed to look at, doing what one has been told to do? Is it a special cognitive capacity or some type of ability? Actually, since attention is a hypothetical construct, it is anything that a researcher or theorist wishes it to be. In IPP research it has been studied as a cognitive process that significantly affects the operations of other cognitive processes (Torgeson, 1981, p. 52) Lack of attention and impaired attention have been indicated as major causes of faulty information processing. Along these lines Torgeson (1981) has stated that "attention deficits are really deficiencies in information processing behaviors . . . a failure to apply efficient strategies and control processes for processing information, or a lack of organized cognitive schemes and production systems that can direct appropriate information processing for a given task" (p. 58–59).

Typical IPS Models

There are many different types of IPS models. They range from ones that explain the phenomena in brief sensory experiences to those that explain creative problem-solving activities. We have chosen to devote most of our attention in the rest of this chapter to two general types of IPS models. One is a memory model; the other is a problem-solving one. In understanding these, the reader will be better able to understand IPS models in general.

AN IPS MEMORY MODEL

This model illustrates one way that information arriving at our senses may be processed, stored in our permanent memories, and then recovered for use. (See Figure 7–5.) Our discussion represents a distillation of several views.

As we review this model, we should keep in mind that even though we do not discuss them here, the IPS central processing units and other control mechanisms and processes manage the flow of information through an IPS memory system.

Short-Term Sensory Store (Buffer)

We are constantly being stimulated by information though our sense organs can register only a certain amount and type of it at any given moment. This information is registered in sensory registers or buffers that altogether make up our short-term sensory store (STSS).

The events that affect the selection of information for registration in the STSS are determined in great part by the nature of our physical receptors. These respond only to certain types of stimuli, and they record information from these stimuli in ways that are specific to their nature. We can thus talk of different sensory stores for each of our senses, each of which registers and codes information in ways specific to that sense.

Sensory information entering our short-term sensory stores first registers there in pre-conscious or "preattentive" fashion; we are not aware of the information. The information that first registers in the STSS is of an analog sort. That is, it corresponds in some way to the physical nature of the stimulus. This sort of information is sometimes described as being *iconic* for the visual buffer (*icon* being a Greek name for *image*), and *echoic* for the auditory buffer.

Once information is registered in the STSS, certain control processes set to work and select out certain types of information from it for special coding. Various feature detectors located in our visual pathways, for example, extract significant features from a visual stimulus input. Thus, some visual images or aspects of visual images are attended to more closely, while others are neglected or suppressed. Sensory preselection plays an important role in the STSS information processing. It decides in large part what information will be processed further.

The STSS continuously communicates with the other IPS components. It constantly sends information to and receives information from these components, and it monitors and is monitored by such information. The IPS often attends to or selects information items for further processing in the STSS because it is cued by information from its other memory components. We are more likely to respond to the information created by certain stimuli if we have been attending to the particular sensory channel in the STSS on which the stimuli are impinging. For example, we are more likely to be aware of changes in a fireworks display if we have been watching it than if we are casually conversing with our friends while it is going on. We are more likely to respond to stimuli that are important to us; for example, we may hear many names called out in an airport but we don't usually "hear" any until our own or that of a friend is called out. We are more likely to respond to a particular stimulus if a stimulus impinging on another sensory channel alerts us to it; for example, an elevator chime (an auditory event) is often used to alert passengers to watch out for the opening of the elevator's doors (a visual event).

The STSS appears to have an unlimited capacity in the sense that everything our senses are physically exposed to initially registers on them. Mayer (1981) describes the visual information registered at any given moment in the STSS "as being exact and complete . . . as a snapshot" (p. 24). The information in the STSS, however, undergoes rapid time decay. That is, STSS can hold information only for a very brief period, e.g., no more than half a second in the iconic buffer. Sensory information decays or drops out from the STSS almost instantly unless it is processed and passed on to the next information-processing stage.

Whether information is passed depends on a number of factors: the duration that the information remains in the STSS; the information's accentuation by control processes; the speed and accuracy with which the STSS creates internal codes for that information; and the nature of the sensory buffer dealing with the information; for example visual and auditory sensory buffers code information more effectively than do tactile or kinesthetic ones.

Individuals may differ significantly from one another in one or all of these factors. Children with learning problems and handicapped pupils are likely to be deficient in a number of them.

Short-Term Memory Stores

The internal codes for sensory information created in the STSS are passed on to and entered into the short-term memory (STM). The STM is the active part of our memory system. It is that part of our mind where we can exercise some voluntary controls over our cognition. Part of the STMS is usually considered synonymous with what we call the *conscious mind*. When we become aware of new stimuli impinging on the STSS, our awareness is in the STM. When we recall a memory, we remember it consciously by picturing it, hearing it, feeling it, etc., in the STMS. When we solve problems, we call up information and procedures from long-term memory into the STMS, where we can apply them to the problem.

The STM has fast access to items of information it receives. Information is manipulated in the STM with greater ease and rapidity than in other IPS components.

Information entering the STM is often described as entering into separate and distinct memory slots. The STM appears to preserve the temporal order of the incoming symbols (coded information) that it receives in its slots. This can be observed by asking someone to repeat digits backward; it is much more difficult to do than saying digits forward.

Information entering the STM remains there for a much longer duration than it does in the STSS. Nevertheless, it still does not remain there long. Old information items in the STM are constantly being bumped out of their slots by new information items, or they drop out on their own after a while.

Unlike the STSS, which has unlimited information acquiring capacities, the STM has a distinctly limited capacity. It doesn't ordinarily appear to be able to hold more than four to nine symbols or coded items at any given moment.

The control processes that operate at the STM level provide it with some flexibility in dealing with information. Some of these control processes focus attention on particular types of information in the STM. Some manipulate information so it will remain in the STM longer. Other control processes apply STM information to problems. Still others organize and encode information for storage in the long-term memory. Others assist in retrieval of information from the long-term purposes. Most operate automatically. Some are subject to conscious voluntary control. Let us look at several that may be of particular interest to remedial and special educators.

Chunking

The STM can manage a limited amount of information at any given moment. Its capacity is best described in terms of units or chunks of information. This capacity is relatively constant for any individual. The average capacity for humans ranges between four and nine units, seven being the average.

A *chunk* has been described as an integrated information unit. It can also be described as a stimulus pattern or sequence that we can somehow cognitively identify or recognize as a single unit. Thus when we see a friend, we don't respond to the person in terms of isolated features, i.e., eyes, nose, brow, but rather as a person we know—as a single unit. When we read a word, we usually read it and think of it as a word—a single unit—rather than as a collection of separate letters. When we read a sentence, it too can become a single unit or chunk of information under certain conditions.

Our STM can handle more bits of information when that information is organized into larger, more inclusive units (chunks) since it reduces our memory load. STM control processes can put a variety of strategies to work that help us chunk information more effectively. While we often use these strategies automatically and unconsciously, we can be taught to use them consciously. By so doing, we can improve our memory. It is possible to train pupils with poor memories to improve them through improved chunking procedures. It has even been demonstrated that when chunking is guided in an organized way, a person with a normal memory can remember and repeat back as many as 82 digits after hearing them just once.

Rehearsal

Information items remain in short-term memory only for a brief period. They are quickly bumped out by new information items or otherwise fade away. The longer that information remains in the STM, the greater the chance that it will be properly chunked, that it will be systematically stored within long-term memory, and that it will be more accessible for later retrieval (remembering) and meaningful use. Rehearsal is a means of retaining information in the STM for longer periods.

Rehearsal is essentially a matter of repeating or rehearsing information we have in the STM—of going over it in our minds, trying to remember what we have experienced or been taught. We may repeat information to ourselves, orally under our breath, or perhaps try to visualize and auditorize the appearance and sounds of things we have seen and heard after they have faded away (disappeared from the STSS). By rehearsing information we can maintain it in our STM for longer periods. Information that is not rehearsed is likely to drop out of the STM rapidly. Rehearsed information is more likely to be processed better and to be stored more effectively in long-term memory.

There are different ways of rehearsing information. Some appear to be more effective than others. Craik and Watkins (1973) distinguish between mechanical rehearsal and meaningful rehearsal. In mechanical rehearsal we organize the information as we rehearse it or associate it with other information in ways that make it more meaningful. Both types of rehearsal help us retain information longer in the STM. Meaningful rehearsal, however, improves the chances of that information being more efficiently stored in our memories and of being more easily remembered later.

Most of the research done on rehearsal has been with verbal materials. It is easier to rehearse verbal information than to rehearse nonverbal events such as visual scenes, sounds, and smells. It is possible, however, to rehearse the latter to some degree through the use of imagery (Paivio, 1975), e.g., picturing things or activities in our minds, "reauditorizing" statements that we have heard. Many remedial and special educators believe that rehearsal training can be beneficial to students with learning problems (Belmont & Butterfield, 1971).

Organization

Organization is still another critical control process partly under STM control. Good STM organization allows information to be chunked, rehearsed, coded, and stored more effectively in long-term memory for later recall.

One way of organizing information in STM is to think about it in systematic ways. Another way is to associate it with related information or experiences that anchor it within specific cognitive contexts.

Organization of information in the STM can be accomplished in a variety of ways. When teaching in a systematic fashion, a teacher helps pupils to organize STM information. Pupils can also organize information on their own, e.g., by studying in a systematic fashion.

Coding

One of the major operations within the STM is the recoding of the information within it for the purpose of storage in the LTM. Proper chunking, rehearsal, and organization improve coding. Most of our coding activities are not subject to control but rather determined by the nature of our cognitive structures. Some, however, are governed by control processes.

Working Memory

Some theorists believe that memory information-processing systems include another stage of memory between short-term and long-term memory components. This stage is sometimes called the *intermediate memory store* (IMS). It is more usually known as *working memory* (WM).

When the concept of working memory is employed, it is often considered an extension or appendage of short-term memory (Mayer, 1981) and assigned some of the functions otherwise attributed to short-term memory. It has been described as the IPS center of consciousness. It has also been described as the STM tool box, the place where it stores its control processes, programs, and plans (Bower, 1975) or as the STM scratch pad, an area in which the STM can try out conscious mental manipulations, e.g., using its control processes (Mayer, 1981). It has also been described as a frame of reference for the STM, consisting of "memory structures which maintain information about the local context of what is being learned, information which is neither in the focus of active (short-term) memory nor in the distant edges of short-term memory" (Bower, 1975, p. 53). According to this latter view, information in the WM updates information in the STM by constantly freshening it with new information items from the STSS. According to this perspective, WM is also the means through which perceptual information and long-term memories enrich abstract ideas with which the STM deals.

Some theorists disagree with the concept of an intermediate type of memory. They believe that it is an unnecessary conceptual addition to IPS models and that the STM constructs can account effectively for all the operations attributed to working memory.

Some theorists identify what we have discussed as short-term memory as working memory and identify the STSS as short-term memory (Moates & Schumacher, 1979).

Long-Term Memory

Long-term memory (LTM) store is assumed to be a permanent repository of all the information that we possess but are not immediately using. It stores perceptual and motor skills, spatial models of all sorts, verbal concepts, mathematical formulas, our knowledge of laws and properties, even our beliefs (Bower, 1975).

Information stored in long-term memory is considered relatively permanent in nature. That is, it doesn't fade from long-term memory or is ever lost except perhaps as a result of illness or deterioration of the nervous system. What goes into the LTM is in a sense there forever.

The long-term memory system can best be conceptualized as a sort of organized, spatial storehouse of information. Information that is read into the LTM is classified, categorized, cross-indexed, and stored there in a variety of ways. Bower (1975) says that "the LTM is to be considered as conceptual network into which information (propositions) is inserted through the working memory (or short-term memory) and from which the central (an executive) supervisor processor retrieves answers to questions" (p. 57).

This process of storage in the LTM is sometimes compared to the cataloguing and cross-indexing of books in a library. At other times it is compared to the entry of data items into the electronic memory of a computer. The degree to which information in the STM is efficiently coded, organized, and enriched increases its chance of being properly stored within the LTM and of it being later recalled (remembered).

The exact nature of the storage in the LTM is of particular fascination to IPP theorists. This is quite natural since what we call *knowledge* is ultimately explained by LTM codes.

Models have been used to explain storage in the LTM. Network models (e.g., Anderson & Bower, 1973; Quillian, 1968) have been the most popular type. Other kinds of models have been proposed. These include set theory models, feature comparison models, and models developed within the framework of schema theory.

In this chapter we restrict our interpretation of long-term memory within the framework of network models. We attempt to explain memory in order to provide the reader with a general understanding of network models and theory. Any network conception of long-term memory merely represents one of a number of ways in which memory may be conceived.

A Network View of Long-Term Memory

In a network model, long-term memory is conceived of as a vast network of nodes and links. The nodes represent concepts, e.g., symbol codes. The links or associations between the nodes interrelate the concepts (nodes) and provide them with their properties or characteristics. The nodes and their connecting links in the LTM constitute the permanent knowledge (memory) base that guides our thoughts and actions.

A variety of links connect our concepts. Some links establish a concept (symbol) as belonging to a particular classification or category; for example, the concept of dog is likely to be linked with a particular animal species; it has linkages that establish it (the dog) as being canine in nature. Other links attach a concept to superordinate or subordinate concepts. The dog symbol (concept) is thus likely to be linked to other memory symbols in memory in a way that establishes it within hierarchies of concepts, e.g., dog-canine-mammal-animal. Still other symbol links provide additional information about the symbol (concept) or modify what it means. We are likely to remember a particular dog or a particular instance involving a dog because of these types of personal linkages.

Depending on the linkages established, any particular information item stored in the LTM can mean different things on our remembering or thinking about it. Different types of information lend themselves to different kinds of storage. Perceptual information and items of an emotional nature are likely to be stored in the LTM in less structured ways, i.e., in the form of simple symbols loosely related to others. Abstract information, such as scientific concepts, is likely to be encoded in more structured ways, i.e., within elaborate symbol structures, organized in categorical or hierarchical ways.

Quillian's Hierarchical Model of Semantic Memory

Quillian has provided a classic model illustrating hierarchical storage. This model is presented in Figure 7–4.

Looking at Quillian's tree model, we see how particular concepts or symbols are defined by their associations or links. *Canary, ostrich, salmon* and *shark* are concepts or symbols whose associations give them particular meanings as specific types of animals.

In Quillian's tree model the canary, ostrich, salmon, and shark symbols are linked to superordinate concepts that represent broader classifications, i.e., the bird symbol for canary and ostrich, the fish symbol for salmon and shark. Still higher in the Quillian tree model, the symbol for animal represents a still more extensive concept, to which those for bird and fish are subordinate.

This model has a number of implications (see Figure 7–4). We limit our concern to only one consideration, however. It is the types of meanings assigned to the specific animals in the symbol hierarchy by their linkages. Thus, at the one (the lowest) level of the hierarchy, the symbols for canary, ostrich, salmon, and shark have quite specific meanings; e.g., a canary is yellow. However, because of the linkages with the superordinate concepts of bird and fish, these specific symbols can also be identified in terms of other more extensive attributes. Thus, at the second level in Quillian's model, canary, ostrich, salmon, and shark are classified as either birds or fish and are assigned meanings attributed to birds or fish. And at the highest level of Quillian's hierarchy the specific animals take on meanings identified by their participation in (linkage to) the broader concept (symbol) of animal.

Beyond the information suggested by Quillian's model, we should remember that such symbols as canary, ostrich, salmon, and shark have a wide variety of associations that individualize them for particular people. The symbol for canary may also be associated with information about a particular pet, that for ostrich with remembered information from a trip to the zoo with one's parents, that for salmon with a dinner at a special restaurant, that for shark with a variety of frightening films. It is the total of linkages that make a symbol what it is.

Semantic and Episodic Memory

A major distinction in LTM information storage is made between semantic and episodic memory. Semantic memory involves organized retrieval of meaningful information. Episodic memory involves memory of specific events in one's life.

Underwood (1978b) has observed that semantic memory "is the organized [categorical] repository of rules, concepts, and relationships between words and other symbols" (p. 238). Semantic memory items can be readily stored both categorically and associatively in the LTM. Items of episodic memory on the other hand are most likely to be stored associatively in the LTM. That is because the episodic memory items develop from personal events, e.g., sensory, intuitive, emotional experiences. They are not usually well organized or systematically related to other types of information.

Episodic memory items are less likely to be recalled voluntarily than semantic memory items because they are not systematically organized. On the other hand they are more likely to be evoked by circumstances: The scent of a particular perfume brings back an image of a person we knew, the taste of a type of food brings back memories of a particular country we visited. Since episodic memory items are so often linked to semantic items, they serve as cues or triggers for the latter and help us to recall them. Sometimes episodic memories accumulate to the point where they themselves can create semantic memory items.

Analogical versus Propositional Representation

In earlier discussions of coding we discussed disagreements about the nature of codes. Most IPP theorists allow that there are differences at early stages of processing, e.g., during sensory processing; that there may be a distinct iconic code for visual information, an echoic one for auditory information. There are more disputes about storage in long-term memory. Is all information stored there in the same type of code?

For some theorists the answer is yes. After all the computer can represent all information, whether mathematical, verbal, graphic, music, etc., by identical electronic on-off states.

Is this also true of the IPS? It is not necessarily true. Some theorists have suggested that information is stored in long-term memory within two separate and distinct systems. The first is an imagery system of some sort; it stores analog information, i.e., information that is directly representative of something. The second is a semantic system that stores abstract codes, e.g., about verbal and numerical information and the propositions that assign them meaning (Paivio, 1975).

Remembering a car provides an example of how information about an object can be stored in both systems: (1) analogically, in the form of images, and (2) semantically, in terms of language codes. We can remember a car by picturing it in our minds (figurally) the way we last saw it. We can also remember it (semantically) through the propositional (verbal) statement: a Chevrolet, 1978, blue, four-door, dent in front fender, that belongs to me.

Those who opt for such dual systems of storage (Paivio, 1975, 1979) argue that analogically stored information need not consist of exact images of objects or situations but simply must represent them in some direct fashion rather than by means of abstract symbols. After all we don't need a perfect photograph to identify a person we meet for the first time; for that matter even a simple caricature of the person might do. Supporters of dual-memory systems argue that the systems, though independent of each other, are interconnected so that activity in one system can set off activity in the other and that the two systems exchange information and support each other. Those who disclaim the dual-system conception believe that one type of LTM code ultimately represents figural as well as semantic-propositional information (Newell & Simon, 1972).

Procedural versus Declarative Knowledge Systems

Just as distinctions have been made between LTM information of an analogical and propositional sort, so has one been made between declarative and procedural information systems stored within and accessed from the LTM (Anderson, 1976). This distinction doesn't necessarily imply different types of codes, but it does imply separate knowledge systems that are different in their nature and functions.

According to this view argued by Anderson and his colleagues, *declarative knowledge* is what we usually consider to be *information*. This could be information we recite or hear about a movie playing at the Bijou, our friends' addresses, somebody's birthday, the main character in a novel, and the contents of a text we have studied. *Procedural knowledge* can perhaps best be identified with performance skills, e.g., with how we decode words, apply algebra algorithms, solve chess problems, follow through on a golf swing, tie a shoe lace, or start on the opposite foot for a backhanded tennis stroke. Moates and Schumacher (1979) describe declarative knowledge as being communicable to others, while procedural knowledge isn't. Declarative knowledge is used in different ways—e.g., you discuss poverty from a variety of standpoints—but procedural knowledge is usually applied in one particular way—e.g., you follow through on a certain type of golf shot.

Remembering

A number of factors govern our remembering and they differ from person to person. There are limits to the rate at which information can be stored within or recovered from the LTM over any given period. Recovery of information from the LTM (remembering) is limited by the LTM's storage capacity. Recall is dependent on the efficiency with which stored items are organized when entering the LTM. Recall is determined by the types of networks into which the stored information has been entered. Recall is dependent on avenues of access to LTM information; thus, when external cues entering the STSS are related to LTM information, they may trigger recall of that information. Recall is dependent on passage of time; newer items stored in the LTM may obscure older items, become confused with them, or otherwise block their retrieval.

Recall

How does one proceed to remember, i.e., recover information from the LTM? What is the nature of recall? There are a number of theories. Some of them are clearly based on computer analogies.

Memory Tags

A number of different theories or models have been proposed to explain how it is possible to recover stored memory items. Anderson and Bower (1973, 1974) suggest that each information unit is given a "memory tag" when it is placed in storage. This tag identifies it as having a particular location in the LTM. Retrieval of that information from the LTM begins with a search for its tag. This leads to a location in the LTM where the information is stored with other types of tagged information. Various information tags in the LTM are mentally examined till the one that identifies the information item is found. After that it can be retrieved, i.e., remembered.

An everyday analogy to this process is that of retrieving luggage from a checkroom. We give our check to an attendant, who searches for a corresponding tag on the pieces of luggage in the checkroom and after finding one that corresponds to our check, retrieves our suitcase. If the tagging theory of memory is correct, remembering (information retrieval) is a two-stage process: (1) a tag search or identification (recognition stage) and (2) a separate (recall) retrieval stage. It also suggests that we can help ourselves to remember things by entering new information items into the STSS that match up with the tags on the information we are trying to recall.

Prompting of Recall

Information (memories) can be recalled in a number of ways. This is often accomplished through the use of various sorts of prompts. As we have observed, some of these prompts cause recall without any intention on our part. Indeed, sometimes they may bring back memories we should just as soon not remember.

There are external prompts. Information entering the STSS links up somehow with information stored in the LTM and triggers its recall into consciousness (the STM). Often the simplest external cues can do this. The smell of a particular cologne, the taste of a particular item of food, the sound of a song—all can bring back memories. The power of STSS-LTM linkages is perhaps best demonstrated by the déjà vu phenomenon. In a déjà vu experience, we see something and feel that we have experienced it once before, even though this isn't the case. The feeling of reexperience is possible because the present scene triggers memories (thoughts, attitudes, emotions, even actual physical sensations) stored in the LTM that are associated with a particular experience to which the present experience is linked in some fashion.

Internal prompts can also assist memory. An example of this is when we provide ourselves with mental cues that help us to remember something better. Thus, if you have misplaced something on entering your home, it may help if you review everything you did when first entering. When you do this, certain items that you recall may prompt you to remember where you placed the misplaced object you are seeking (because of their linkages with it).

The use of mnemonics also demonstrates the use of internal prompts. Trying to recall a person's name, we may first conjure up some images we have learned to associate with that name, trying to recall the latter through its linkages to those images. Thus, picturing a fish being carried out by a man may help us recall the name of *Fischman*. Still another way of providing ourselves with internal prompts is to search consciously a list of items in the LTM; this may help us recall the particular item we are searching for; it will often pop into mind.

An Address Register Component

Broadbent (1971) has suggested that the recall of information is helped along by a special address register component that is located in the IPS between the STM and the LTM. This address register doesn't hold any information by itself. Rather it attaches labels or addresses to information moving from the STM into the LTM. These addresses, then, can be used later to identify the information we wish to recall. When we try to recall information from the LTM, we first "review" their addresses, which tell us where to search for the information.

Other theorists write about codes in the STM that facilitate retrieval of information from the LTM or of STM information templates that when they correspond to ones in the LTM, recall information from the LTM (Moates & Schumacher, 1979).

The Memory Search Process

What goes on when we try to recall things deliberately? Atkinson and Shiffrin (1968) have suggested that deliberate recall is carried out by a central processor seeking out stored information in the LTM.

It may be that the central processor recalls information by carrying out intentional memory searches, i.e., by examining all of the items in a particular tagged sample of LTM information one at a time, until wanted information items are found. This has been compared to a child having a particular marble in hand (the STM) and pulling other marbles one at a time from the bag of marbles (the LTM) until finding another that matches it (Houston, 1976). Atkinson and Shiffrin (1968) have suggested that the central processor tries to match information from the STM with information in the LTM. Recall is achieved when the appropriate match is made.

Recall and Recognition

Distinctions have been made between recall and recognition. Recall involves both identification of the LTM information and its retrieval, often by an active search. This is a two-step process. Recognition, however, is a simpler, one-step process. It bypasses the retrieval process, since in order for us to recognize an information item, we don't have to find an information item in the LTM that corresponds to one in the STM. We merely have to decide whether the items in the STM and LTM correspond. In our previous checkroom analogy, in recognition the attendant simply must know that our luggage is in the checkroom; he doesn't have to find it. In recall he not only must know the luggage is there but he must recover and give it to us.

Some theorists consider recall and recognition as distinct independent processes (Flexser & Tulving, 1978). Others insist that they are essentially the same (Rabinowitz, Mandler, & Patterson, 1977). Craik has suggested that it may be a matter of similar processes applied to different tasks (1979).

Reproductive and Reconstructive Memory

Distinctions are sometimes made between the reproductive and reconstructive memory. The first duplicates or repeats information in more or less exact form; i.e., in recalling information from the LTM we retrieve it in the same form it was originally stored. The second reconstructs the original information into new forms. That is, in reconstructive memory retrieval the information coming from the long-term memory is modeled and reshaped as it moves into short-term memory.

Loftus (1973) has carried out a considerable amount of research showing that much of what we remember is actually reconstructed, i.e., changed from its original form. She has carried out research to show that when we recall something, we reconstruct it according to other information stored within the LTM and by our thoughts, feelings, and attitudes at the actual time of recall. Thus the information we are recalling is often changed significantly as it passes into the STM, where it is consciously remembered. This is why eyewitnesses are so often inaccurate in their reports even when they believe they are remembering things exactly.

Levels of Processing versus Levels of Memory

Most IPP theorists conceive of memory as consisting of a number of separate and distinct components or stages; they believe that information processing proceeds from memory stage to memory stage (component to component).

However, a small group of theorists believe that the idea of stages may actually be a misinterpretation of memory events. They consider memory to be a unitary system and believe that what appear to be different types of memory storage systems really are different events within the same (single) memory system. One of the most prominent of such views is the levels of processing theory (Craik, 1979; Craik & Lockhart, 1968).

According to the levels of processing theory, information doesn't proceed through different IPS memory stages, such as the STSS, STM, LTM. Rather a single system processes the information at different levels. It is the way that information is processed, i.e., the levels at which it is processed, that gives the impression of different memory stages.

Thus, at the most superficial level, information processing is essentially unelaborated sensory processing. At a deeper level, processing becomes more selective and organized. At a still deeper level there is encoding in terms of associations and categories that create meaningful information, i.e., what is usually known as *semantic memory*. The deeper and more meaningful the level of processing carried out by the IPS, the better our retention of information is.

The effects of different types of rehearsal are readily explained by the levels of processing theory. The reason why rote rehearsal of information is considered of limited value for later retention is that it processes information at a superficial level. Elaborative rehearsal on the other hand is deep rehearsal that enriches, chunks, organizes, and stabilizes information before its storage. There are those who disagree with the value of this type of explanation.

Observations on the IPS and Memory

Because memory is an integral part of learning, it continues to be front and center in the concerns of IPS researchers. We have been able to touch on a few of the many IPP memory concepts. Many books deal with this topic. We recommend the following: Anderson (1980), Howe (1980), and Kintsch (1977).

PROBLEM SOLVING

IPS researchers are showing increasingly greater interest in the study of problem solving. IPS researchers are studying a wide range of human problem-solving efforts, many with implications for school learning.

Some cognitive research into problem solving has unfamiliar names, e.g., Game Theory, The Prisoner's Dilemma, and Towers of Hanoi. Nevertheless these involve problem-solving issues similar to those facing schoolchildren in a variety of situations. Much of this problem-solving research is being carried out along IPP lines.

Problem Solving As Decision Making

An organism dealing with a problem must make decisions and choices. It must decide or choose among alternative courses of action. Problem solving and intelligent behavior can be defined in terms of decision making and choices (Lachman, Lachman, & Butterfield, 1979).

We are inclined to think of problem solving as a peculiarly human activity requiring conscious voluntary decisions and choices. Nevertheless it can go on at all levels of human behavior and cognition. Indeed most of our problem-solving activities are carried out in an unconscious, involuntary, even automatic fashion. Our neurons make decisions, i.e., whether to fire or not to fire. Our retinas decide whether to let in or to shut out light. Our neuromuscular apparatus makes automatic choices in adjusting our movements when we walk or perform other physical acts.

For that matter, machines also solve problems. A car's automatic transmission decides what gear it should go into. A thermostat decides whether a house is too hot or cold and chooses to turn a furnace on or off. A toaster makes its mind up when the toast is done, a space rocket whether it is accelerating properly. Even though we are specifically concerned with human problem solving in this chapter, it will help us to remember the broad nature of decision making and thus of problem solving.

Human Problem Solving

Newell and Simon are leading IPP researchers in the problem-solving field. They have studied both human and simulated (computer) information problem solving (1972).

In some of their earlier research Newell and Simon studied the ways students solve problems through protocol analysis. They first asked the students to explain the procedures they used when solving problems, and they were able to use this information to create computer programs that simulated the students' problem solving procedures. They also developed procedural models that demonstrate the ways that the student problems might best be solved. Figure 7–6 shows one such model. It is a spatial model of problem solving.

In Figure 7–6 we find that the solution to a problem has been conceptualized as a goal-directed search through a problem space. The search involves the selection of operations at specific points within the problem space that will solve a series of subproblems (achieve subgoals or substates). Achieving all of the subgoals means the achievement of a terminal goal state and the solution of the problem.

Problem solving, expressed in these terms, involves movement from an initial (problem) state, through intermediate (problem-solving) states, to reach a final (goal) state. Inability to proceed through these states to the ultimate goal state or termination of efforts to reach the latter constitutes a failure.

Newell and Simon have developed problem space strategies that teach computers to solve problems. Some of these programs can also be used by humans (1972). One of the most powerful of these strategies is means end analysis.

Means End Analysis

Means end analysis requires that the problem space be clearly defined. Its premise is that when all of the possible problem states in a problem can be specified, all of the operations to solve the problem can also be specified.

Using means end analysis, the IPS proceeds to solve a problem by instigating a series of successive productions that go on till the problem is solved or the person stops trying to solve the problem. These productions are governed by programs stored in the LTM and activated by IPS control processes.

Let us examine how means end analysis works in a problem-solving sequence; we examine only part of the process (see Figure 7–6). In this sequence the IPS is presumed to strive toward the solution of a problem by using three general subgoals. Each of these subgoals may be addressed any number of times in attempting to solve the problem. But only one subgoal may be addressed at any time.

- Subgoal 1. Transform State A to State B. This means you are at one state (A) in trying to solve the problem and you are trying to move to the next state (B), to achieve subgoal 1. The first step is to compare State A to State B. If both states are the same, you have already achieved Subgoal 1 and should go on to achieve the next state (C) in the problem-solving space. If, however, State A and State B are different, you must determine what that difference (D) is and then move to Subgoal 2.

Figure 7–6 Spatial Model of Problem Solving

1. Transform state A into state B

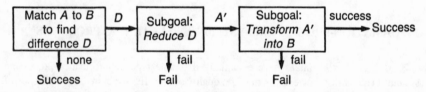

2. Reduce difference D between state A and state B

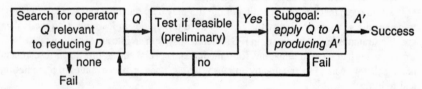

3. Apply operator Q to state A

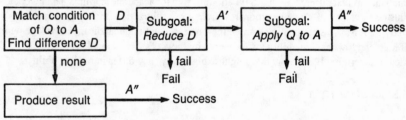

Source: Adapted from *Human Problem Solving* by Allen Newell and H.A. Simon, p. 417, with permission of Prentice-Hall, Inc., Englewood Cliffs, N.J., © 1972.

- Subgoal 2. This subgoal is to make the difference between State A and State B less. In order to do this, you search for some operator (Q) that you expect will do the job. An operator is any information, plan, strategy, technique, or skill that may help to reduce the difference between states A and B. Finding one, you proceed to Subgoal 3.
- Subgoal 3. Having found an operator (Q) that is expected to reduce the difference between A and B (eventually to reach Subgoal B), you apply it to State A. If it works as expected, you will achieve a new state of A, which satisfactorily approximates or is identical with State B. If the operator is not successful, you return to Subgoal 2 and try to identify another operator that may be successful in reducing the difference between A and B. Eventually, if adequate operators are applied, State A will be transformed into State B or the equivalent of State B, and you will have accomplished a particular step in solving your problem. You can then go on to attempt another step, e.g., to transform State B to State C, and so on.

This type of means end analysis is to be used throughout a particular problem-solving effort until all the subgoals in the problem space are reached and the entire problem is solved. Programs for means end analysis, though originally developed for computer use, have been a source of insight into the ways the human mind works; they have also served as guides to help humans solve problems.

INFORMATION-PROCESSING SYSTEMS AND LEARNING PROBLEMS

As discussed, all humans have essentially the same type of information-processing systems. They differ, however, in the size, quality of their IPS structures, the efficiency of their architectural arrangements, the effectiveness of the control mechanisms and processes that govern the speed and accuracy of information flow, coding, retrieval, etc., and in the power of the executive processes that regulate the IPS.

It would seem that an understanding of the IPS may help remedial and special educators to determine some reasons why their pupils have difficulties in learning. Can we isolate specific strengths and weaknesses in IPS structures, system architecture, control processes, etc., in ways that have implications for remedial and special education? Some researchers believe that we can do so and that by doing so, we can open up new avenues of remediation and training.

Keeping this in mind, we examine some IPP research into individual differences by Earl Hunt and his associates. These investigators have been particularly interested in the implications that differences in IPS functioning hold for academic learning. Their work also illustrates values of decomposition research, i.e., subtraction and addition methods in studying IPS. We specifically examine their research with nonhandicapped college pupils of high and low reading ability (as measured by the *SAT*s). Hunt and his associates (1975) tried to determine IPS factors that might explain why they differ in reading ability.

A Study of the LTM

In letter recognition the student must search the long-term memory to identify the letter; this requires a search for that letter in the LTM and the retrieval of the meaning from the LTM.

To study letter recognition in high and low verbal ability students, Hunt and his associates applied subtraction methods developed by Posner and his associates (Posner, Boies, Eichelman, & Taylor, 1969). Two letters are shown on a screen, e.g., *A* and *a*. The student presses a yes button if both are the same, a no button if they are different.

In a physical match task, the student must press a yes button when both letters flashed on the screen were physically identical (e.g., *a, a*) and a no button when they were not identical (e.g., *a, b*). In another name match task the pupils had to press a yes button when the letters have the same name (whether or not they were physically identical), e.g., *A, a*, and a no button if they did not have the same name.

From an information-processing standpoint the requirement of a physical match and a name match task are quite different. When simply asked to perform a physical match, the student must move the letters from the STSS into the STM, use control processes in the STM to make a decision as to whether they are physically identical, and issue a command (to self) to execute a response, i.e., press button yes or button no. In performing a name match, there are different as well as more complex tasks to be performed. The subject must enter the letters into the STM, look up (retrieve) the names for each of the letters from the LTM, make a decision whether these names match the letters in the visual display, and finally decide whether to press button yes or button no. By subtracting the time for a physical match from the time for a name match, we are able to determine the additional time required to look up the name of the letters in the LTM in the latter task.

Groups of low verbal ability students tested in this experiment didn't differ significantly from high verbal ability students in the times they needed to make physical letter matches. This means that the two groups were equally able to move letters from the STSS into the STM, to make decisions about the equivalence of the letters, and to execute responses. The two groups, however, differed markedly in their times on the name match task. The high verbal ability group showed a time difference of only 33 milliseconds in responding to the physical and name match tasks. The low verbal ability group showed a difference of 196 milliseconds.

The low verbal group was thus considerably slower than the high verbal groups in retrieving information from the LTM. A 0.53 millisecond difference per item between the groups in LTM retrieval, by itself, is not much. However, it rapidly adds up to a substantial difference if there is a good deal of material to read. When we realize that the average short novel has about 500,000 morphemes, it is clear that even the slightest delay in LTM retrieval of an information item can mount up to create a serious time lag in reading.

A Study of Deficiencies in Control Processes

Hunt also studied control process differences in his high and low verbal ability students (1975a, 1975b; Hunt, Lenneberg, & Lewis, 1975). In order to comprehend verbal materials effectively, a student must be able to perform rapid operations on the verbal information entering the STM. The student must form letters into words, words into sentences, sentences into clauses, clauses into sentences, sentences into paragraphs, etc.

Hunt used a modified task developed by Sternberg (1969) to study the speed with which high or low verbal ability students operate on verbal information in short-term memory. The students were presented with one to five target letters; the letters *Y, R, D, N, S* were shown on a screen one at a time, a second for each. After each letter was shown, a probe letter was flashed on the screen. The students were then required to press a yes button when the probe was the same as the target letter and a no button when it was not. What is involved in this particular task? It requires the subject to put the target letter into the short-term memory, hold it there, move the probe letter into the STM, make a mental comparison between both letters, and then execute a response (pressing either the yes or no button) that indicates whether the letters are the same.

This task becomes considerably more complex and thus more time-consuming if two target letters are flashed on the screen before the probe letter, for the subject is then required to make two comparisons. When there are three target letters, the complexity of the task again increases, and so on. We can determine the additional times required for each additional mental comparison (as the number of the target letters increase) by subtracting the time required for simpler comparisons from those required for more complex ones.

Hunt found that high and low verbal ability student groups were about the same in their reaction times on this task when only one target letter was involved. But high verbal ability students required only an additional millisecond to respond for each additional target letter that was introduced, while low verbal ability students needed about 80 milliseconds for each additional one. Low verbal ability students were clearly less effective than the high ability ones in the efficiency and speed of their STM control processes. This may have accounted for some of their verbal problems.

STM Capacity

Information entering the STM must be held there for a sufficient time if it is to be processed effectively. In reading, one must be able to maintain the first words of sentences being read in the STM long enough to make sense of the final word. Otherwise one can't understand the entire sentence. If a pupil's STM has a limited holding capacity, the student is likely to have difficulties in reading comprehension. Hunt and his colleagues adopted a Peterson and Peterson task to study the STM capacity of high and low verbal ability students.

The subjects in this task were shown four letters on a screen, one at a time. Then they were engaged in a distractor task that required them to read numbers flashed on the screen for a few seconds. After the distractor task, the subjects were asked to recall and name the four letters they earlier saw in their original order. This task requires that the subject hold the earlier information (the letters) in STM storage while mentally attending to a newer task (the numbers). This is similar to what takes place in reading; one is required to retain the first part of a sentence in the STM while the latter part is being entered.

Hunt's low verbal ability students generally made more errors on this type of recall than did high ability students. Indeed they made three times as many errors in short periods of exposure to the original letters. Their STMs appeared to have lesser holding capacities than those of high verbal ability students. It is a limitation that may account for their low verbal ability.

IPP IN REMEDIAL AND SPECIAL EDUCATION

The studies just reviewed show some of the reasons why IPS theories and models have affected research into learning. It is also easy to see why the IPP has become influential in remedial and special education. It has provided us with new ways of studying cognition and cognitive problems.

Instead of conceiving of pupils with learning problems as simply being deficient or impaired in respect to their general abilities, IPP researchers try to identify the causes for this. Their approach is quite different from the specific ability approaches reviewed in Chapter 2. The implications of saying that a pupil has deficiencies in the STM have different implications than that of simply identifying the student as having a poor memory or as being deficient in perception. New conceptions in remedial and special education are emerging thanks to the IPP. On the other hand the usual words of caution are in order. Thus recent research has suggested that differences of the sort Hunt found can be explained by differences in general intellectual ability (Carroll, 1976a, 1976b).

IPP AND THE MODIFIABILITY OF COGNITIVE FUNCTIONING

The degree to which children can be modified by their experiences is one of the great continuing debates in remedial and special education. Are children basically programmed by heredity so that they *must* cognitively develop in predetermined ways? Or are they essentially free to developing a great variety of different ways, depending on their experiences? This debate, frequently called the *nature-nurture controversy*, has never fully been resolved.

Cognitive theorists, more than behavioral ones, are likely to believe in the hereditability of cognition and behavior. Nevertheless, they often sharply split on the nature-nurture issues. Some, like Eysenck (1973) and Jensen (1973, 1979), strongly believe that much of what we call *intelligence* is inherited and cannot be changed to any great degree. Others like Feuerstein (Feuerstein et al., 1981) are convinced that education can greatly improve, if not entirely modify, children's intellectual functioning.

In recent years a somewhat different perspective on the modifiability of cognition has emerged, guided by the information-processing paradigm. This new perspective no longer seeks to determine how much of cognition is determined by inheritance or by the environment or as a result of the interaction of the two. It tries instead to distinguish and separate the structural characteristics of cognition from the ways in which these characteristics can be used.

Thus two levels of intelligence can be distinguished. One level is that of a biologically based cognitive architectural system. This includes such components as STM capacity, the rate at which information is lost from STM, the efficiency of storage in LTM and its later retrieval. The second level is that of an environmentally developed executive program whose processes regulate and direct the architectural system.

This theory is obviously based on computer analogies. We see this in the first level of intelligence. Computers have basic structural components that are organized in predetermined architectural patterns. These determine its information-processing capacities. The human nervous system also has basic components "hard wired" in predetermined patterns. These determine the way it processes information to a large extent.

The computer analogy is also evident in the second level of intelligence. The computer's executive programs command or control the functioning of the computer's structures. They also make it possible to program the computer's capacities in ways that compensate for, and even overcome, some of the computer's structural deficiencies. Many cognitive scientists believe that we can also program humans so as to overcome their cognitive (structural) deficiencies. Chapter 8 is based on this assumption.

CONCLUSIONS

The information-processing paradigm is the dominant one in cognitive studies. It has been applied to almost every issue of human cognition. There are good reasons for its popularity. It has provided us with new insights into cognition and has proven a valuable conceptual tool for studying many topics important to psychology and education. Another reason is the influence of the computer age. IPP models of cognition have employed knowledge of computer operations to explain cognitive functioning. The computer and computer science provide metaphors of cognitive functioning that make the IPP scientifically respectable. A less obvious reason for the IPP's popularity is that it is relatively easy to translate older theories of cognition into IPP terms. It has been done for Guilford's (1981) and Cattell and Horn's (1981) theories. It can also be done for specific abilities. It has been done for Piaget as well (Case, 1978b); a number of IPP theorists find many of Piaget's ideas quite compatible with their own. Nor is the IPP incompatible with behaviorism.

In education a great number of IPP models and theories dealing with all aspects of academic work have helped to understand learning and instruction better (Reid & Hresko, 1981). There are many models for all aspects of reading (Farnhan-Diggory, 1978). IPP theories and models lend themselves well to research and intervention with almost any kind of population, from young children to mature scholars, from the mentally retarded to the gifted.

Perhaps the surest testimony to the IPP's success is the new IPP intelligence test developed by Kaufman and Kaufman (1983), which emphasizes distinctions between serial and simultaneous cognitive processing.

The IPP has also cast new light on old problems in remedial and special education. Efforts to overcome deficiencies in cognitive capacities by improving or remediating coding processes, chunking, rehearsal, and using external and internal prompts such as imagery to access information are but a few of the ways that IPP has influenced cognitive remediation.

However, current views and models of information processing are under constant revision, and the newer models that will undoubtedly emerge will most likely have different implications than present ones. For one, some cognitive theorists believe that the current approaches are excessively influenced by the computer and research laboratory models (Neisser, 1976a).

What this means is that we should not commit ourselves blindly to the IPP in its present form. It is premature to explain the reasons pupils fail to learn or why they develop cognitive handicaps purely from an IPP point of view. This being said, we remain enthusiastic about the value of the information-processing paradigm in understanding cognition and in assisting us in remedial and special education.

Chapter 8

Cognitive and Learning Styles

What are cognitive styles? The simplest way to explain them is that they are constructs that help to explain the ways that personality differences influence cognition and, through cognition, influence behavior. Two individuals with identical IQs, with the same configurations of specific abilities, or with exactly the same type and strength of information-processing capacities may nevertheless be quite different in the ways that they perceive things, think, solve problems, recall events, come to decisions, play musical instruments, swing baseball bats. They differ in their cognitive styles.

For such reasons many cognitive researchers recommend the study of cognitive styles. An understanding of the latter may help to explain why particular students think and act in particular ways, even though appearing similar on the basis of our tests or experiments. For these reasons we have chosen to review cognitive styles at this particular juncture of our text.

HISTORICAL PERSPECTIVE

Like most other psychological phenomena, the construct of cognitive styles has a long and elaborate history, stretching to antiquity. An in-depth study of this history is beyond the scope of this book. An understanding of some of its recent events, however, is essential to understanding this chapter.

Before World War II the study of cognition was usually restricted to the study of intelligence and of group abilities. Psychologists were largely interested in the use of cognitive tests to predict success in school or on the job. Cognitive assessment was thus carried out to select individuals for inclusion in or exclusion from various school programs, employment classifications, and the like. While the industrial, clinical, and school psychologists who studied cognition recognized that personality characteristics affected cognition, they made little effort to investigate the ways that they did so.

World War II aroused considerable interest in personality factors. This was partly due to the fact that many war casualties were psychiatric in nature, i.e., due to mental or personality breakdowns. Following World War II the federal government committed a great deal of resources to the care of psychiatrically disabled veterans and trained large numbers of psychiatrists, psychologists, and other mental health personnel to work in its hospitals and clinics. Also following World War II there was a great deal of interest in personal self-development. Psychological therapies, which promise to improve personality functioning, particularly psychoanalysis, became popular.

Along with these trends, and partly as a consequence of them, there was increased interest in the use of tests to assess personality characteristics and to determine how the latter affected cognitive functioning. It was thus inevitable "that new constructs . . . [would be developed] . . . to account for the form and manner [i.e., the personal characteristics] of cognition rather than [just] the sheer skill of [cognitive] performance" (Kogan, 1980b, p. 64). Researchers interested in the form and manner of cognition began to open new areas of investigation into the ways that personality affected perception, memory, thinking, and problem solving during the late 1950s. Among the most prominent of these was that of cognitive styles, in which "the interface between cognition and personality is studied" (Kogan, 1980b, p. 64).

The topic of cognitive styles has become an important one in cognitive literature. This chapter should provide the reader with a basic perspective on cognitive styles and on learning styles, which is a related area of study.

Cognitive Styles

Before presenting cognitive style definitions, we should like to remind readers of what they already know. Any separation of personality from cognition is artificial. We function cognitively as persons, rather than as collections or combinations of cognitive factors on one hand and personality ones on the other. And while the concept of cognitive styles is intended to emphasize the "togetherness" of cognition and personality, it also makes a distinction between the two that cannot be made in real life.

DEFINITIONS OF COGNITIVE STYLES

A variety of cognitive-style definitions prevail in the literature. According to Messick (1976), cognitive styles include a person's typical modes of perceiving, remembering, thinking, and problem solving. Kagan, Moss, and Sigel (1963) have defined cognitive styles as representing "stable individual preferences in the mode of perceptual organization and conceptual categorization of the external environment" (p. 8).

Coop and Sigel (1971) define cognitive styles as denoting consistencies in individual modes of functioning in a variety of behavioral situations. Goldstein and Blackman (1978) define cognitive styles as referring to "the characteristic ways in which individuals conceptually organize their environment" (p. 2).

Kogan's (1980b) definition is perhaps as useful as any: "Cognitive styles reflect individual variations in *modes* of attending, perceiving, remembering and thinking . . . [they] represent an] . . . interface between cognition and personality" (p. 64).

Witkin and his associates (Holland, 1982) listed three essential characteristics that define cognitive styles: "(a) Cognitive style refers to process, not product, (b) cognitive style dimensions cut across traditional and perhaps inappropriate learner characteristics (such as IQ), and (c) the learner's cognitive style remains stable though not necessarily unchangeable" (p. 8).

Other investigators provide definitions that emphasize the following:

- Cognitive styles represent individual differences in cognition rather than particular motivational, emotional, or biological states.

- Cognitive styles are concerned with the style rather than the content of cognition.
- Cognitive styles are related to the individual's other personality characteristics.
- Cognitive styles are traits. That is, they are enduring, consistent characteristics that manifest themselves across a variety of behaviors and situations. A particular cognitive style means that the individual will consistently perceive, think, remember in certain ways under most circumstances (Kogan, 1980a, 1980b; Holland, 1982).

CATEGORIES OF COGNITIVE STYLE

Cognitive styles may be classified from a number of standpoints, and often the same cognitive style can be classified several ways. A particular three-way classification scheme suggests itself to us:

1. A cognitive style may simply identify particular characteristics or traits that a person possesses in more or less greater degree. This is true of a cognitive style like authoritarianism; some individuals are more authoritarian than others.
2. A cognitive style may indicate placement at a particular point on a cognitive/ personality dimension whose opposite poles indicate opposing cognitive orientations; this is true for a number of styles including the popular ones of field independence versus dependence and conceptual tempo (reflection versus impulsivity)—the very inclusion of the word *versus* in the names of the styles suggests opposing positions.
3. Certain cognitive styles place an individual within a particular cognitive category; this is true of conceptual styles according to which individuals may be classified as being analytical, categorical, or relational in their thinking.

Kogan (1980b) has suggested another type of classification of cognitive styles. It is one based on their evaluative implications. He has distinguished three distinct types depending on whether identification according to a style has positive or negative connotations.

Type I. Certain cognitive styles resemble cognitive abilities in the sense that they imply good or poor cognitive performance. Thus one of the most famous of cognitive styles, Witkin's field independence versus dependence dimension, is assessed on the basis of tests of perceptual accuracy. Field-independent individuals necessarily score higher on these tests than do field-dependent ones. Their higher scores of perceptual accuracy imply higher levels of cognitive efficiency. And indeed a considerable body of research suggests that field-independent individuals are cognitively superior to field-dependent ones in a number of important ways.

Type II. The second type of cognitive style, according to Kogan (1980b), does not specifically identify individuals as superior or inferior to others in a direct way. Nevertheless this type of style is still "characterized by an explicit or implicit evaluative dimension" (p. 64). That is, while Type II cognitive styles are not identified or assessed in terms of accuracy, certain styles of this type are usually considered superior to others, though the decision as to which ones are superior is often a matter of personal or theoretical bias.

Conceptual styles provide an example of Type II styles. Kagan, Moss, and Sigel (1963) proposed three such styles in order to describe the ways that children group objects:

1. Children who favor analytic modes of thinking tend to group objects on the basis of similar features. They might thus group a number of objects on the basis of the fact that they all have handles, regardless of other ways that they could categorize them.
2. Children who favor a categorical cognitive style are likely to group objects because they are representatives of a particular class or category. They might thus group objects because they are all foods or all vehicles.
3. Children who are relational thinkers are prone to group objects on the basis of their relationships to each other. They might thus place together a match and a pipe, a small dish, and a table on the basis that the match lights the pipe, the pipe's ashes go into a small dish, and the dish belongs on a table.

None of these conceptual styles is inherently superior to the others. Accuracy of performance is not involved. Any of the three types of cognitive styles may be appropriate or inappropriate, accurate or inaccurate in various degrees, depending on the situations in which a grouping is made and its particular purpose. Yet Kagan and his associates made an explicit or implicit evaluation and decided that one type of conceptual style is better than another. They decided that the analytic one is the most advanced of the three because it involves cognitive differentiation. They regarded relational conceptual style to be indicative of cognitive immaturity because it involves grouping of objects on the basis of their most "obvious and compelling . . . qualities" (Kogan, 1980b, p. 65). Other cognitive-style researchers, taking a somewhat different position, believe that the categorical conceptual style is likely to be the superior one because it represents an application of abstract thinking (Gardner & Schoen, 1962).

Type III. The third type of cognitive style is one in which "neither accuracy of performance or value judgments are implicated" (Kogan, 1980b, p. 65). This type of cognitive style is thus "stylistic in the purest sense" (p. 65).

An example that Kogan gives of this Type III cognitive-style dimension is that of preferred breadth of categories. This is also defined in terms of the ways that people group objects. Some individuals set broad category boundaries for themselves when grouping, while others set quite narrow ones. Broad categorizers are likely to group things in an expansive way, which is sometimes vague or tenuous. They might thus group a can opener with a stove and a bottle of sherry on the basis that all three are used in cooking. Narrow categorizers, on the other hand, are likely to exclude from their categories many items that could justifiably be included. Thus when asked to group objects that represent vehicles, they might include tractors, buses, automobiles, and motor scooters in their vehicle category but exclude bicycles because the latter are not powered by engines.

Type IV. Kogan (1980b) also describes certain cognitive styles as cutting across two or more of his types. This is true of the conceptual tempo dimension, which is usually assessed in two ways: (1) the amount of time that a child takes to reflect on (think about) an action before actually carrying it out and (2) the child's degree of accuracy in judgment or performance. Conceptual tempo thus includes both ability (Type I) and evaluative (Type II) components. It also has a "more purely stylistic (Type III) component" (p. 66). One child may score as reflective, another as impulsive. Yet this doesn't necessarily mean one is superior to the other. On any given occasion an assessment of reflectivity may be an indication of maturity and good judgment, but on another occasion it may indicate cognitive slowness or indecisiveness. On any particular occasion impulsivity may indicate poorly thought-out behavior and a proneness to error, while on other occasions it may be indicative of assertiveness and even of leadership.

It is difficult, however, to exclude or prevent value judgments from labels. This is also true of cognitive styles, even for those of the Type III variety. Inevitably cognitive styles tend to develop either positive or negative connotations.

SPECIFIC TYPES OF COGNITIVE STYLES

We review some of the more prominent cognitive styles in this section, though we leave consideration of the two most popular of all, field independence-dependence, and conceptual tempo, to a later section.

Before we begin our review, we would like to emphasize two points made in a number of earlier chapters. The first is that cognitive styles are constructs and are subject to the same limitations as any other type of cognitive construct. Furthermore different investigators identify and describe cognitive styles in ways that depend on their own personal opinions.

The second point is that any given cognitive style or more precisely speaking the implications of particular cognitive style test scores depend on the circumstances under which the style is assessed and validated. An example of what we mean is provided by the study of authoritarianism, which began in earnest at the close of World War II with the work of Adorno, Frenkel-Brunswik, Levinson, and Stanford (1950). Various scales and tests were developed to assess the stylistic variables of what might appropriately be called *right-wing authoritarianism*, since the researchers were interested in the personality factors that influenced the development of fascist or Nazi-like thinking. While we now are all too aware of left-wing authoritarianism, it was not an important issue for cognitive researchers during the early 1950s. As a consequence, the original scales used to assess authoritarianism would not be fully appropriate to assess the authoritarian tendencies of modern left-wing thinkers. While it is true that the authoritarianism of the right and that of the left do have common features, they also present deep differences that make it difficult for a single type of assessment to measure both effectively.

In a similar vein the features of what we in the United States might call *authoritarianism* have different implications in other cultures. Thus using the same type of instrument to assess authoritarian tendencies in both American and Japanese cultures may provide interesting data but may not provide fully accurate insights into Japanese attitudes on authoritarianism. Similarly the results of conceptual tempo tests given to children of different nationalities must be culturally interpreted to make sense. What are considered reflective or impulsive attitudes in one culture are not necessarily such in another culture. Along the same lines, age differences affect the meaning of different conceptual-style scores. A particular conceptual style may be mature and efficient at one particular age but not at another.

COGNITIVE CONTROL STYLES

The cognitive styles that are likely to be of the most interest to remedial and special educators appear to have had their beginnings in George Klein's introduction of cognitive controls, a construct based on his research at the Menninger Clinic and developed within the framework of psychoanalytic theory. Because Klein and his associates first used perceptual tests to study cognitive controls, he originally defined the construct as consisting of perceptual attitudes. He later changed their name to *cognitive attitudes, cognitive system principles,* and *cognitive control principles.* The latter were interpreted as "enduring cognitive structures that presumably emerge from the interaction of genetic and experiential determinants" (Goldstein & Blackman, 1978, p. 5). Among the specific cognitive control mechanisms studied by Klein and others who had worked or been influenced by his work were conceptual differentiation, constricted-flexible control, leveling-sharpening, scanning-focusing, and field articulation. Gardner, Jackson, and Messick (1960) have attempted to distinguish such cognitive controls from cognitive styles on the basis that the former are specific cognitive dimensions while the term *cognitive style* should refer to their organization within a person. This distinction, however, has not really caught on and is not used in this chapter.

The reader will find that some cognitive controls overlap conceptually even though they also have specific cognitive style implications. It is easy to see why. They are often studied in similar ways.

Leveling-Sharpening

The *leveling-sharpening* cognitive control dimension has been defined by Gardner, Jackson, and Messick as representing "the characteristic degree to which current percepts and relevant memory traces interact or assimilate in the course or registration of the current percepts and memories" (Goldstein & Blackman, 1978, p. 8).

An examination of one of the principal procedures used to assess this construct will help us to understand the latter. This is the schematizing test. In the schematizing test, subjects are first placed in a dark room and given time to adapt visually to it. They are then required to judge squares of light that are of increasing size. With this test it was found that subjects usually underestimate the size of later (larger) squares because their judgments have been influenced by the size of earlier ones. As the researchers put it, there generally tends to be an assimilation among percepts of new squares. *Levelers* are individuals who are particularly prone to assimilation. Thus they are inclined to underestimate significantly the size of later (larger) squares because of their experiences with earlier ones. *Sharpeners* on the other hand are better able to resist the influence of earlier experiences and to assess more accurately the size of the later squares. Comparisons between levelers and sharpeners on other tasks usually favor the latter. Their judgments are more realistic. They do better in problem solving.

Scanning-Focusing

The scanning-focusing cognitive control dimension is one that remedial and special educators are more likely to be familiar with than the leveling-sharpening one, which it resembles to some degree.

Scanning and *focusing* were originally defined in terms of the extent to which an individual attempts to validate the judgments made (Gardner & Moriarity, 1968). Size-estimation tests are used to assess the degree to which an individual scans or focuses. In one of these tests, subjects are required to match a projected circle of light to each of three disks. In another test they are required to adjust a circle of light so that its size matches that of other projected circles. A paper-and-pencil version of these tests called the Circle Test has been developed for use with children.

Accuracy in matching on these tests has been correlated with an individual's tendency and ability to "verify" experiences. Focusers, who score high on these tests, are more likely to be more accurate in making decisions than are scanners, who do poorly on the tests. Scanning and focusing constructs have become popular ones in learning disability literature. They have received considerable attention in the study of attention problems. They have also been studied in the context of cognitive strategies (see Chapter 9).

Conceptual Differentiation

This cognitive control dimension was originally described as *equivalence range* and defined in terms of people's consistency in what they will accept as similar or identical in a variety of tasks (Gardner, 1953). It was later redefined by Gardner, Jackson, and Messick (1960) as "the degree of differentiation in an individual's experiences of similarity and differences." It was then renamed by Gardner and Schoen (1962) as being a dimension of *conceptual differentiation*, the name it now bears.

An object-sorting test was originally used to assess the conceptual differentiation dimension. In this test, subjects are required to develop their own categories for sorting and then to sort some 73 objects accordingly. The more categories a subject creates and uses, the more conceptually differentiated the thinking is considered. The reasons why the name *equivalence range* was originally chosen for this dimension are clear, for the test used to assess the cognitive control dimension assesses the degree to which an individual regards things as equivalent. An individual who has a low equivalence range is an individual who makes many conceptual differentiations. An individual who has a broad equivalence range is low in conceptual differentiation. A high degree of conceptual differentiation is usually regarded as an indication of conceptual sophistication and flexibility.

Constricted-Flexible Control

Smith and Klein (1953) first reported on this cognitive control dimension. They originally assessed it using Thurstone's (1944) version of the *Color-Word Test* and later with another version called the *Stroop Test*. The latter uses types of cards colored red, blue, green, or yellow. A single color name—red, blue, green, or yellow—is printed on each of these cards. These color names, however, differ from the color of the cards. Thus the word *blue* may be printed on a red card, the word *red* on a blue card, the word *green* on a yellow card, the word *yellow* on a green card. The subject's task is to identify correctly the card's color while disregarding the conflicting cues provided by the color names. The extent to which a person can do this task quickly and accurately is a measure of the subject's cognitive flexibility. The *Stroop Test* was also later used by Broverman to develop two additional cognitive styles: perceptual motor-conceptual dominance and automatization.

The results of the *Stroop Test*, which was originally developed for use with normal reading adults, must be interpreted differently for younger children or for older ones who have reading or other learning difficulties. Whereas the adults are ordinarily more inclined to respond to the color names on the cards rather than to the cards' colors, the children might be expected to do the opposite, i.e., respond more readily to the colors of the cards than to the color names.

Santostefano and Paley (1964) developed the *Fruit-Distraction Test* to provide a measure of constricted-flexible control specifically for children. The *Fruit-Distraction Test* consists of three large cards. Fifty drawings of fruit are depicted on each. On the first (the control card) the fruits are appropriately colored. The child is required to identify each of the fruits by name. The second card shows pictures of the same fruits but with a variety of achromatic line drawings dispersed among them to distract or confuse the child otherwise. As with the first card the child is required to name the fruits. The fruits on the third card are colored inappropriately. This time the child must identify an appropriate color for each of the fruits. There are three scores derived from this test: (1) the speed of naming the fruits, (2) the number of errors in naming the fruits or in identifying their correct colors, and (3) the number of achromatic objects that the child is later able to identify after seeing them on the second card.

Using this test to study groups of good and poor readers, Santostefano, Rutledge, and Randall (1965) found that poor readers took longer than good ones to identify the correct colors for the inappropriately colored fruits on the third card; this suggested that they had difficulties in coding information. The fact that they were better able to name the achromatic distractors on the second card than were the good readers, also suggested that they were more prone to distraction. Both good and poor readers did equally well in respect to the numbers of fruit pictures they were able to identify and to their general error rate.

Denney (1974) repeated Santostefano-Paley's study and in so doing substantiated many of their earlier findings though he also found that the good readers in his study also did better than poor ones in identifying the fruits on the first card.

It seems to be somewhat difficult to identify the *Fruit-Distraction Test* as one that assesses constricted-flexible controls. It appears to be just as much a test of cognitive efficiency and ability or perhaps one of focal attention. In any case the test clearly provides a measure of cognitive control.

Field Articulation

Field articulation is a cognitive control dimension. An individual high in field articulation is presumably able to attend to relevant stimuli selectively even when there are compelling irrelevant ones around to attract attention (Gardner, Jackson, & Messick, 1960). The construct is not heard much now. The reason for this is that it is quite similar to, if not entirely identical with, the field independence-dependence cognitive style, which was once identified with it but is now the best-known and -researched cognitive style. Indeed the assessment of field articulation is based on very much the same tests as is the field independence-dependence cognitive style. Nevertheless, Gardner and Long have maintained that the field articulation dimension is a broader concept than that of field independence-dependence (Goldstein & Blackman, 1978).

OTHER EARLY COGNITIVE STYLES

While cognitive control studies were the source of many of the more important cognitive styles, some of the latter derived from other avenues of investigation. Among them are conceptual styles and category width.

Conceptual Styles

The construct of conceptual style was developed by Kagan, Moss, and Sigel (1963) on the basis of work with his *Conceptual Style Test*. This test initially consisted of 44 triads of pictures, though shorter versions are usually used. The subject is asked to select two pictures that go together from each triad. On the basis of the results from this test, children are categorized as using analytic relational or inferential conceptual styles. Kogan (1976) has reviewed the topic of conceptual styles, and again more recently (1980b) in his examination of relationships between cognitive styles and reading.

The original construct of category width and the instrument to measure it were developed by Bruner, Goodnow, and Austin (1956). They were seeking to determine the consistency and range of conceptualization used by people in making decisions. In order to do so, they used a type of estimate test. Specifically, subjects were required to assess samples of actual windows provided them with a factual basis for their estimates. A paper-and-pencil version of this test was later developed. In its 20-item final form it presents the subject with a control measure and requires the individual to choose one from four alternatives at the lowest end of the range and another from four alternatives representing the highest end of the range. These tests are presumed to provide a measure of consistency of judgment. Additionally, broad categorizers are supposed to be willing to risk being overinclusive in their judgments, while narrow categorizers are inclined to do the contrary. Category width styles are similar to some of the cognitive control dimensions discussed earlier, particularly those of conceptual differentiation.

Field Independence-Dependence and Conceptual Tempo

The two cognitive styles most likely to be of interest to the readers of this book are field independence-dependence and conceptual tempo (reflection-impulsivity). Blackman and Goldstein (1982) state that these two cognitive-style dimensions are of particular interest to learning disability specialists because of the easy availability of instruments to assess them and because instruments to measure them have been specifically developed for children.

There are other reasons for interest in these styles. The field independence-dependence cognitive style is the most heavily researched of any style. The conceptual tempo cognitive style is relevant to many issues of childhood behavior—and misbehavior.

FIELD INDEPENDENCE-DEPENDENCE

Over three thousand studies are available on the topic of field independence-dependence. Many of these relate to academic learning, some specifically to academic problems and handicaps. Because of its general importance we devote much more time to the discussion of this particular cognitive style dimension than to others. First let us review the four basic ways that this construct has been assessed.

Tilting-Room Chair Tests (TRCT)

In these tests a chair is suspended in a small room. Both the chair and the room may be tilted either to the left or right. In the *Room-Adjustment Test (RAT)* the room is tilted to

56 degrees and the chair, 22 degrees. With the chair remaining tilted, the subject must direct the examiner to reorient the room to an upright position. The test consists of eight trials. In four of them the room and chair are initially tilted in the same direction. In another four they are tilted in opposite directions. The degree of success with which the subject directs the examiner to reorient the room determines the scores as being field independent.

In the *Body Adjustment Test (BAT)* the room remains tilted and the subject directs the examiner to move the subject to an upright position. Once again the success with which this is done determines the subject's field-dependence score.

Rod and Frame Test (RFT)

This was the major instrument used in early field-independence research. The subject is seated in complete darkness and looks at a luminous rod that is suspended in a lighted frame. Both rod and frame can be tilted independently. The subject directs the examiner to adjust the rod to a position believed to be vertical. The degree to which the subject succeeds determines the degree to which the person is field dependent. If a subject orients the rod in relation to the frame, the individual is considered field dependent because the perceptions have been influenced by the field (frame), i.e., environment. To the degree the subject orients the rod vertically, despite the position of the frame, the person is identified as field independent.

Embedded Figure Test

This test requires that the subject locate a simple figure that is more or less hidden or obscured within a complex perceptually confusing background. Witkin used 24 figures originally developed by Gottschaldt and then superimposed color patterns on the pictures to make them even more difficult. Subjects were originally allowed five minutes to identify the figures within each of the pictures. The higher the score, the more field independent the subject was judged to be. This test has gone through several modifications. It is a popular one with children because it is easily given and is nonthreatening.

Other Types of Field Independence–Dependence Tests

These tests described so far are spatial-perceptual in nature, as indeed are many other cognitive-style measures. That they should be so is a natural consequence of the fact that cognitive styles were originally discovered in the context of perceptual experiments. Nevertheless concerns have been raised as to whether the construct of field independence-dependence is overly dependent on perceptual measures. As a consequence some researchers have attempted to study this stylistic dimension using other means. Thus Bruninks (1971) developed a language test of field independence-dependence. Subjects are shown ambiguous sentences (the field) and are required to select and interpret their structures or meanings. The degree to which they can do this is interpreted as assessing their degree of field independence. Scores on this test have been found to correlate well with scores from the traditional perceptual field independence-dependence tests, supporting Witkin's contention that it is a dimension that "pervades the individual's perceptual, intellectual, emotional, motivational . . . and social operations."

Implications of Field Independence-Dependence

Field independence represents the ability to resist inaccurate perception. Field independence-dependence researchers have almost inevitably favored field independence as being a positive attribute and regarded field dependence as being a negative one. Field-independent people almost always come out better than field-dependent ones on intellectual, emotional, social, academic, and achievement comparisons. Field-independent pupils are usually described as being brighter, more cognitively efficient, better able to solve problems, and better able to learn from their mistakes. They are also described as being more organized and definitive in their thinking and less distractible or suggestible. They are supposed to perform better on the job, be more emotionally stable, and suffer less psychiatric problems than do field-dependent individuals (Kogan, 1980a, 1980b).

In instructional situations field-independent students are described as being generally superior to field-dependent ones. Thus field-independent pupils are described as being intrinsically motivated, and field-dependent ones as learning best under conditions of external reinforcement. Field-independent pupils can supposedly provide their own structure to learning experiences and learn well using discovery methods. Field-dependent pupils on the other hand require more external guidance and appear to learn best in situations when instructional objectives are used.

Field-independent individuals have been found to be better readers in a number of investigations, both in terms of decoding and comprehension. They also appear to be better in mathematics and science. The research on these and other issues of education is, however, confounded by other factors associated with poor academic preparation, bilingual backgrounds, cognitive handicaps, etc. (Kogan, 1980a). Unless such factors, and in particular general ability factors, are carefully controlled in research (and often they are not), much of the evidence supporting the superiority of field independence over field dependence can be explained as matters of low ability, poor academic preparation, and even cultural disadvantages. We should not forget that the tests used to assess field dependence-independence are above all else tests of accuracy and judgment.

Witkin and other field independence-dependence researchers have tried to soften somewhat their earlier enthusiasm and theoretical favoritism for field independence and to reduce the negative implications of field dependence. Many normal and competent people are field-dependent according to Witkin's criteria. Thus there have been reports that field-dependent individuals may be better than field-independent ones in humanities and certain language arts and that they tend to be more intuitive and holistic in their thinking. There have, of course, been the inevitable linkages of field independence-dependence to differences in left- and right-brain functioning.

CONCEPTUAL TEMPO (REFLECTION-IMPULSIVITY)

If the field independence-dependence has been the most widely studied of all cognitive styles, it is also true that conceptual tempo has proven to be the most popular of styles for those whose interests lie with children. In fact its constructs, unlike those of field independence-dependence, were originally developed on the basis of research with children (Kagan, Rosman, Day, Albert, & Phillips, 1964; Kagan & Kogan, 1970).

Reduced to its essence, tests of this cognitive conceptual tempo assess children in respect to the different speeds with which they make decisions, usually under uncertain or ambiguous conditions. There are a number of ways in which conceptual tempo may be assessed, including teacher observation. Let us, however, examine the ways in which the construct was originally studied to understand the origins of the construct.

Kagan et al. used the *Matching Familiar Figures Test* originally to assess reflection-impulsivity. Pupils are presented with a series of 12 test pictures. They are also shown a number of alternative pictures and required to choose from among them the one that most exactly matches the ones selected by the examiner. This task requires a pupil to scan the alternatives, to make a decision as to the one that best matches the examiner's picture, to verify it to oneself, and then to respond (a situation somewhat similar to the IPP research reported in Chapter 7). The time each child takes to respond to this test is considered a measure of the tendency to reflection or impulsivity. Another measure used to assess conceptual tempo is error rate. Kagan and his associates found that both length of time and error rate correlated well with each other in an inverse direction; i.e., the more time a pupil takes to respond on this test, the less errors are usually made in identification. This tends to be true even when the pupils' verbal abilities are statistically controlled. Kagan and his associates then diagnosed pupils who responded rapidly and made numerous errors as being impulsive, while those who responded slowly and made few errors were assessed as being reflective.

When Kagan and his associates studied the relationships of conceptual tempo scores to reading test scores, their not unexpected finding was that reflective pupils did better than impulsive ones. Further research, however, showed that this relationship held only for those pupils who had good verbal ability. Pupils of low verbal ability who had general difficulties in mastering the mechanics of reading were little affected in their reading performance by conceptual tempo. Being reflective or impulsive made little difference to a pupil with poor reading skills. In contrast these styles clearly appeared to affect the performance of the high verbal ability pupils who were ordinarily competent in reading. Reflective high verbal ability pupils did better than impulsive ones on the reading tests. Pupils with impulsive high verbal ability were both hasty and inaccurate in their answers.

Following Kagan and his colleagues' original studies was a lag of interest in conceptual tempo. Then interest in the reflection-impulsivity dimension picked up and has continued despite concern about the validity of the tests used to assess it and about the dimension's dubious reliance on both error and rate of responding scores for evaluating conceptual tempo. The utility of the dimension in explaining school success and failure and its demonstrated relationship to positive and negative behaviors appear to assure its continued popularity in school and clinic (Blackman & Goldstein, 1982).

Implications of Conceptual Tempo

As might be expected, research into conceptual tempo generally favors reflection over impulsivity. A reflective cognitive style is usually found more compatible than an impulsive one with school achievement and good adjustment achievement. In academic performances the impulsive child is frequently described as confusing speed with achievement, as acting on hunches with little thought, and of responding to superficial or misleading cues. This child is also described as being an uncritical thinker, of formulating superficial answers, of being deficient in problem solving. Perhaps most important of all, impulsivity has been found to characterize many behaviorally disturbed children (Meichenbaum, 1977).

In contrast, reflective children are described as being thoughtful, persistent, and careful in their schoolwork. Though typically slower than impulsive children, they carry out their assignments more systematically and are more successful in achieving their goals. They have also been found to be superior over impulsive children in respect to a variety of specific cognitive measures including visual discrimination, serial learning, inductive learning, word recognition, and intelligence. Behaviorally, reflective children are more likely to be well adjusted than impulsive ones are (Blackman & Goldstein, 1982).

However, in support of Kogan, who advises that what may appear impulsive under one set of circumstances may in fact be associated with superior achievement, not all rapid responders after all are deficient cognitively or behaviorally. Furthermore, impulsive, unthinking behavior and a high error rate are sometimes more indicative of cognitive impairments than of a particular cognitive style.

Recent Trends

As discussed in Chapter 3, there is intense interest in the distinctions between left-brain and right-brain functioning. Some researchers believe differences in the functioning of the two cerebral hemispheres may be associated with difference in cognitive styles. Thus we read of right-brain persons being more intuitive or global in their thinking and of left-brain ones being more logical and rigid in theirs (Bogen, 1977; Alesandrini, Langstaff, & Wittrock, 1984).

The 1983 emergence of the *Kaufman Assessment Battery for Children* has brought an effort to differentiate serial from simultaneous information-processing styles. There have also been efforts to convince teachers that they should teach their pupils differently, depending on their processing preference, i.e., whether they tend to emphasize serial or simultaneous processing of information when they learn (Reynolds & Miller, 1984).

ALTERING COGNITIVE STYLES

It is human nature to seek improvement. Certainly remedial and special educators are loath to accept an evaluation of a pupil's weaknesses or deficiencies without making efforts to correct them. Definitions of cognitive styles emphasize the fact that they are enduring characteristics. They also emphasize that cognitive styles are created through the interaction of hereditary and environmental factors. Since environmental influences are important in determining cognitive styles, it would also appear that they might play an important role in changing them. And indeed many efforts have been made to alter specific cognitive styles, e.g., to make a pupil more field-independent or reflective or more differentiated conceptually—depending on what a particular researcher, teacher, or therapist deems important (Blackman & Goldstein, 1982).

One of the problems confronting efforts to change cognitive styles is misidentification of changes in test scores with actual cognitive-personality alterations. It is possible, for example, to train a pupil to do better on various field-independent tests. But has the pupil become more field independent? More likely than not, we have simply taught the pupil to perform better on a particular type of test without increasing field independence.

Nevertheless, successful efforts in changing cognitive styles have been reported, though success is more likely with some cognitive styles than with others. It appears easier, for example, to help pupils develop more reflective cognitive styles than it is to help them become truly more field independent. The latter may be more deeply based on inherited cognitive structures (Kogan, 1980a).

APTITUDE TREATMENT INTERACTION

It would be an impossible task to try to improve all of a particular pupil's cognitive styles. It is also unlikely that we can change any one of them beyond a certain point. Thus some researchers have sought ways to individualize instruction according to particular pupils' cognitive styles in the hopes that this might help them become better learners. Such efforts often proceed under the aegis of aptitude treatment interaction (ATI) studies. For example, ATI efforts have been made to determine whether there are whole word–part whole reading approaches interacting with conceptual tempo. It would seem that impulsive children should do best in a whole word approach, while reflective ones would do better on part–whole training efforts. The results of such studies do not offer any great hopes of an instructional breakthrough. True, the impulsive pupils were found to do as well as reflective pupils on whole word recognition training. And the reflective pupils were found to do better on part–whole word recognition training. Nevertheless, impulsive pupils did just as well in part–whole training as they did in whole word training (Kogan, 1980b).

A major problem with cognitive-style ATI studies is the overwhelming influence of general ability factors (Messick, 1976). Nevertheless it would appear reasonable to expect that remedial and special education teachers become generally conversant with their pupils' cognitive styles if for no other reason than to anticipate variations in their academic performances.

LEARNING STYLES

Frequently, a distinction has been made between learner styles and cognitive styles. The distinction between the two is arbitrary. What we called *learner styles* encompass cognitive styles, and cognitive styles constitute learner styles. Learning style constructs, however, are much more classroom-oriented, more instruction-oriented, than are traditional cognitive styles. Unlike cognitive styles, which have been studied in and applied to a broad variety of conditions outside schools, learner styles are almost always identified with schools and in instructional contexts. There is considerable literature on the implications of cognitive style for personal adjustment, psychiatric disorder, job success, achievement in the armed services, etc. Learner styles are not ordinarily related to such areas. They tend to be school-bound.

Another way that learning styles can be differentiated from cognitive styles is that they—at least most of them—are more oriented to environmental events. While cognitive-style researchers study the particular ways in which individuals respond to their environments, learning-style researchers are more likely to study the ways that these environments affect the individual. One does not often read of cognitive-style researchers being concerned with the effects of such situational variables as the warmth of a classroom or the hardness of a pupil's seat or the quality of lighting when studying. Learning-style researchers, in constrast, are often interested in such environmental features. And learning styles are often defined in terms of the ways that pupils respond to such external aspects of learning.

Still, cognitive-style researchers usually study a particular cognitive style in depth to the exclusion of others, while learning-style researchers are often found to concern themselves with large numbers of stylistic variables and their interrelationships.

Finally, and most important of all, learning styles are specifically studied for the purpose of improving instruction. Whereas cognitive styles are also sometimes studied for this purpose, this has usually been secondary to their study as psychological characteristics. To put it in other terms, the study of cognitive styles is typically carried out for descriptive purposes, i.e., to understand the individual, while learning styles are usually studied prescriptively, i.e., to determine how best to help that individual succeed in school. Research into learning styles is thus not a matter of abstract scientific interest but rather a way "to make decisions about what students would learn and which methods would most effectively accomplish the desired outcomes" (Holland, 1982, p. 8).

How many learning styles are there and how important are any of them? The numbers are many. Rita Dunn (1983), in a recent review of "Learning Styles and Its Relation to Exceptionality at Both Ends of the Spectrum" wrote that most people have between 6 and 14 learning-style elements that affect them strongly.

DEFINITIONS OF LEARNING STYLES

Learning styles can be defined simply in terms of the way that a pupil's characteristics, including needs and preferences, stylistically affect learning, or even more simply as ways that a pupil learns. Bennett (1979) and Dunn and Dunn (1975, 1977, 1979) provide more elaborate definitions. According to Bennett, learning style may be defined as a "student's preferred way of learning. It represents a cluster of personality and mental characteristics that influence how a pupil perceives, remembers, thinks and solves problems" (Holland, 1982, p. 8). According to Dunn and Dunn learning style is a phenomenon that "(a) varies among individuals, (b) is identifiable, and (c) requires complimentary [i.e., individualized] instructional methodology as to . . . teaching styles" (Holland, 1982, pp. 8–9).

A more recent definition from Rita Dunn (1983) is that learning style represents "the way individuals concentrate on, absorb, and retain new or difficult information or skills" (p. 496). In keeping with the information-processing vogue, Dunn (1983) goes on to say that "style consists of a combination of physical, psychological, emotional, and widespread elements that affect the ways individuals . . . receive, store and use knowledge or abilities" (p. 496–497).

Learning styles can be defined in terms of "accessibility characteristics, i.e., particular cognitive and motivational orientations which can be aligned with optimal instructional approaches" (Hunt, 1974).

TAXONOMIES OF LEARNING STYLES

As discussed, the topic of learning style is a broader, more encompassing one than that of cognitive styles. Indeed taxonomies of learning styles often include traditional cognitive styles. Our review of learning styles, guided by Holland's exposition in the *Journal of Special Education* (1982), reveals an extraordinary range of variables that have been studied as part of this topic.

Cognitive Learning Styles

Cognitive-style variables have been used to individualize instruction. While Ausburn and Ausburn (1978) advise against efforts to alter cognitive styles because they are so resistive to change, they suggest "planned *supplementation* involving overt alteration of the task requirement [so as to make it more compatible with the pupils' cognitive style] with which the learner is having difficulty" (Holland, 1982, p. 8).

Ausburn and Ausburn (1978) provide the following list of cognitive styles that should be studied for this purpose. These include styles that are quite familiar, while others are of the same or similar vintages: field independence–dependence, scanning, breadth of categorizing, conceptual styles, reflectivity-impulsivity, cognitive complexity, leveling-sharpening, constricted-flexible control, tolerance for unrealistic experiences, risk taking-cautiousness, and visual-haptic perceptual-type.

Geogoric (1979) has also identified a number of cognitive learning styles that he believes are directly related to the demands of instruction. They indicate a student's preference for a particular learning source and whether the pupil prefers to learn through concrete or abstract means. Four types of learning styles can thus be distinguished:

1. Abstract-sequential. Pupils of this type prefer to deal with abstract concepts and symbols and prefer to do so through formally organized and systematically paced instruction.
2. Concrete-sequential learners. Pupils of this sort prefer learning through concrete experiences, such as sensorimotor supports. Like abstract sequential learners, they learn better in a systematic, sequential way.
3. Abstract-random learners. This type of pupil prefers abstract conceptual modes of learning but prefers to learn in unstructured unsystematic ways.
4. Concrete-random learners. This sort of pupil prefers concrete learning experiences and wishes to learn through trial-and-error methods.

D.L. Hunt (1975a) has proposed a conceptual levels (CL) learning-style model that embodies dimensions of cognitive complexity, maturity, independence, and adaptability to social environments.

Status Variables

Status variables are learner characteristics that "correspond to a person's membership in different social groups" (Holland, 1982, p. 10). The stylistic aspects of learning created by status variables are, with the exception of age, assigned by birth. For example, sex and race are status variables.

A great deal of research has been devoted to the influence of status variables on learning. There are also major debates as to their importance and whether they are amenable to alteration. These have been both recommendations for and protests against different types of instruction for different types of racial or social groups. Since the 1960s the issue of gender-based learner characteristics has become a topic of increasing debate. Questions have been raised as to whether mathematical ability is a sex-linked ability, i.e., a status variable.

The relationship of age to learning status has been a less controversial topic than either race or sex, but it too is an unsettled topic. Does the nature of cognition, a child's learning styles, and what the child is able to learn, suddenly and dramatically shift from one age or from one developmental level to another as Piaget (1952) has advised? Or is it rather as Bruner (1966) at one time suggests—a matter of a child being able to learn particular things at any age, if taught properly and appropriately? Must younger or developmentally less able pupils necessarily solve problems differently from older, cognitively able ones, as again Piaget indicates, or can they be taught to function as well cognitively with proper training as some cognitive strategy researchers appear to suggest (see Chapter 9)?

Environmental Factors

While traditional cognitive-style researchers do not overly concern themselves with environmental influences on cognition, learning-style researchers tend to take them quite seriously. Dunn and Dunn (1979) have identified four major environmental learning-style elements: (1) sound, (2) light, (3) temperature, and (4) design. Based on their research and observations they have concluded that these elements can play a significant role in learning regardless of a pupil's ability or socioeconomic or achievement level since "students respond uniquely to their immediate environment" (Holland, 1982, p. 11).

Dunn and Dunn (1979) believe that sensitivity to light is a major environmental learning-style characteristic. A particular pupil may be unable to study well under strong lights, while another cannot do so under dim lighting conditions. Some types of pupils are affected by variations in light that most other pupils ignore.

Dunn and Dunn also identify sound variables as important learning elements perhaps equal to the theory of light. Sound variables also affect learners differently. Some pupils become distracted at the slightest noise. Others actually seem to benefit from noisy surroundings; we all know of pupils who study well listening to rock music. Some pupils benefit from certain types of sound, i.e., "white sound" that appears to block out distractions or otherwise stabilize them when they are trying to learn. Music may facilitate routine learning but interfere with the learning of complex materials.

Dunn and Dunn (1977) also determined that there are stylistic differences in the way that pupils respond to temperature while learning. Some pupils are most attentive in a cool environment, while warm surroundings impair their concentration. Other learners become tense and irritable if the immediate environment is overly cool; a warm room makes them less distractible, more attentive.

As to design variables, Dunn and Dunn make a major distinction between informal and formal physical designs for learning. Some pupils learn best under informal conditions—lying on a carpet, flopping about in a lounge chair, or sprawling on a bean bag. Others need formal physical conditions to remain on task. They seem to learn best when seated at a desk, perhaps on a hard-backed chair, or under library conditions.

As the case for most learning-style elements, different environmental factors affect individuals differently. Some pupils are barely affected by any of the factors discussed. For others, they may be important learning-style variables.

Personality Factors

Cognitive styles first emerged from concern about the effect of personality factors on cognition. It was inevitable that they incorporated personality factors, including those of an attitudinal and emotional nature. Many learner styles also incorporate personality factors.

Hunt's complexity (CL) model developed with older learners takes into consideration such personality-emotional factors as level of independence, level of achievement motivation, need for affiliation, anxiety level, and locus of control, all of which have been areas of intensive investigation for researchers interested in the influence of personality on cognition and performance.

Dunn and Dunn have reported four emotional elements of learning style that appear to be particularly relevant to basic education. These are (1) motivation, (2) persistence, (3) responsibility, and (4) structure. Motivated learners are usually persistent and assume responsibility; they impose structure on learning tasks or seek it out; i.e., they try to obtain explanations and to determine the resources available to them. They are likely to welcome praise and teacher feedback after they have accomplished their tasks.

Unmotivated learners are usually not persistent and are less responsible. They benefit from shorter assignments and fewer objectives. They respond best, when learning, to a great deal of teacher supervision and clearly defined objectives.

Sociological Needs

Dunn and Dunn believe that pupils' ability to learn is also partly determined by sociological patterns (Holland, 1982). Some students do better cognitively when working alone. Others do better working with one or two friends. Still others learn more effectively in small groups or as part of a team. Some pupils learn better in relationships to adults, others through relationships with peers. Some pupils function at their best cognitively in a direct-line relationship with a teacher or other authority. There are pupils who need varying combinations to do their best.

Physical Needs

Dunn and Dunn have delineated a number of physical need variables that they also believe are important to academic functioning. These include modality factors. They believe that perceptual preferences play an important role in learning. They believe that 20 to 30 percent of pupils are auditory learners, approximately 40 percent are visual learners, and the remaining 30 to 40 percent are either tactual kinesthetic or visual tactual in preference or learn best through a combination of four senses. From this standpoint lectures and teaching through lectures (an auditory approach) are not appropriate for many students.

Dunn and Dunn also observe that other physical characteristics or needs neglected by most teachers may nevertheless influence cognitive functioning and through it academic learning. Thus some students have a need to eat, chew, drink, or smoke when studying. Some students learn best in the norms, others must move about during periods of learning; the latter are often judged hyperactive.

Contextual Characteristics

While some learning styles are stable across all types of cognitive functioning, others are situational in nature and are chosen for particular purposes. Thus students may study some types of materials for purposes of understanding them, others simply for the purpose of providing answers that satisfy the teacher. Pupils study differently for one type of test than for another; we all have heard of multiple-choice mentalities. The style through which a pupil learns may thus be adapted as a particular learning or cognitive strategy (see Chapter 9).

ASSESSMENT OF LEARNING STYLES

Cognitive styles are typically assessed through tests of various kinds. Some of these tests are of a laboratory variety, such as Witkin's rod-and-frame test. Others are paper-and-pencil tests, e.g., the *Hidden Figures Tests*.

Learning-style researchers and theorists certainly have relied upon such types of instruments. In addition, however, learning-style investigators also obtain information for learning-style constructs from behavioral checklists, inventories, and questionnaires. One of these is the *Edmond Learning Style Identification Exercise (ELSIE)* (Reinert, 1976). It identifies four major avenues through which students acquire information: (1) visualization, (2) written word, (3) listening, and (4) activity. Pupils identify their own needs and learning-style profiles to discover the way their styles are patterned or combined.

Another instrument is the *Learning Style Inventory (LSI)*, which was developed to determine pupils' learning preferences for 24 different elements of learning style, many of which we have studied in this chapter (Price, Dunn, & Dunn, 1977). They follow along the theoretical lines formulated by the Dunns. There are four major groupings, according to four basic learning "stimulants": (1) environment and the student, (2) emotional, (3) sociological, and (4) physical learning patterns. The responses from the *LSI* tend "to reveal highly personalized characteristics that, when combined, represent the way in which an individual learns with maximum ease" (Holland, 1982, p. 11).

Some researchers have studied pupils' language as a means for determining their learning styles. Along these lines, others have carried out research that suggests the language people use is indicative of the ways they process information; i.e., learners use words that are related to their preferred ways of responding to information.

Learning-style researchers are clearly making efforts to develop not only reliable and valid assessment learning-style instruments but also ones that have practical usefulness. The same cautions must be raised about their efforts as for tests used to evaluate cognitive styles. One cannot be sure the results from particular assessment results mean the same thing for different pupils at different ages or from different cultures or of different cognitive abilities. Teachers interested in assessing learning styles will surely want to become knowledgeable about learning-style assessment. But they should rely on their own observations and judgments to evaluate their pupils' learning styles.

TRAINING AND REMEDIATION IN LEARNING STYLES

Most cognitive remedial approaches attempt to correct deficient cognitive characteristics, whether of structure, process, or content, or to develop new ones. Another approach to cognitive remediation of which aptitude-treatment interaction is an example is to adapt instruction to meet or match the pupil's characteristics. Hunt has thus defined *learning styles* as representing "accessibility characteristics" against which "may be aligned a particular teaching approach that is attuned to the learner's needs." This is the type of remedial intervention that is most likely to be attempted on the basis of learning styles.

Fantini (1980) has sounded the call to action in respect to this in his statement that "we appear to be at a stage presently in which the notion of designing programs to fit learners is replacing the older notion of fitting learners to standard programs." Learning-style researchers thus write of tailoring instructional approaches to fit individual pupils, even of matching teachers' teaching styles to pupils' learning styles, of adjusting instruction and teaching styles as the pupils' learning styles change. The executive director of the National Association of Secondary School Principals Scott D. Thompson hailed the mapping learning style as the "most important development in curricula and instruction in a generation . . . and the most scientific known to individualized instruction" (Dunn, 1983, p. 805).

Efforts to match instruction to learning style are nothing new. Educators have been trying to identify individual pupil differences and to adjust instruction to them for many years. Many of the learning-style enthusiasts simply do not appear to be aware of the history of similar efforts when putting in their claims for identifying a new and pioneering way of education individualization. They do, however, appear to be unique with respect to the fact that they so frequently address a multitude of learning characteristics that affect instruction, and in learning style their radiating of environments towards different learner characteristics so as to take into consideration the full range of classroom events.

When learning-style interventionists claim positive results for their methods (Dunn & Dunn, 1975), they nevertheless appear more successful in changing emotional attitudes and behaviors than in dramatically improving academic achievement.

CONCLUSIONS ABOUT LEARNING STYLES

Interest in learning styles is another modern recognition of individual pupil differences. This interest encompasses an extraordinary range of pupil characteristics. It is also different in the emphases it gives to the influence of environmental factors. To make these points, the readers need only compare the research efforts of learning-style researchers to those of cognitive-style researchers.

Many cognitive theorists claim that their methods have special implications for education and for remediation. The claims of learning style researchers to have developed particularly powerful new tools of cognitive management must be interpreted in this light. These claims must also be called into question on other grounds. Though learning-style researchers can reliably assess a variety of learning-style characteristics in a statistically reliable way, it is questionable whether many learning style elements are practically reliable. That is, it is doubtful whether they are reliable guides under conditions of either classroom instruction or remediation. Statistically significant results in an experiment don't necessarily have implications for classroom practice. Broad cognitive variables are usually more useful in predicting relevant achievement than are specific ones. This also seems true for learning-style variables, of which there are so many.

Second, many of the learning-style characteristics may be reliable in the sense that they help us to discriminate one pupil from another. But that doesn't mean they are important. Does the need to chew gum play an important role in learning? Does sitting on a soft chair versus a hard one significantly affect learning? Is there any definitive evidence that pupils learn better at one time of day than another even though they may feel more comfortable at different times or that learning in groups of two rather than in those of three will significantly improve academic achievement? Attention to too many learning styles may distract teachers from the most important of them.

Third, isn't it essential that pupils learn to adjust to situations with which they may not be stylistically comfortable? Should we let girls, let us say, who tend to be less comfortable with mathematics shirk advanced algebra because it doesn't fit in with their learning styles, when we know that if they stick with it, they can master it as well as boys, who are more positively oriented to mathematics? Do we want our pupils to expect that the world will always adjust to them?

Finally, there are limits to which schools, teachers, and instructors can be accommodated to individual pupil needs. It thus would appear to behoove teachers to identify the most important of learner-style elements, which are likely to be few, and to make modest educational adjustments for their pupils according to them, rather than to offer instruction on the basis of a laundry list of learning styles.

CONCLUSIONS

Teachers should become knowledgeable about their pupils' cognitive and learning styles in the most expeditious ways possible and use their knowledge to become more aware of the pupil as a particular learning person rather than the styles as specific guides to alter their instruction. Because they usually work with small groups or on an individual basis, remedial and special educators may be better able than a regular classroom teacher to apply this knowledge. Thus a remedial reading teacher might be able to adjust remedial efforts according to information about their pupil's cognitive and learning styles, while a special education teacher could use them as guides for individualizing educational programs. There is much work to be done, however, before knowledge of either cognitive or learning styles will do more than provide general hints for such purposes.

Chapter 9

Cognitive Strategies and Metacognition

The study of cognitive strategies and metacognition (a particular type of cognitive strategies) is proving a most active and productive area for modern cognitive education (Sternberg & Wagner, 1984).

What are *cognitive strategies* and what is *metacognition*? We try to provide precise definitions of both. For the moment let us content ourselves with a general explanation. They represent "executive" cognitive processes that we can use to monitor, control, and manage our cognitive functioning. They are mediators of learning and performance (see Chapter 2).

Cognitive strategies have been studied under various names for a long time. Among early-twentieth-century investigators are Duncker (1945), Bruner, Goodnow, and Austin (1956), Polya (1957, 1968), and Wertheimer (1959). Among post–World War II pioneers the names of Miller, Galanter, and Pribam (1960) stand out. To Bruner and his associates may belong the credit for first using the term *strategies* in the sense that it is interpreted in this chapter. Piaget's work also has been inspirational to the study of strategies (Brown & Palincsar, 1982). It appears, however, that the information-processing paradigm has influenced the course of cognitive strategy research and training.

FIXED AND MODIFIABLE COGNITIVE CHARACTERISTICS

Perhaps the most important contribution that information-processing theory has made to the study of cognitive strategy is its distinctions between fixed and modifiable cognitive characteristics. IPS structures such as the STM, WM, and LTM and their component parts represent fixed unmodifiable cognitive capacity variables, while such IPS cognitive processes as attention, chunking, rehearsal, organization, and imagery represent modifiable control processes.

The distinction between fixed and modifiable cognitive characteristics is clearly an important one to remedial and special education. It makes the point that cognitive functioning is determined both by inherited characteristics, which place limits on what we can do, and by modifiable characteristics, which are affected by our experience and training. Second, it poses a challenge to remedial and special education to distinguish between the types of cognitive dysfunctioning that are actually attributable to unalterable cognitive deficiencies or defects, and the ones that are due to modifiable inadequacies that can be corrected through training and remediation. The ability to distinguish between fixed and modifiable cognitive characteristics can be important in determining whether pupils are doing poorly in school because of a handicap or because of cultural deprivation or poor instruction.

The distinction between unmodifiable capacities and modifiable process variables opens special avenues of intervention to remedial and special educators. The specific ability approaches reviewed in Chapter 5 usually attempt to improve cognitive disabilities by directly training or remediating the pupils' abilities or capacities. The approach suggested by the IPP is quite different: It acknowledges that unalterable cognitive limitations are sometimes responsible for academic difficulties; it suggests (conversely) that some pupils who have perfectly adequate cognitive capacities will still do poorly academically because they have problems in controlling their cognitive functioning; it proposes that pupils who have cognitive limitations can sometimes compensate for them or even overcome them by learning to control and direct their cognitive processes strategically; and cognitive strategies of various sorts have been proposed to help them do this.

DEFINITION OF COGNITIVE STRATEGIES

The *Random House Dictionary of the English Language* provides a useful general definition of strategies that will help us understand cognitive strategies somewhat better: "[Strategy] 4, a plan, method, or series of maneuvers or stratagems for obtaining a specific goal or result" (1966) ed., s.v. "strategy"). Strategies, according to this definition, are planned ways of doing things. Thus, cognitive strategies are planned ways of using one's cognitive abilities to achieve specific goals or results. These are the ways that cognitive researcher Underwood (1978b) interprets cognitive strategies:

> When information is presented to an individual the sequence of processing is not pre-determined, but the individual is able to select certain processes and reject others. The view here is that the individual's response may be structurally limited, but that in the strategies used by the processor—the individual plays a vital role. (p. 2)

Young (1978) states:

> The notion of strategy is intimately bound up with fact that many tasks can be carried out in several different ways. . . . [It may be supposed] that . . . every-one has at his command a number of different strategies from which he chooses according to the occasion. . . . Each strategy is seen to be a self-contained module of problem-solving ability, pertaining to a particular task or part of a task. . . . [There is an] . . . analogy between strategies and the subroutines used by computer programmers to organize [their] programs." (pp. 357–358)

Cognitive strategies and metacognition are closely related; indeed, the latter is really a special variation of the former though we distinguish between both for purposes of research and training. Since cognitive strategies are the more basic of the two, they are discussed first.

COGNITIVE STRATEGIES

From an educational standpoint, cognitive strategies are types of procedural knowledge or cognitive techniques to guide pupils in their use of cognitive resources. They are to be distinguished from the pupils' abilities (structural capacities) and background of knowledge. They are rather the means by which those abilities and that knowledge are channeled, directed, and expressed. The cognitive strategies a pupil uses are a matter of choice (though not always consciously chosen or used). The pupil chooses to apply abilities and uses particular types of information in certain ways to solve particular problems.

Interdependence of Cognitive Strategies and Cognitive Capacities

Earlier in this chapter we distinguished between cognitive capacities (structures) and cognitive strategies (processes). It would be a mistake, however, to assume that the two operate independently of each other.

For one, the nature of our cognitive capacities ultimately determines and limits the cognitive strategies that we learn and our ability to use them. As Underwood (1978b) has pointed out, "structural limitations can only be overcome by the strategical manipulation[s] within those limitations" (p. 3). A child will use different strategies than does an adult because its cognitive capacities are less developed. A gifted child has a wider and more sophisticated variety of cognitive strategies at its disposal than does a mentally retarded child. The child who is deaf may be deficient in certain cognitive strategies because of language deficiencies. If Piaget is correct, a physically impaired child will have problems in developing cognitive strategies because the child is unable to develop comprehensive sensorimotor schemata. It is doubtful that teaching profoundly retarded pupils reading strategies will ever help them to become proficient in reading.

On the other hand the nature of our cognitive strategies determines in large part how our capacities are used. It would be a mistake to assume that a pupil will do well in school simply because of a high IQ. It is equally a mistake to believe that a pupil of lower ability, or with special disabilities, will necessarily do poorly in school. The strategies that these pupils use, as well as their abilities, will play major roles in determining how well they perform.

An Overview of Cognitive Strategies

Cognitive strategies are of particular interest because they suggest ways of modifying the cognitive functioning of pupils who have learning problems or handicaps. They have, however, much broader implications, for they encompass all of the ways that people think and solve problems.

All of us—the gifted, the underachiever, the handicapped—are constantly using cognitive strategies to direct our thinking and behavior. The carrying processes a pupil chooses in simple addition are strategic in nature. Checking one's schoolwork or accuracy is a strategic approach. The way a pupil takes notes or studies for a test is selectively determined by particular strategies. We use some strategies because we are genetically programmed to do so. We use other strategies because of the ways our personalities work or because of our special cognitive styles. We learn some strategies in an informal way. We learn others in formal training.

Some cognitive strategies are general. We apply them to a variety of situations; attentiveness and good study habits are among these. Other cognitive strategies are applicable only to special academic tasks, e.g., phonic skills, learning to carry, knowing how to apply algebraic algorithms. We sometimes use long-term strategies, as when we make systematic plans to go to college. And there are short-term ones, as when we figure out ways to answer multiple-choice test questions. Training in cognitive strategies may thus range from teaching general "thinking skills" to teaching "splinter" academic ones. Good learning is dependent on good strategies. So is good teaching, for that matter.

Not all cognitive strategies are helpful or effective. Some are incorrect or inadequate. Others are actually maladaptive. Many errors in schoolwork can be attributed to the use of improper cognitive strategies. If we wish to train children to use good strategies, it is often necessary to train them to stop using poor ones. Indeed the training of cognitive strategies is frequently a matter of replacing ineffective or even harmful cognitive strategies with others that work. Finally, some pupils don't use good strategies even when they know how to use them; this is often true of poorly motivated underachievers.

Awareness of Using Cognitive Strategies

Underwood's (1978a, 1978b) definition of cognitive strategies might suggest that they are purposely and knowingly applied and with conscious intention in mind. This is sometimes the case, but most often not. Most of us are not aware of using cognitive strategies even as we use them. And we rarely become conscious of using them unless they are called to our attention. Indeed we appear most often conscious of strategies when we first acquire them. They then move to subconscious levels, where they tend to monitor our performances without any further awareness on our part, though we may become conscious of them again when we are confronted with a novel or perplexing problem.

A concert pianist utilizes cognitive strategies when playing. It is often a pianist's superior strategies that distinguish   the artist from the technician. Both types of pianists might have equal technical skills, but the former possesses a greater (strategic) grasp of the music and directs playing skills to greater advantage. In any case, while a pianist may be conscious of strategically controlling playing during practice, this is not true during an actual concert. Otherwise, the person would be too self-conscious to play effectively. In fact the best cognitive strategies may be the ones that we are able to use without being conscious of them.

Automatizing cognitive functioning, i.e., as a means of making it more efficient, is a topic of increasing importance for cognitive remediation (Samuels, 1979; Sternberg & Wagner, 1981). This might be one of the reasons that Young (1978) suggests Newell and Simon's concept production systems be used along with cognitive strategies: "Production systems . . . [are to be defined as automatically analyzing] . . . problem solving into components which specify . . . what the child does . . . [utilizing a particular] set of production [strategies]" (p. 397).

Role of Strategies in Cognitive Difficulties

Baron (1978) has attempted to clarify the different types of cognitive limitations that affect a child's performance of school tasks. Failure to achieve may be due to failure to use appropriate cognitive strategies, inadequate proficiency in the use of strategies, or limited cognitive capacities.

In respect to the first of the limitations, Baron suggests that many cognitive failures, and seeming cognitive impairments, are attributable to the fact that a pupil hasn't yet acquired proper cognitive strategies. For example, older children who are instructed to learn a list of items usually rehearse the list's items in order to remember them. In contrast younger children and the mentally retarded rarely employ rehearsal strategies unless they are specifically trained to do so. They may thus fail on memory tasks that they are able to perform. By teaching younger children and mentally retarded pupils to use appropriate cognitive strategies, we can improve their "memory" to a considerable degree.

In respect to the second type of cognitive limitations, Baron states that training a child to use cognitive strategies may not be enough to improve the child's functioning. Children who know strategies equally well often differ in their ability to use them. It is necessary, then, not only to teach our pupils the cognitive strategies they need. We must also help them become proficient in their use. Repetitive training and extensive practice under a wide range of conditions help to achieve this goal.

As to the third type of cognitive limitation, a child, though proficient in the use of cognitive strategies, eventually reaches a level where the pupil cannot improve performance of a task. This is likely to be an indication that the child has reached the limits of cognitive capacities. Capacity limitations play a dual role here. These, Baron, points out, not only set a ceiling on a child's achievement; they also determine how effectively the child can use particular cognitive strategies. Nevertheless Baron appears to believe that most academic failures can be attributed to surmountable strategy difficulties rather than capacity limitations.

CLASSIFICATION OF COGNITIVE STRATEGIES

Cognitive strategies can be classified in all sorts of ways. We can do it in terms of the particular areas we are studying, e.g., perception or memory. We can do so along particular theoretical lines, e.g., IPP or Piagetian. We can also do it in terms of academic application, e.g., reading strategies, addition strategies, spelling strategies. Our interest in this section is in the broader issues of classification.

Along these lines Baron (1978) has suggested that we categorize strategies in three ways: (1) central strategies, basic to the development of others; (2) general strategies, applicable to a variety of situations; and (3) specific strategies, pertaining to particular types of application.

Newell (1979), an IPP theorist, has addressed the classification of strategies somewhat differently, using the metaphor of an inverted cone of strategic skills. At the bottom of this cone are large numbers of solutions or strategies, each of which applies only to specific types of problems. These strategies are powerful, and when properly used, they should solve the problems to which they are applied. However, they have only limited applicability; i.e., they apply only to special types of problems or work only under specific conditions.

As one moves up Newell's hypothetical strategy cone, there is a trade-off between strategies' power and their generalizability. At the cone's tip (on top) are a few highly general strategies. These are applicable to almost any kind of problem-solving situation. But they are as weak as they are general. One by itself is inadequate to solve any specific problem. Thus the general strategy of checking schoolwork is useful in many areas of schoolwork. But it isn't sufficient by itself to solve any specific problem. A pupil can't solve an algebra problem simply by checking the work. That pupil must also apply strategies that apply specifically to algebra problems.

Is it better to teach general or specific strategies? Both types of training may be needed. Training in study skills is a type of general strategy training that will help most students in most situations. Training in the application of specific strategies, e.g., algorithms, is needed to help pupils deal specifically with algebra problems. Cognitive-strategy researchers and trainers are confronted with many problems when they study or train specific strategies. This is because there are many different strategies that pupils can use when dealing with the same academic tasks. The computer is increasingly being used to assist in the identification of specific strategies and strategy deficiencies (Brown & Burton, 1978).

It may be that remedial and special educators will find it is most useful to train intermediate-level cognitive strategies. These strategies possess moderate generality, yet have some relatively specific applications (Brown & Palincsar, 1982). Proper left-to-right reading procedures are examples of this sort. So are the rules that govern addition-carrying procedures.

AGE AND ABILITY DIFFERENCES IN COGNITIVE STRATEGIES

While age differences obviously influence cognition to an enormous degree, we have not given it much attention in this book except in Chapter 6. Its importance in this particular chapter is due to the fact that a number of cognitive theorists believe that younger children often are at a disadvantage in learning compared to older pupils because they haven't learned to use strategies effectively, rather than because they lack ability (capacities) (Brown, 1978; Loper, 1982).

When younger children are compared to olders ones on a variety of memory tasks, e.g., requiring them to learn a list of pictures for later accurate recall (in the same order), a number of differences are found. Kindergartners don't typically rehearse the information they are learning nor do they chunk it or check on their performances. They sometimes don't even seem to be able to orient themselves to school tasks. Normal fourth-graders can carry out all of these (chunking, checking, orienting) strategies effectively. Their recall is thus much better than that of kindergartners. Yet it has proven possible to train kindergartners to use cognitive strategies so effectively that their memory performances can be quite similar and almost equal to that of older children, though this has been done under research rather than real-life situations. This has raised expectations that similar successes can be achieved with cognitively impaired pupils. Indeed researchers have found that mentally retarded learners who are taught the right cognitive strategies can improve their functioning on certain tasks to a level where it is about as good as that of normal learners (Belmont & Butterfield, 1971; Zeaman & House, 1963).

The success of strategic training with developmentally mature and developmentally handicapped pupils has encouraged many cognitive educators to believe that cognitive strategy training can improve or overcome many, if not most, of the cognitive deficiencies that learning disabled and retarded pupils suffer from (Cavanaugh & Borkowski, 1980).

TRAINING OF PUPILS IN THE USE OF COGNITIVE STRATEGIES

The goals of cognitive strategy training include the surmounting of cognitive limitations and impairments, compensation for cognitive limitations or impairments, and more efficient academic learning by pupils with or without cognitive or academic problems.

A great deal of research is going on to determine how cognitive strategy training can be carried out, and a number of researchers have offered guidelines for the teaching of cognitive strategies. Belmont and Butterfield (1971) have provided the following suggestions:

- The trainer must be able to describe accurately the strategies that pupils need to solve the problem (cognitive task analysis is a way of doing this; see Chapter 11).
- The strategies and behaviors a child uses to perform a particular task must be directly measurable.
- The trainer must be able to specify how well the pupils should do in order to conclude that a particular type of cognitive strategic training is successful.

Hagen and colleagues (1982) suggest that the following procedures are required for the successful implementation of cognitive strategy training program:

- selection of task-appropriate problem-solving strategies
- implementation in use of selected strategic routines for problems of a similar nature
- on-line adjustment and revision of strategic behaviors to accommodate changes in task demands
- monitoring to determining how well the use of the strategies is proceeding

The following are recommendations for the training of strategic trainers (Brown & Palincsar, 1982; Cavanaugh & Borkowski, 1980):

- The specific task that is performed should be divided into capacity and strategy requirements.
- The instructor should determine whether the pupils can spontaneously use the strategies necessary to perform the task. If essential strategies are missing or deficient, the pupils should be trained in their use.
- Once pupils have learned a strategy, they should be trained so that they will be able to use it effectively whenever conditions warrant.
- Pupils should be trained to transfer or generalize the strategies they learn to a variety of tasks (other than those on which they were originally trained).
- Pupils should be taught or trained to monitor their strategy production and the ways that strategies interact with and affect the use of their abilities (capacities and skills) so as to understand how to best cope with school tasks.
- Pupils should be motivated to use their strategies. They may even need motivation training to help them learn the proper use of strategies and to be willing and ready to apply the strategies as needed.

Blind and Informed Cognitive Strategy Training

There is a distinction between blind and informed cognitive strategy training. The term *blind* is not intended to suggest that cognitive trainers do not know what they are doing. That is not at all the case. Blind training programs are usually well engineered and have shown good results (Belmont & Butterfield, 1971; Borkowski & Wanschura, 1974). The word *blind* simply means that the subjects don't know the purpose of the training they are undergoing.

The typical procedure in blind training is to teach the trainees to perform particular strategies without understanding the purpose or value of their activities. They are thus told or otherwise induced by the trainer to carry out certain strategies without being informed why, when, and where the use of these strategies may help them. Some children manage to figure out the significance of the strategies on their own. Most do not.

One of the weaknesses of blind training is that pupils trained blindly often do not use the strategies they have learned once their training ceases. Another weakness is that blindly trained pupils don't seem to be able to apply their strategies in situations that differ from the training conditions.

Informed training in the use of cognitive strategies also prepares pupils to use cognitive strategies, but it goes beyond blind training in that it helps pupils understand the purpose of their training and the usefulness of the strategies they are learning. There is evidence to suggest that it is more successful than blind training in promoting the effective use of strategies. This is in terms of both the pupils' continual use and generalization of their strategies (Ryan, Ledger, Short, & Weed, 1982). Kennedy and Miller (1976) found that pupils taught rehearsal (memory) strategies are more likely to continue to use them if they are shown that the strategies actually work. Kendall, Borkowski, and Cavanaugh (1980) showed that mentally retarded and normal pupils who understand the usefulness of elaboration (memory strategies) employ them more effectively and continue to use them more frequently after their training than do blindly trained pupils.

Paris, Bewman, and McVey (1981), as reported by Brown and Palincsar (1982), have compared strategy training under informed and noninformed (blind) conditions. Groups of pupils trained under either conditions were taught to use various types of memory strategies, e.g., grouping, labeling, rehearsal, and recall. Pupils in the informed training groups were also provided with a brief discussion of the reasons why they were being taught these strategies and given feedback as to the ways that the latter would help them to remember better. They outperformed the blindly trained group both during the initial training sessions and in later posttraining probes of memory ability.

COGNITIVE STRATEGIES AND CHILDREN WITH LEARNING DISABILITIES

Many cognitive researchers believe that deficient cognitive strategies are largely responsible for poor school performance (Baron, 1978). Many underachievers have not learned useful cognitive strategies, don't know when to apply them, or are unmotivated to apply them (Brown, 1978; Sternberg, 1981a). LD children are often found deficient in both general, intermediate-level, and specific cognitive strategies.

Baron (1978) has observed that mentally retarded pupils are almost always deficient in the use of cognitive strategies. He believes, however, that their deficiencies are often amenable to correction. He states that there is no convincing evidence that retarded pupils' limited capacities are directly responsible for the poor school performance. He believes that effective cognitive strategy training may overcome what were previously thought to be uncorrectable "ability" or "capacity" limitations.

The classic study that supports Baron's statement and appears generally to have inspired the efforts of cognitive strategy trainers is Zeaman and House's investigation of the role played by attention in discrimination learning (1963). In discrimination learning, subjects are shown stimuli that differ on a number of dimensions such as color, size, and form. They are then asked to point to the stimulus that the experimenters have designated as the correct one. An analysis of such discrimination learning reveals that it involves two distinct tasks: (1) attending to the correct dimension and (2) learning which type of response is correct.

When Zeaman and House compared the performance of retardates to normals, they found that the former were deficient only in respect to the first task, i.e., attending to the correct dimension. Apart from attention they could learn the second task about as readily as did the normal subjects. Furthermore their attention deficits appeared to be due to strategy rather than capacity deficiencies. That is, they were not able to direct their attention strategically as well as did the normals and, as a consequence, attended to fewer stimulus dimensions and learned fewer relationships. When the trainer helped mentally retarded subjects to correct their strategy deficiencies, they were able to attend about as well as did normal ones. Such work has inspired cognitive educators to believe that strategic training can overcome what were once thought to be permanent cognitive disabilities.

Cognitive Strategies Curriculum

It is possible to develop cognitive strategies curricula (Borkowski & Cavanaugh, 1979). Winschel and Lawrence (1975) have recommended that strategy training be part of the daily curriculum in EMR classrooms. Their curricular approach emphasizes strategies such as labeling of objects and groups of objects in terms of time sequences, classifying complex materials, learning to observe more than one dimension of an object at a time, and learning to understand and reproduce sentences that employ all types of linguistic patterns. In still another approach Ross and Ross (1978) developed the Pacemaker Primary Curriculum for EMR pupils. It teaches following directions, listening, remembering, planning, and problem solving.

Prosthetic Cognitive Strategies

Ideally pupils would be able to learn the cognitive strategies they need and be able to apply these strategies appropriately and effectively whenever necessary. It is unlikely, however, that this ideal state can ever be achieved. It is unrealistic to believe that we can teach our pupils all the cognitive strategies they need or that we can ever completely remediate their deficient ones.

Despite our successes in training pupils to use cognitive strategies, the improvements we achieve are often limited. It is one thing to train a pupil to use a strategy successfully in a particular situation. It is far more difficult to assure that the pupil will apply the strategy successfully in a variety of school situations. It is thus necessary that remedial and special educators concerned with cognitive efficiency should also try to utilize instructional techniques that lessen the demands on the pupil's strategies or compensate for their weaknesses.

Certain proponents of perceptual training, e.g., Cruickshank (1961), have recommended that stimulus information be diminished when teaching a learning disabled or brain-injured child. This is supposed to reduce demands on children's cognitive abilities and make it easier for them to learn. This sort of perceptual control system is really a type of prosthetic cognitive strategy imposed by the trainer. Behavioral educators also prosthetically structure the school environment, e.g., provide special external cues and prompts to pupils with behavioral learning difficulties to assure that their pupils appropriately respond. Many of their procedures can be viewed as trainer-imposed strategies that lessen the need for pupils to use their own. Good instructional objectives, too, structure subject matter so as to reduce the cognitive demands made on pupils. This is a major reason why they help them to learn more effectively.

Other approaches may be considered to serve prosthetic strategic purposes. Cognitive psychologist David Ausubel (1968, 1969) introduced an instructional approach in the 1960s that can help pupils who are deficient in cognitive strategies. It is the use of advanced organizers. Advanced organizers often introduce pupils to an instructional topic on a general level. Thus, the pupils may be provided general concepts before reading particular facts or ideas. This provides them with a particular mind set or frame of reference that enables them to learn the specifics of the topic more easily. Or before learning a topic, the pupils may be taught key words, sentences, or concepts. These, too, reduce their need to use their own cognitive strategies.

Markman (1979) has reviewed ways of remediating problems in reading comprehension. He shows that many textbooks are deficient in the cognitive guidance that they provide their reader. Markman also discusses ways of improving textbooks so as to reduce the cognitive demands they make on the reader. Such efforts can be considered prosthetic since they relieve pupils of the need to develop or use cognitive strategies.

By this time it is clear that much of what is good instruction represents the teacher's use of instruction to help pupils to develop and use cognitive strategies on their own or on the other hand to reduce pupils' needs for them.

QUESTIONS ABOUT COGNITIVE STRATEGIES

Schoolchildren do employ cognitive strategies in their schoolwork. It is also clear that pupils with learning problems and handicaps differ from and are usually deficient compared to academically successful pupils in respect to the effective use of cognitive strategies. Learning handicapped pupils often lack adequate strategies. Sometimes they have adequate strategies at their disposal but use the wrong ones for particular situations. Sometimes they don't know when to use one strategy or another. They have been found to be deficient or inefficient in their use of cognitive strategies, at all levels of generality and specificity.

Nevertheless several questions must be raised: Can cognitive strategies be distinguished from cognitive capacities? Might the lack of strategies or the use of poor ones be symptomatic of basic cognitive deficiencies, rather than being important in their own right? Does the training of cognitive strategies accomplish a useful purpose? Do strategies make a difference in everyday schoolwork?

Let us examine these questions from the standpoint of cognitive strategy researchers or theorists. Almost all of them would answer yes to the first question. Responding to the second question, most would agree that problems in the use of cognitive strategies may reflect basic cognitive (capacity) deficiencies but that they can be distinguished from the latter and should be dealt with separately. Responding to the third question, most cognitive strategy researchers and theorists believe that pupils can be trained to use cognitive strategies in ways that really improve their academic performance (Baron, 1978; Borkowski & Cavanaugh, 1979; Brown, 1978).

This brings us to another issue, which concerns generalizability. This is a great challenge to all educational and training efforts. While we sometimes wish to teach our pupils to do one specific thing well, and that one thing only, we more often wish to teach them generalizable knowledge and skills. Among the major criticisms of both behavioral and cognitive skill training approaches is the frequent lack of generalizability. Indeed one of the major reasons for current interest in cognitive strategies is that cognitive strategies appear to provide the means of assisting pupils to generalize the use of their knowledge and abilities.

But to do this, the cognitive strategies themselves must be generalizable. By and large cognitive strategy trainers are optimistic on this score. Borkowski and Cavanaugh (1979) claim that when optimal training is provided, the strategic behaviors taught to retarded pupils can and do generalize effectively. They also state that it is the amount and the appropriateness of the strategy training that determines a strategy's generalizability, and they believe that the failure to generalize cognitive strategies can usually be attributed to inadequate training. They advise that the chances for generalizability are increased if strategy training is carried out in a variety of settings and by a variety of people. They also advise that the chances of generalizability are improved if the use of strategies is supported by natural contingencies in the environment. Above all, Borkowski and Cavanaugh advise that strategic training must be long and persistent to assure generalizability.

METACOGNITION

Metacognition is one of the most interesting of the new areas of cognitive investigation. It is another aspect of cognitive strategy research and theory.

First, let us consider what the prefix *meta* means. In the *Oxford English Dictionary* the term *meta* can be used in two ways. The first is as "a designation for a higher science of the same nature but dealing with ulterior or more fundamental problems" (3rd. ed., s.v. "meta").

Another definition in the *Oxford English Dictionary* is that it refers to "later, subsequent, or more developed processes" (3rd. ed., s.v. "meta").

Metacognition is interpreted by educational and psychological researchers as involving cognitive self-awareness and regulation and control of the strategic aspects of cognition. This is indicated in the definition provided by Flavell (1976), the individual most responsible for recent interest in the topic:

> [Metacognition] refers to one's knowledge concerning one's own cognitive processes and products or anything related to them, e.g., the learning of relevant properties of information or data. For example, I am engaging in metacognition (metamemory, meta-learning, metattention, metalanguage, or whatever) if I notice that I am having more trouble learning A than B; if it strikes me that I should check C before accepting it as a fact; if it occurs to me that I had better make a note of D because I may forget. . . . Metacognition also refers . . . to the active monitoring and consequent relation and orchestration of these process[es] in relation to the cognitive objects on which they bear, usually in the service of some concrete goal or objective. (p. 232)

Flavell (1979) also distinguishes between cognitive strategies and metacognition. He observes that while the former are necessary to make cognitive progress, the latter must monitor and direct them.

Brown (Brown & Palincsar, 1982) has also discussed the implications of metacognition. She says that it "involves conscious access to one's own cognitive operations and reflections about those others. . . . It requires that learners step back and consider their own cognitive processes as objects of thought and reflection'' (p. 1–2). She believes metacognition is involved in almost every aspect of cognition. It consists of knowing about what we know, knowing about our cognitive activities, i.e., how our minds operate, and ultimately knowing the way to direct our minds' operations.

It is easy to see why Brown (1978) has also called *metacognition* a concept that serves to integrate a variety of cognitive constructs and considers the "developing child as a whole person rather than as a repository of fragmentary skills in various stages of development" (p. 81). It is also easy to see that the concept of metacognition is so broad and encompassing that it can easily become vague and unfocused.

DISTINCTIONS IN METACOGNITIVE FUNCTIONING

Flavell has attempted to make some distinctions in the conceptualization of metacognition by creating a metacognitive taxonomy. He and Wellman (1977) have thus divided metacognition into the broad categories of metacognitive sensitivity and metacognitive variables.

Metacognitive sensitivity refers to those metacognitive operations through which a child learns about the types of situations in which internal directed learning is required.

Metacognitive variables can be categorized in three ways: (1) person variables, i.e., knowledge about one's own cognitive capacities (their strengths and weaknesses as manifested in learning, memory, problem solving); (2) task variables, i.e., knowledge about the nature of the tasks to be learned and the difficulty level of particular problems; and (3) strategy variables, i.e., knowledge of different types of cognitive strategies that may be applied to particular tasks and knowing which ones are most appropriate for a given purpose in a given situation, e.g., to facilitate learning, memory, and problem solving in particular areas of academics.

METACOGNITIVE AWARENESS AND REGULATION

Perhaps the most important distinction to be made in metacognition is between its awareness and control aspects. While Flavell made this distinction in his original definition of metacognition, he did not elaborate on it in his taxonomy and it is often overlooked. Brown has tried to make the distinction more explicit: She states that "metacognition has been used to refer to many aspects of active cognition . . . but two broad definitions can be distinguished, namely knowledge [self awareness] about cognition and regulation of cognition'' (p. 1).

The self-awareness or knowledge aspects of metacognition have their roots in Piagetian thought. Piaget devoted much of his research to the study of how children developed cognitive self-awareness. He believed that it was present from infancy. Nevertheless he did not believe that self-regulation of cognition in a conscious, i.e., metacognitive sense, is possible before an individual achieves the formal operational stage.

In contrast, researchers and theorists who are interested in the regulatory aspects of metacognition believe that conscious self-regulation is possible even during the early years of life. Indeed they consider young children and mentally retarded pupils to be capable of metacognitive regulations even though they haven't achieved formal operational status. Russian psychologists have played an important role in the development of this point of view. Major Soviet researchers such as Vigotsky (1962) and Luria (1982) emphasize the early development of inner cognitive controls in children. The IPP is another major source of inspiration to regulatory conceptualization in metacognition. IPP theorists as a rule do not concern themselves with developmental status when they study control and executive processes.

IMPLICATIONS OF METACOGNITION FOR SCHOOLWORK

In school situations, metacognitive awareness refers to a pupil's knowledge of what the individual is learning, i.e., the knowledge of tasks assigned, the solutions to be achieved, the ways to achieve it, and the cognitive strengths and weaknesses. Few pupils at any age possess broad powers of metacognitive awareness. Indeed, full metacognitive awareness may not always be necessary or even helpful in school. Many pupils successfully apply cognitive strategies to academic problems without being aware of doing so. And it may not be advisable to make such pupils self-conscious about their thought processes. On the other hand other pupils appear to be unsuccessful in school because they are not knowledgeable about the ways they think,   what they know and do not know, or how to apply strategies. Such pupils may well benefit from increased cognitive self-awareness. They may be helped by metacognitive awareness training that teaches them methods of self-appraisal, self-recording, and self-questioning (Loper, 1982).

Metacognitive self-regulation, i.e., the control of one's own cognitive processes, directly affects a pupil's school performance. As such it is of particular interest to remedial and special practitioners. Metacognitive regulation can be carried out in an unconscious way, i.e., automatically. However, it often requires metacognitive awareness. Actually it is difficult to distinguish or separate metacognitive self-awareness completely from metacognitive self-regulation. Such metacognitive activities as planning, monitoring, self-checking, self-correction, and cognitive self-management involve both metacognitive awareness and regulation, though in different degrees at different times.

The following are some aspects of metacognitive awareness and metacognitive self-regulation that appear to be particularly important to instruction :

- Metacognitive planning. Pupils should cognitively prepare themselves to deal with particular tasks or problems. Metacognitive planning includes cognitive anticipation of strategies that may be research in schoolwork. It also includes cognitive trial and error, e.g., trying cognitive strategies to see if they work.
- Monitoring. Pupils should engage in strategic monitoring activities when carrying out their work. This monitoring includes self-testing, revising work procedures, and rescheduling learning activities as might be required by changing circumstances.
- Checking outcomes. This is also a form of monitoring. Pupils should evaluate the effectiveness of their strategic actions when trying them.
- Correcting or changing strategies. Pupils should correct faulty cognitive strategies or substitute new ones for them as the occasion demands.
- Self-direction. This encompasses the metacognitive activities already listed. It also implies the intentional conscious application of one's cognitive abilities and knowledge to achieve one's purpose in school and elsewhere.

METACOGNITION AND LEARNING PROBLEMS

It has also been found that while many poor readers lack effective cognitive strategies, others may be fully capable of exercising strategies but do not know when or how best to use them. These readers are metacognitively deficient. They don't understand that different strategies are needed to achieve different goals. They read at the same rates for materials of low and difficult levels. They read in the same ways for trivial and important information. They read the same ways when they try to get a general overview of a topic and when they try to learn specific details. They also read uncritically and are unable to focus on relevant information. They often cannot evaluate new material they read in terms of what they already know.

A state of learned helplessness may metacognitively orient a pupil to avoid the use of positive cognitive strategies. It may also cause a pupil to use strategies that are ineffective or self-defeating. The pupil in either case is likely to attribute the outcomes of learning to circumstances beyond personal control, either internal, e.g., ''I'm just too dumb, so why bother trying,'' or external, e.g., ''The teacher is unfair so why should I try.'' The pupil may be unwilling to learn better ways of solving problems because of this learned helplessness. The pupil may set low standards for achievements and refuse to raise them even when able to do better or may carry out academic assignments any which way just to get them over with.

Children who are doing poorly in school, whether they are underachievers, poor readers, or handicapped, tend to develop inaccurate causal attributions and inappropriate attitudes of learned helplessness. Thus, a pupil may develop realistic negative attributions after prolonged academic failures in a certain area of schoolwork.

These negative attributions may carry over into other situations where the child can succeed, and they may stop the child from succeeding in these situations. They may also cause the child to engage in compensatory negative behaviors so as to deny perceived limitations.

Concept of the Inactive Learner

All educators know that many children fail to learn because of personality problems, disinterest, lack of motivation, etc. Piaget (Chapter 6), information-processing theorists (Chapter 7), and now cognitive strategy theorists have stressed that learning does not simply result from the passive associations of stimuli and responses or because of reinforcements. Rather learning is viewed as achieved by the learner through active participation in learning situations. Active learners are likely to employ appropriate cognitive strategies effectively. Inactive learners are likely not to use, or to underuse, cognitive strategies. They may thus fail to learn despite having adequate ability and receiving good instruction (Torgeson, 1982).

Multiple factors dispose one child or another to become an inactive learner. For example, the child may be passive by nature or impaired by illness. Nevertheless pupils usually become inactive learners because of faulty attributions or because of learned helplessness. While it is a difficult task to change inactive learners into active ones, some success has been reported through altering the learner's causal attributions. Thus, metacognitive training may be most appropriate when used with pupils who are failing in their problem-solving efforts. It can be most successful when applied to specific problem areas and then faded out, allowing automatized functioning to take over as soon as possible.

Still another question might be raised about metacognitive training. Might it be counterproductive because it uses up some of the time and energy the pupil might otherwise devote to actual school learning? This question may be asked of any type of intervention, cognitive or otherwise. The question is perhaps a more pressing one for cognitive trainers, however, in the light of the limited success that cognitive training has achieved. It is incumbent on metacognitive trainers to show that the time spent in metacognitive training justifies itself by enhanced or accelerated achievement in academics or other areas of importance to the pupil.

Chapter 10

Cognitive Behavior Modification

The term *cognitive behavior modification* (CBM) suggests a reconciliation between cognitive and behavioral points of view. It may seem a contradiction in terms. Behavioral and cognitive points of view are, after all, considered to be opposite points of view, and one of the major justifications for behavior modification is that it deals with observable behavior rather than with inferred cognitive states.

But it is also true that from the beginnings of behaviorism some behaviorists have made various efforts to reconcile the two points of view. For example, Watson (1925), the father of modern behaviorism, tried to reduce thinking to muscular movements associated with speech. Later Hull (1952), Spence (1950), and Kendler and Vineberg (1954) explained cognition in terms of S-R variables. On the other side of the Atlantic, Pavlov (1927), the great Russian physiologist who discovered the conditional reflex, conceived of language (a cognitive construct) as constituting a second (inner) signal system (the environment being the first) controlling behavior. Such explanations of cognition in physiobehavioral terms died down for a while when Skinner's radical behaviorism took hold. They have, as seen in Chapter 2, been renewed.

THE BEHAVIORAL CHALLENGE TO PSYCHOTHERAPY

The term *psychotherapy* is by its name cognitive. That is, it implies therapy of the spirit, soul, or mind—the psyche. Here too behaviorists have made efforts to explain its phenomena in behavioral terms, e.g., Holt (1914) and Dollard and Miller (1950). Nevertheless, until behavioral therapies became popular, most people who worked with people's problems did not think in behavioral terms.

Psychotherapy may be broadly defined as efforts to correct people's thought and emotional processes through verbal (language) interchanges between the therapist and the patient or client (Ledwidge, 1978). It is often employed to cure mental and behavioral problems, neuroses and psychoses. Sometimes it is directed to solve problems on a conscious basis, i.e., to help patients develop more appropriate mental perspectives or to learn how to handle their problems better. Aaron Beck's (1976) cognitive therapy is a recent example of this type of approach. There are, indeed, many varieties of psychotherapy. They almost all seek to change psychological (cognitive processes) through the use of language (Ledwidge, 1978; McMullen & Giles, 1981).

There have always been questions and doubts about the value of psychotherapy. The modern behavioral challenge to psychotherapy was inaugurated with Skinner and Lindsley's introduction of the term *behavioral therapy* in 1954. It then heated up as a consequence of Eysenck's 1958 review of psychotherapeutic results. In his review Eysenck criticized psychotherapy as being both unscientific and ineffective. He declared that the principles of S-R conditioning could explain all so-called psychopathology and emotional problems and that they could also serve as a basis for a behavioral therapy. In attempting to clarify the distinctions between the latter and psychotherapy, Eysenck (1959) stated:

> We are dealing [when treating emotionally disturbed patients] with unadaptive behavior conditioned to certain classes of stimuli [requiring] no reference . . . to any underlying disorders or complexes in the psyche. . . . [Furthermore, unlike psychotherapy which seeks mental changes] . . . behavior therapy concentrates on actual behavior . . . [or] conditioned responses. (p. 66)

Eysenck (1959) observed that behavior therapy demystifies the treatment of psychological problems: "From the standpoint of learning theory, treatment is . . . a very simple process. In the case of surplus [unadaptive or maladaptive] conditioned responses treatment should consist in the extinction of these responses; in the case of deficient conditioned responses treatment should consist in the building up of the missing stimulus-response connections" (p. 65). As Ledwidge (1978) has described it, behavior therapy seeks to modify a patient's responses (behavior) to specific stimuli "rather than to modify with words [his/her] faulty thought processes" (p. 353).

DISTINCTIONS BETWEEN PSYCHOTHERAPY AND BEHAVIOR THERAPY

The management of a child's aggressive behavior may serve as one example of how behavioral therapy approaches are different from those of psychotherapy. As psychotherapists we would try to help the child develop insight into the reasons for aggression, to work through the child's emotional conflicts, and perhaps to persuade the child verbally to act more positively. As behavior therapists we would rather try to reduce or extinguish the child's surplus aggressive responses and to help the child respond with more positive behaviors (Rs) to situations (Ss) that elicited aggressive behaviors (Rs).

The management of school phobia can provide us with another example of how behavior therapy differs from psychotherapy. In traditional psychotherapy with a school-phobic child we would try to help the child understand the reasons for anxiety about attending school and to resolve the emotional conflicts. From the behavioral point of view, anxiety represents an amalgam of negative responses that are activated by the child's prospects of school. These include muscular tensions, heightened gastrointestinal activity, excessive perspiration, avoidance behavior, and behavioral agitation. A behavioral therapist treating school phobia would use behavioral modification techniques to extinguish these negative responses to school and to develop positive responses on the child's part.

DEFINITION OF BEHAVIORAL THERAPY

Early behavioral therapies were based on traditional S-R conceptions (see Chapter 2). These are well exemplified in methods that psychiatrist Joseph Wolpe (1978) continues to use. Wolpe claims to be able to apply successfully the principles of S-R conditioning to many psychiatric disorders. In dealing with a phobic patient, he first finds out the types of situations to which the patient responds phobically, i.e., with anxiety behaviors. He then has the patient engage in experiences (thoughts, images, etc.) that initiate or create anxiety stimuli (Ss). When these evoke anxiety responses on the patient's part (Rs), e.g., muscular tension, palpitations of the heart, Wolpe uses conditioning methods, e.g., systematic desensitization, to reduce them. He also conditions the patient to respond positively to situations (Ss) that previously made the person anxious, e.g., through reciprocal inhibition.

Since operant behaviorism has become popular, behavior therapists have tended to be less concerned about identifying the precise stimulus-response relationships that might be involved in psychological problems; they have instead concerned themselves primarily with efforts to modify behavior through control of subsequent contingencies, e.g., reinforcers. Gearhart's (1976) definition of behavior therapy makes this clear. It is, he writes, an approach that involves "the planned, systematic arrangement of consequences to a given response" (p. 51).

BEHAVIORAL THERAPIES AND BEHAVIOR MODIFICATION

The term *behavior modification* has come to be preferred in many circles over that of *behavioral therapy*. This is particularly true when children are concerned. The preference for the term *behavior modification* seems to be due to the fact that it doesn't have medical implications. It thus seems to be a more appropriate term for use in schools. The two terms, *behavior modification* and *behavior therapy*, however, for most purposes may be considered synonymous. They include a variety of methods that are quite familiar to remedial and special educators. These include contingency management, behavioral modeling, token economy, and reinforcement. They also include methods that are less familiar to educators such as implosion, covert sensitization, and stimulus satiation (Ledwidge, 1978). Such methods focus on overt behavior, and they seek to change maladaptive behavior (Ullman & Krasner, 1968). The terms *behavior therapy* and *behavior modification* are used interchangeably in this chapter, though the use of *behavior modification* is preferred when discussing children.

As remedial and special educators well know, behavioral techniques have been successful in helping children with problems. Remedial educators have found behavioral analysis to be a most useful tool in treating learning problems. Great advances in helping the mentally retarded have been achieved primarily through the application of behavioral technologies.

A COGNITIVE DIRECTION

Despite the great achievement of behavioral methods, their success with educational and emotional problems has been a qualified one. Behavior modification has proven more helpful in dealing with problems in narrow areas of functioning than with those of a complex nature and more effective in managing lower-order behaviors than with those of a more advanced nature. It is easier to extinguish a single type of aggressive behavior than it is to create positive attitudes. Reinforcement schedules are more helpful in teaching decoding than in teaching reading comprehension. Furthermore, research on behavior methods suggests that their results often do not last long or generalize well. They may prove effective as long as treatment continues, but their effects do not always last. They may work in the school where the child was trained but not in a different type of environment.

Behavioral therapists, wrestling with these problems, have explored a variety of ways to improve the power and effectiveness of their methods. Some of them have turned to cognition for help. Indeed as Ledwidge (1978) has pointed out, "slowly but surely over the years behavioral therapy has become more cognitive" (p. 354).

The behavioral drift into cognitivism can partly be attributed to the increasing willingness of behaviorists to use cognitive terms. Thus Rimm and Masters (1974) state:

> We include under the label behavior therapy any of a large number of specific techniques that employ psychological (especially learning) principles to deal with maladaptive human behavior. The term "behavior" is interpreted broadly, encompassing covert responding (for example, emotions and implicit verbaliza- tion), when such can be clearly specified in addition to overt responding. (p. 1)

Further evidence of the role that cognition came to play in behavioral therapy is exemplified by the works of Joseph Wolpe. Wolpe is a pioneer behavior therapist who is strongly opposed to psychotherapy and insists that he is purely a behavior therapist. Yet he constantly deals with cognitive states therapeutically. Thus Wolpe requires a patient to introspect, i.e., "look into his mind," to "introspect, think, reason, judge, discriminate, image, and to purposefully control the actions of his own mind" (Ledwidge, 1978, p. 363). He has the patient describe experiences and problems so as to evoke images, thoughts, and emotions associated with the problems. While this would seem to make his approach a cognitive one, Wolpe and his followers insist that it is completely behavioral.

Let us study Wolpe's therapeutic methods more closely. Wolpe attempts to weaken negative S-R associations in his patients, in effect to condition stimuli that elicit negative responses from the latter so that they cease to elicit negative responses or at least   elicit them less intensely. Wolpe also tries to condition stimuli so that they elicit positive behaviors in place of negative ones.

Wolpe interprets *cognition* as constituting a source of stimuli (S). Patients are viewed as responding to the stimuli (S) generated by their thoughts, images, memories, etc., with undesirable responses, i.e., behaviors (R). These responses may be excessive sweating, muscular tension, or gastrointestinal discomfort. He tries to recondition the patients' behaviors (responses) so that the negative responses to these stimuli are replaced by desirable ones, e.g., muscular relaxation.

Wolpe justifies his methods as being purely behavioral, on the grounds that the aim of his treatment method is entirely that of behavioral improvement. In his treatment approach the behavior itself is considered to be the therapeutic agent. He doesn't attempt to modify directly his patients' cognitive states, e.g., thought processes, emotions, and attitudes. He rather tries to recondition the responses (behaviors) that the patients make to the stimuli caused by these states. Thus he trains his patients to stop responding with gastrointestinal stress to the stimuli-caused worries and instead to relax in their presence. He does not seek to help his patients understand the psychological causes of these problems.

Wolpe has further defended his claim to being a behavioral therapist on the basis that cognitive behavioral distinctions are irrelevant (see Chapter 2). Cognition and behavior, he says (1978), are essentially equivalents since "thought obeys the same 'mechanistic' laws as motor or automatic behavior and results from the same of neurological activity" (p. 438). Cognitive problems are simply "wrong habits of thought," which like wrong habits of behavior are created by faulty S-R associations. What is called *cognitive behavior therapy* (modification) is quite different from Wolpe's methods. For cognitive behavior modification actively seeks cognitive change as a priority to achieving behavioral change, and it seeks to modify cognition (thinking) so as to modify behavior.

SIMILARITIES AND DIFFERENCES BETWEEN PSYCHOTHERAPY AND COGNITIVE BEHAVIORAL THERAPY

In order to understand better cognitive behavioral therapy (modification), we must first attempt to understand better the similarities and distinctions between psychotherapies and behavioral therapies. There are actually cognitive and behavioral components in both (Ledwidge, 1978; Strong & Claiborn, 1982).

The behavior therapies used to help severely autistic or profoundly mentally retarded children weigh in heavily on the behavioral end, while the psychoanalytic treatment given neurotic adults is essentially cognitive. But in between we find psychotherapies and behavioral therapies sharing many elements. Examining some of the points of difference and commonality between the two types of therapy in closer fashion will help us to understand better some of the characteristics of cognitive behavioral therapy.

The Focus of Treatment

As discussed, traditional behavior therapy typically focuses on maladaptive behaviors, while psychotherapy usually focuses on the cognitive states that mediate problematic behavior. Behavior therapies consider behavior itself to be the therapeutic agent. That is, behaviorists consider positive changes in behaviors to be therapeutic. Cognitive therapies on the other hand emphasize cognitive changes. They aim "at modifying behavior and emotion by influencing the client's patterns of thought . . . [by helping the patient] . . . to recognize that some of his . . . cognitions (premises, assumptions, attitudes) are faulty . . . and by helping him to correct them" (Ledwidge, 1978, p. 356).

Despite these distinctions, behavioral therapists often seek cognitive changes in their clients, while psychotherapists clearly want their patients to change their behaviors as well as their thought processes.

Methods of Treatment

Behavioral therapists traditionally emphasize nonverbal means of treatment. Traditional psychotherapists employ language (speech) as their primary method. Thus behavioral therapists may apply or withhold physical reinforcers, or use physically aversive stimulation, while psychotherapists deal with their patients' problems verbally. Nevertheless, it is almost impossible to divorce entirely language from behavioral therapy (Ledwidge, 1978). Behavioral therapists frequently use verbal methods with their subjects. They give them oral directions; they use verbal statements to encourage certain behaviors and to serve as reinforcers or as aversive stimuli. Behavioral therapies thus have cognitive elements. Similarly psychotherapists use nonverbal methods such as gestures and other types of body language that cue, prompt, reinforce, or otherwise direct their patients to carry out certain behaviors and to desist from others.

Criteria for Improvement

Behavioral therapists insist that their interventions are intended to improve their clients' behaviors rather than their cognitive or emotional states and that the results of behavioral therapy are to be judged on the basis of how a patient behaves rather than on how or what the person thinks or feels (Ullman & Krasner, 1968). Psychotherapists on the other hand seek to improve their clients' mental and emotional stability. Yet behavior therapists certainly want their clients to become effective and positive thinkers, while almost all psychotherapists wish their clients to behave better as well as feel and think better.

The Model Guiding Therapy

Behaviorists emphasize the use of objective, laboratory-based (and hence scientific) means of guiding their therapies, while psychotherapists are more prone to emphasize personal and clinical relationships. Yet behaviorists often adapt their methods in a rather casual way to classroom needs and deal personally with their clients. Many psycho-therapists try to control their interactions with their clients and to evaluate the therapeutic process objectively.

Summation

All in all, it does not appear possible to separate cognition from behavior in either psychotherapy or behavioral therapy. Nevertheless there are clear distinctions in emphasis between the two therapeutic approaches. Psychotherapy primarily seeks to alter cognitive states through cognitive means (typically verbal) while behavioral therapy "concentrates on the maladaptive behavior itself using behavioral means to alter it" (Ledwidge, 1978, p. 355). In this sense cognitive behavioral-therapies represent a new type of cognitive-behavioral synthesis since they attempt directly to alter (mediating) cognitive states with the intent of modifying behavior.

COGNITIVE BEHAVIOR MODIFICATION

Cognitive behavior modification, broadly speaking, represents an effort to enrich and improve behavioral therapies through cognitive means. More precisely, it is an effort to modify behavior and to control behavior through cognitive change. Cognitive behavior therapists still use behavioral methodologies and demand behavioral change as evidence of therapeutic improvement and are almost uniformly insistent in their reliance on active motoric performance in therapy.

Nevertheless cognitive behavior therapists also assign a key role to cognition in their therapies. In particular they employ such cognitive elements as imagery, thought, attitudes, motivation, and particularly language to change and control behavior. "Cognitive change is the active ingredient in the treatment" based on the premise that "the human organism responds to cognitive representations of the environment rather than to those environments per se" (Mahoney, 1974, p. 7).

Cognition is important to cognitive behavior therapy from the standpoint of the mediating roles it plays in behavior (see Chapter 2). First, it can transform the nature of the stimuli to which the client responds. A phobic patient who is afraid of dogs, after all, is responding with fear to the cognitive implications of the dog rather than to the dog itself. One way of changing the fear behaviors with which the person responds to the dog is to change the cognitive implications of dog stimuli. This is what Mahoney means by his statement about the human organism responding to cognitive representations of the environment.

Next, cognition can produce mediators that control behavior. Thus while an aggressive child may be brought under control through behavioral modification methods, the child may be better helped if we alter the cognitive states that mediate the behaviors. For example, by using cognitive behavioral modification, one may be taught to delay impulsive behaviors by reminding oneself to think things over before responding, to improve test performances by reminding oneself to "think before I do," or perhaps to decrease aggressive behaviors by considering alternative nonaggressive ways of responding to frustration. A variety of methods are used to do this. But all of them "appear to have one distinctive feature. The child is taught to employ mediating responses that exemplify a general strategy for controlling behavior under various circumstances" (Hobbs, Moguin, & Troyler, 1980, p. 148).

Cognitive behavioral modification approaches include coverant control, (verbal) misattribution therapy, rational-emotional therapy, emotional response routine, problem-solving training, and self-instruction (self-talk) training (Ledwidge, 1978). Although such therapies are cognitive to a great degree, they are also intended to change behavior, and they regard behavioral rather than cognitive improvement as the criterion of successful intervention. It is not enough then for a client to tell a CBM therapist that one feels better, has improved the outlook on life, or is feeling more relaxed after therapy. The client must also act better. In contrast to psychotherapists, cognitive behavior therapists do not accept a patient's statements that the person is more stable psychologically or feels better as an index of improvement, if there are no demonstrable changes in their behavior.

HISTORICAL INFLUENCES IN THE DEVELOPMENT OF CBM

The vein of historical development in CBM as used with children can be distinguished in some ways from that which has led to the use of cognitive therapies with adults, at least to some degree. Donald Meichenbaum (1980), one of the most distinguished of CBM researchers, has defined three distinct areas as having contributed to the initial development of "cognitive behavioral training approach with children" (p. 1). One of these areas is that of social learning theory. During the 1960s and 1970s social learning investigators studied the use of self-applied cognitive strategies by children in a number of laboratory investigations and found that they played an important role in developing self-control in children.

A second influence on the development of CBM for use with children was the work on mediation and mediation deficiencies (see Chapter 2). The results of such research, Meichenbaum (1980) points out, suggest that the "production of mediators, and the use of such mediators [are important] to control nonverbal behavior" (p. 2). When studying children with "self-control problems," Meichenbaum came to the conclusion that such children weren't necessarily impulsive by nature but rather that they couldn't deal effectively with task demands. "Their disruptiveness was seen as secondary to deficient cognitive strategies" (p. 2), i.e., as due to mediation deficits. Indeed a considerable amount of research in the 1970s suggested that mediational difficulties might be responsible for children's failures in impulse control and be a major cause of childhood behavioral disorders. Meichenbaum and others thus concluded that teaching children to produce and use mediators might help them to improve behaviorally.

The third set of influences in the development of CBM derives from Soviet psychology, some of whose major researchers were interested in the role that verbal (speech) processes played in controlling motor behavior. It was in this tradition that Soviet psychologists Vigotsky (1923/1962) and Luria (1961) concluded the notion that speech controls behavior in stages. This has been a major theoretical cornerstone for CBM.

Soviet Theories of Language Mediation

Pavlov, the father of modern Soviet psychology, described two signal systems as eliciting and controlling behavior. The first signal system is shared by animals and humans. It consists of physical stimuli that elicit behavior either directly or as a result of conditioning. The second system is speech, which as it develops, constitutes a second signal system that is internalized within the functioning of the brain as a form of "higher nervous [neurological] activity" (1927). Pavlov believed that this second signal system (inner speech) eventually comes to control much of voluntary behavior. In essence he appears to have identified inner speech with what we call *cognition* and to have credited it as an essential mechanism of behavioral control.

Pavlov's theories were extended by Vigotsky, who elaborated on the ways that *socialized* speech directs behavior. Vigotsky, who developed his theories and wrote about them in the 1920s and 1930s, developed a number of critical themes respecting the role of cognitive processes in regulating behaviors. Like Pavlov, he emphasized the importance of speech to these processes and insisted that speech was not to be interpreted in mere stimuli-response terms; i.e., speech is endowed with special properties by the nervous system.

Vigotsky proceeded further and insisted that the development of cognition (and speech) must be interpreted in cultural-historical terms, that cognition is more than a biological development. Its growth also represents an internalization of a society's social and cultural percepts and values. Cognition thus becomes an internalized means through which society may control the individual. Vigotsky believed that human psychological processes originate in and develop through social interactions. They begin with mother-child relations and mature in later social interaction with parents, family, friends, teachers, etc.

Vigotsky made a distinction between overt and inner speech. The latter is not simply a matter of saying words under one's breath. It is rather an internal representation of what has been learned (procedures and knowledge) from social interactions. And it is the means through which thought and social interactions are linked and turned into inner purposeful regulative mechanisms. In order to understand another person's speech, it isn't enough simply to understand the words but "we must also understand his thought. But that isn't enough—we must also know its motivation" (1923/1962, p. 151).

The most important thing about Vigotsky's theories from the standpoint of cognitive behavior modification is that he believed that speech is first used by society to regulate the child but is eventually used by the child to self-regulate.

Luria's Theories of Language Mediation

Luria (1961) elaborated on Vigotsky's theories. Like Vigotsky he stressed the social nature of speech, its complex nature, and its broad implications. Using Vigotsky's concepts as a springboard, Luria demonstrated how external speech develops into internal controls that regulate voluntary behavior. The ability to perform voluntary acts, he observed, is "formed by the child in her/his concrete contacts with adults" (p. 89). It is the child's mother who originally "organizes the child's motor act initiating it through speech" (p. 89). Indeed a baby's voluntary movements can be considered to be a shared mother-child experience. As the child matures other adults also stimulate, regulate, and monitor the child's movements.

At the second stage of development one learns to give oral commands to oneself, responding, as it were, to one's own speech signals. The child talks to oneself and tells oneself what to do.

At the third stage of development the child's speech is internalized. The child then responds to this inner speech. In this way the original interpsychological activities of speech become transformed into intrapsychological processes that permit self-regulation (voluntary behavior). Along with the "cognitive function of the word and its function as a means of communication, there is a directive function. The word not only reflects reality, it also regulates reality" (Luria, 1961, p. 89).

Luria explained the limited control that young children have over their own behaviors as due to their limited ability to regulate themselves through speech. The inability of some mentally retarded individuals to regulate themselves effectively is due to their speech limitations.

Luria's theory contradicts Piaget to a considerable degree. Piaget minimizes the importance of speech and language in cognitive development, while Luria appears to have minimized the importance of physical activity.

Researchers who extended Luria's ideas to the study of aggressive pupils found them useful. In this vein, Meichenbaum and Goodman (1977) discovered that impulsive children who made a greater number of errors on tasks than nonimpulsive ones also had less verbal control over their behavior. Furthermore when such impulsive children used verbal self-directions, it was more often on a stimulus level rather than on a mediational basis. Similarly, Douglas (1972, et al., 1976), when comparing hyperactive children who appeared to lack the ability to stop, look, and listen to normal ones, found them not only to be more impulsive but deficient as well in their production of covert speech. It was a logical step, then, to assume that deficiencies in verbal mediation may play a major role in behavioral disorders and that the Vigotsky-Luria speech mediation model might guide efforts to modify these disorders. As Meichenbaum and Goodman (1977) have written, "from [the Vigotsky-Luria] hypothetical development sequence, we developed a treatment paradigm to train impulsive children to talk to themselves as means of developing self-control."

As a consequence of the acceptance of the Vigotsky-Luria concept of speech mediation, the field that has been identified as cognitive behavior modification assigns a major role to speech processes (and self-statements) as mediators between the environment (S) and behavioral responses (R) and as means of altering S-R relationships so as to bring behavior under better cognitive control.

Rise of CBM Procedures

These events set the stage for developing new types of approaches to the management of children's problems. Thus the field of cognitive behavior modification developed. Providing an additional impetus to the development of these new approaches was "the increasing concern about the *inability* of earlier behavior management procedures such as operant conditioning programs to foster changes that were generalizable and durable" (Meichenbaum, 1980, p. 3).

TYPES OF CBM APPROACHES

Three general types of cognitive behavioral modification approaches employed with children have been distinguished (Hobbs et al., 1980):

1. Problem-solving techniques. The child is presented with "an oral or written description of the controlling or coping strategy, e.g., the instructions 'look and think' before answering."
2. Self-instruction training. The children are taught verbal self-coping strategies. Thus the child is taught to repeat statements to self, to rehearse them actively for use in problem situations, e.g., "If I keep on going as I'm told I'll do it right."
3. Cognitive modeling. The child is exposed to the teacher, therapist, or peer who exhibits particular behaviors and says certain things that the child is supposed to imitate. The model demonstrates what the child should do and say to direct control of the child's own behavior.

Modern CBM approaches reveal the presence of one or more of these approaches. All of them are characterized in some fashion by the conceptualization of cognitive mediation as a means through which behavior can be brought under self-control, whether through oral speech, silent speech, written language, or thought about what to do (the equivalent of inner speech). When used for school tasks a pupil may be taught through CBM to use speech to orient toward a task ("What's the job?"); to define the task ("What do I have to do to get it right?"); to focus attention ("Do it carefully"); a self-correcting mechanism ("Check that answer," "Oh, I made a mistake, I better watch the next one"); or as self-reinforcement ("Good, keep it up").

In areas of behavioral management the child may be taught to self-talk into acting friendly to other children, not to hit others, to slow down in making decisions, to reassure oneself that the child is not afraid or anxious or that the child can succeed.

Meichenbaum's Self-Instruction Approach

CBM is most prominently identified with Meichenbaum, who has done much to popularize it. A CBM training sequence developed by Meichenbaum follows:

- Cognitive modeling. The child observes an adult performing a particular task while talking aloud describing what the person is doing.
- External guidance. The child performs the same type of task according to the model's instructions.
- Covert self-guidance. The child performs the task, instructing oneself.
- Faded overt self-guidance. The child whispers the instructions to oneself while performing the task.
- Covert self-instruction. The child performs the task using inaudible or silent speech to give oneself instruction.

Meichenbaum has observed the following points about these procedures. By observing the model and then by using the model's statement to guide oneself, the child learns to define the problem, to ask questions about the tasks and the goals valued, to carry out self-instruction that focuses attention on the task, to guide the behaviors that are required for the task's achievement, to develop self-evaluation skills, to reinforce behaviors when correct, and to employ "error correcting options." Meichenbaum also observes that the child must be given adequate practice both in the use of self-instructional methods and in the task itself, in order for such self-instruction to be successful.

While Meichenbaum's methods are intended to integrate the cognitive and behavioral aspects of performance and to help the children more effectively control their behavior, its treatment focus is cognitive. That is, it attempts to teach children how to think and through improved thinking to control better and improve their behavior.

The close affinity or even identification that cognitive behavior modification has to metacognition may be shown by its application to a classroom-related task, i.e., one in which the child learns to copy line patterns. The examiner first performs the task for the child "cognitively modeling" it by speaking out loud as follows:

> Okay, what is it I have to do? I have to copy the picture with the different lines. I have to go slowly and carefully. Okay, draw the line down, good; and then to the right, that's it; now down some more and to the left, good, I'm doing fine so far. Remember, go slowly, Now back up again, No, I was supposed to go down. That's okay. Just erase the line carefully. . . . Good. Even if I make an error I can go down slowly and carefully. I have to go down now. Finished. I did it. (Meichenbaum & Goodman, 1977, p. 117)

Meichenbaum describes this thinking out loud behavior by the model as being important in a variety of ways. First, the model actually performed the task so that the child could learn how to do it. Second, and most importantly from a CBM point of view, the model's discussion prepared a set of cognitive (verbal) structures that the child could adopt to direct, monitor, and improve one's own performance of the task. Thus the model verbally provided the pupil with a problem definition by asking oneself, "What is it I have to do?" The model further directed the child's attention to the task to guide oneself cognitively through such statements as "Carefully . . . draw the line down. Remember go slowly, now go back up again" (in a drawing task). Other statements provided a means for the child of exercising performance options, e.g., "If I make an error I can go on more slowly." The model also provided an example of verbal self-reinforcement by telling oneself "Good, I'm doing fine."

Variations in CBM Methods

Meichenbaum has elaborated the applications of CBM approaches so as to improve their generalizability and utility. He advises that a pupil's CBM training should often proceed in stages—from simple situations to complex ones. For example, the child might begin metacognitive training while working on   simple sensorimotor tasks such as drawing geometric forms or coloring figures within boundaries, using simple verbal self-directions, and then gradually move up in stages till completing complex drawing tasks while self-verbalizing in systematic ways. He also advises that a pupil might be asked to describe behaviors both before and during the performance of the task to bring them under better cognitive control. In more advanced types of CBM training, the model might be dispensed with, or the child could begin work by subvocalizing rather than by speaking out loud.

Meichenbaum (1980) has recently recommended variations that further extend and improve on earlier CBM methods. These include using the child's play medium to provide situations and tasks for training, using tasks that encourage the use of sequential cognitive strategies, using peer modeling, individualizing instruction to meet each child's own particular needs and pace in training, building up the child's package of self-statements to include self-talk of a problem-solving nature to implement those of coping and self-correcting types, guarding against merely mechanical training by using a trainer who is animated and who responds enthusiastically to the child's needs, supplementing self-instruction with imagery practice, and supplementing CBM procedures with additional behavioral modification techniques.

Increasing efforts are being made to adopt CBM to classroom instruction. Indeed Meichenbaum (1980) more and more seems to be orienting to the classroom and has identified his approach as one that teaches children how to think, not what to think.

Applications of CBM

Techniques of cognitive behavior modification are often used to improve academic performances. However, it began as a cognitive therapy to help children with social, emotional, and behavioral problems.

Thus Meichenbaum first used it to help impulsive children learn to control their behaviors better by internalizing self-verbalizations. Others used the paradigm to establish inner speech control over the disruptive behavior of hyperactive children, the idea being in all such efforts to have children stop and think before they act, to assess what they are doing, how it best can be done, what should not be done, and cognitively to guide and support positive behaviors, while correcting or suppressing negative ones.

In a similar vein, emotionally disturbed children were taught to overcome aggressive responses by developing alternative strategies. One study involved hyperactive aggressive and destructive hyperactive aggressive boys in a taunting game, teaching them to cope with self-instruction. Another had pupils write mediation essays on blurting out and making distracting noise in class. Those essays discussed the negative consequence of such negative behavior, the alternative ways of expressing oneself, and the positive consequence of this. Others sought to control negative behavior by teaching children to praise themselves when they didn't behave negatively. Some researchers helped pupils persist in boring tasks by teaching them to think of pleasant events or to say positive things while performing them: "This is fun"; "This is easy!" Still another study helped children who were anxious in the dark to develop greater confidence through making competency statements such as "I can take care of myself," and positive statements such as "The dark is a fun place to be." Others taught preschool children not to litter by teaching them to make statements such as "I like to pick up trash and throw it in a can."

Positive results have been reported for such applications of CBM methods. There have been failures too, and criticisms that the positive results are often circumscribed or superficial. Additionally research supporting CBM has been questioned on methodological grounds (Hobbs et al., 1980).

CONSIDERATIONS ABOUT COGNITIVE BEHAVIOR MODIFICATION

The very idea of cognitive behaviorism indicates how difficult it is for anyone to avoid involvement with cognitive concepts. When we respond to our environment, our behavior is clearly not determined simply by previous reinforcement schedules but also by thought, memories, attitudes, and emotions. We are cognitive organisms. Even the most ardent behaviorists don't usually deny this. They argue instead that cognitive processes are personal events that are not physically verifiable and thus are not fit subjects for scientific study.

Cognitive behavioral modification represents a change in orientation from this position in that it accepts cognition as a topic of scientific study in conjunction with behaviorism. Some CBM researchers, in order to justify doing this, agree that cognition is as physical as behavior or that cognitions are behavioral equivalents. Others have simply decided to accept cognitive constructs as legitimate in their own right with the stipulation that the principles of scientific investigation prized by behaviorism be observed in the joining of cognition to behavior.

Nevertheless the idea of CBM is still a subject of much controversy. Wolpe (1978) has dismissed the idea as redundant and as raising false issues. He (1978) does not agree with Ullman that cognitions are behaviors: "to relabel all cognitive activities—perceiving, imagery, thinking, and the like—does not solve anything and blurs the very distinction that led to the development of behavior therapy as an alternative to psychotherapy in the first place."

Nor does he believe that the situation is improved by trying to justify cognitive activities in behavioral terms as being self-statements. Only if CBM restricts itself to the use of self-talk in a "mindless way," i.e., as a source of physical stimuli, can it truly qualify as a form of behavior therapy, as far as Wolpe (1978) is concerned: "To the extent, however, that the client listens, understands, and believes what he has been taught to say to himself (and surely that is the therapist's expectation) cognition as well as self talk [is going on], . . . and we are dealing with cognitive therapy" (p. 356).

More importantly Ledwidge believes that when they become cognitive, behavioral therapies lose much of their scientific justification while gaining little or nothing in terms of better results. It has also been argued that when cognitive behavioral therapies are effective, it is because of their behavioral aspects rather than their cognitive elements (Kalish, 1981). In a different direction, some CBM pioneers such as Meichenbaum (1980) have voiced concern over the limited generalizability of CBM results and believe that there must be a greater emphasis on its cognitive side—if its effectiveness is to be increased.

Nevertheless it appears that cognitive behavioral modification, for whatever reason, does help some children become better behaved, happier, and more effective in their school and work habits. Because as practitioners we are more concerned with results than we are with the finer points of theory, we recommend trying CBM in remedial and special education. Along these lines such writers as Meichenbaum appear to have been properly cautious about the method, while still remaining enthusiastic.

Chapter 11

Cognitive Task Analysis

Many of the cognitive approaches studied in Chapter 10 involve what may be called *cognitive task analysis*. We have thus seen the analysis of intelligence into different factors (Chapter 4), the identification of specific mental abilities (Chapter 5), the study of cognition according to developmental stages (Chapter 6), and the differentiation of different information-processing states (Chapter 7). Nevertheless it is appropriate to devote an entire chapter to the topic of cognitive task analysis. First, teachers should carry out cognitive as well as behavioral tasks analyses. Second, the cognitive approaches studied in this chapter provide a somewhat different perspective on cognition than those examined in earlier chapters.

BLOOM'S COGNITIVE TAXONOMY

It may be somewhat difficult in this age of behavioral objectives to believe that there was a time when cognitive objectives were more popular than behavioral ones, but this was true before the 1960s. The most prominent of such cognitive objective approaches was expressed in the taxonomy scheme suggested for the cognitive domain by Benjamin Bloom and his associates (Bloom, Engelhart, Furst, Hill, and Krathwohl, 1956). Because it is usually associated with Bloom's name, we refer to it as Bloom's taxonomy. Bloom and his associates developed taxonomies for affective and motor domains but we are not concerned with these. In any case they have not been as influential as those developed for the cognitive domain.

Distinctions between Taxonomies and Hierarchies

Taxonomies and hierarchies have always been popular in cognitive approaches to cognition. How do they differ? Klausmeier (1976) states that a taxonomy involves "inclusive-exclusive relationships among classes of things whereas a hierarchy implies relationships among things ordered by some principle of importance, priority or dependency" (p. 193).

That is, a hierarchy implies a distinct unchangeable order. An instructional hierarchy means that things must be taught and skills mastered in a particular order proceeding from level to level in a fixed and unalterable sequence. In contrast, an instructional taxonomy is a logical system whose interrelated levels and elements do not require any particular instructional sequence. For example, in teaching a topic according to a taxonomy, you can teach its subordinate concepts before its main ones without violating the taxonomy (Klausmeier, 1976). Bloom's taxonomy doesn't prescribe the order in which a pupil should be taught particular competencies. The teacher makes the decisions as to the order of teaching.

The Basic Outline of Bloom's Taxonomy

The following are the six levels of cognitive objectives in Bloom's taxonomy. They relate to the cognitive goals implicit in such academic topics as social studies, science, and literature:

1. Knowledge. This cognitive domain includes memory, i.e., recognition of ideas, and facts, i.e., knowledge that the learner has previously accrued.
2. Comprehension. This domain involves abilities that make use of information but do not necessarily relate this information to other information, nor does it necessarily imply an understanding of the information's implications. In other words a student at this level of cognition understands the material learned but does so in isolation.
3. Application. This area involves the ability to use abstractions, ideas, principles, and methods as they apply to specific concrete types of situations and problems.
4. Analysis. This involves the ability to break information into its various parts or into specific meaningful components.
5. Synthesis. This involves the ability to work with the parts or components of information that have been analyzed. These parts may thus be combined or otherwise joined in various ways to create the new cognitive patterns or structures that are required in order for the pupil to achieve and solve various academic problems.
6. Evaluation. This involves the ability to make qualitative and quantitative judgments as to whether the products created by the previous steps satisfy the criteria for successful performance.

Bloom's taxonomy is quite elaborate, and it is difficult to do it justice in a short review. Interested readers are advised to read the original version (Bloom et al., 1956). There are a number of things to be observed about Bloom's taxonomy. First, it deals with cognition in general or nontechnical terms. Second, the taxonomy is not based on research. Rather it was developed on the basis of conceptual analysis; that is, it represents the ways the authors believed that students should proceed cognitively when dealing with academic learning. Third, it is a very general taxonomy that is intended to provide educators with a cognitive framework within which they can develop their own cognitive objectives for the particular subjects that they are teaching. Thus a social studies teacher might use it to guide development or selection of social studies objectives, a mathematics teacher to select mathematics objectives. The taxonomy was also intended to guide curriculum planners and test developers. The general nature of the taxonomy has indeed encouraged its wide application in education. But the taxonomy is too general to permit precise applications.

Some authors such as Metfessel, Michael, and Kirsner (1969) tried to translate the taxonomy into more precise terms for instructional purposes. It is, however, not precise enough for direct application to particular learning situations or problems.

Remedial or special education teachers will not find Bloom's taxonomy particularly helpful in individualized instruction or for remedial work. It doesn't lend itself well to remediation; that is, it doesn't identify what pupils should actually do in learning, the exact objectives they should achieve, or the actual criteria for successful achievement of particular objectives, though attempts have been made to use it remedially. Most of its value for remedial and special education is to remind us of the richness of human cognition and the many challenges to its exercise that good instruction should provide. The taxonomy can also provide us with a frame of reference for the vast varieties of cognitive goals that we might possibly address. Teachers of the gifted should find this aspect of the taxonomy most helpful.

GAGNÉ'S THEORIES OF LEARNING AND INSTRUCTION

In this section we discuss one of his earlier models, which reflects the traditional "learning theory" outlook of the time (1965) and his later model, which has been influenced by information-processing theory (Gagné & Briggs, 1979; Gagné & Dick, 1983). Gagné is a particularly important person to know since he pioneered in the development of task analysis.

Gagné is perhaps best known to remedial and special educators in terms of his early conceptualization of a model of learning hierarchies (1965), which was quite influential within education for a while and significantly affected thinking in remedial and special education. According to Gagné's learning hierarchy, a number of different types of learning skills must be mastered sequentially (hierarchically) to achieve an instructional goal and the sequence of mastery is invariant; i.e., the achievement of later, succeeding learning skills depends on the successful accomplishment of earlier, preceding ones.

How does one identify a learning hierarchy? It is done, first of all, by developing a broad framework as to how learning proceeds. It is secondly accomplished by analyzing a learning task into the subskills and achievements required to achieve the learning task's terminal objectives. This requires that the instructor observe how students deal with various learning tasks and determine the skills the pupils must demonstrate to perform these tasks correctly.

Gagné's learning hierarchy postulates eight types of learning. It is based on learning theories that prevailed during the 1960s and on the author's logical analysis of learning tasks. While the hierarchy is more or less based on S-R principles, it also deals with broad cognitive realms.

The issue of hierarchism is critical to an understanding of Gagné's learning hierarchy and its influences on task analysis. Gagné at one time believed that all learning is hierarchical. If this is true, pupils must learn in a specified fixed sequence in order to achieve the ultimate (terminal) goals of their learning and instructors must teach in a systematic step-by-step fashion in accordance to the hierarchical principles.

Gagné's development of learning hierarchies proceeded in two related though different ways. The first established a hierarchical model or scheme for general learning. The second called for the application of the hierarchical model to specific areas of instruction. To accomplish the latter, various learning tasks must be (task) analyzed to determine (a) the component skills to be mastered and (b) the specific performances that achieve the desired terminal objectives.

Gagné's Hierarchy of Learning

Gagné's learning hierarchy begins with the most basic, one might say most primitive, of learning skills and advances in stages to the highest of cognitive levels. The components in this hierarchical model of learning, proceeding from the lowest to the highest type of learning, are as follows:

1. Signal learning. This is learning that involves the making of a general type of emotional response or orientation to a stimulus or signal of some sort. For example, a child anticipating a test is somewhat anxious. This represents an emotional awareness of challenges facing the person. A child anticipates going to a circus (looks forward to it) and develops a general happy anticipation, again an orienting response. In school, signal learning is a kind of learning that orients pupils to school tasks and gets them ready to work. As those who work with severely and profoundly handicapped pupils know well, it is necessary that pupils learn to respond to signals before they can be taught other types of behaviors.

2. Stimulus-response learning. This type of learning involves learning to make relatively precise muscle movements in response to stimuli. For example, a child may see a friend approaching and begins to form the mouth in a way that permits the child to say hello. A child asked to write something by teachers begins to grasp a pencil in anticipation of doing so. Stimulus-response learning, i.e., associating responses (R) to stimuli (Ss), is a basic form of learning. It is possible only after a child emotionally responds or otherwise orients to a learning situation.

3. Chaining. This involves the connection of a series of previously independent stimulus-response (S-R) connections so as to coordinate them into meaningful behavioral patterns. Thus, when a student tries to form the mouth to say hello, it isn't enough simply to create a number of different motor responses to stimuli. These responses must be coordinated in a meaningful pattern. Similarly, in order for a pupil to pick up a pencil to write, the child's separate finger movements must be combined and coordinated to create a skillful pattern of pencil movement. In other words, chaining is the combining of separate stimulus-motor responses into meaningful motor patterns. It observes hierarchical principles. First the S-R associations are formed. Then they are chained.

4. Multiple discrimination learning. In this type of learning a variety of stimuli are distinguished from each other so that the pupil can accurately and efficiently respond to one or more of them. A child who calls every animal doggy has not achieved the ability to make multiple discriminations. A child who correctly classifies postage stamps according to the countries that issued them or per denominations is making correct multiple discriminations. The complexities of schoolwork and indeed of everyday living constantly demand multiple discriminations. According to Gagné's hierarchy, effective chaining of S-R responses is essential before successful multiple discriminations can be made.

5. Verbal (symbolic associations). This is an advanced type of chaining made possible once the learner is capable of successful multiple discriminations. Verbal associations are involved when stimuli responses in various chains are of a verbal nature, e.g., words. When we learn the foreign language equivalents of English words, we are making verbal associations. All types of symbolic association, including those of a numerical nature, are included in this category of learning.

6. Concept learning. In concept learning we respond to various things and situations by placing them in their proper classifications or categories. Concept learning is involved when a pupil identifies dogs and cats and whales as all being mammals. It is also involved when a pupil learns that all bodies of water surrounded by land are

continents or that certain rocks are igneous. Such learning is possible only when the pupil is capable of verbal or symbolic associations.

7. Principle learning. Principle learning involves the understanding of relationships among concepts. A pupil is engaged in principle learning when coming to understand cause-and-effect relationships and the various laws of physics. Obviously a pupil must have an adequate number of concepts at one's disposal to engage in principle learning.

8. Problem solving. The pupil applies the principles learned so as to solve problems or to develop an understanding of new and higher order types of principles.

In addition to the vertical learning sequences suggested by the hierarchy, Gagné made the point that a horizontal sequencing of learning should also go on. Thus, at any given level of the hierarchy certain skill units are prerequisite to the achievement of others. For example, at the stimulus-response level of learning, pressing the lips together is a S-R unit that must be learned before the S-R unit of opening the mouth. In learning mathematical concepts, the concept of addition is a prerequisite to that of subtraction. In principle learning, the pupil must understand cause-and-effect relationships before being able to understand energy principles (Gagné & Briggs, 1979).

Gagné's hierarchy is in debt to Piaget in several ways. For example, Gagné's theory is also a stage theory; i.e., Gagné believed that cognition develops from lower to higher levels in an invariant fashion. He also believed that earlier stages of learning must be consolidated as prerequisites to the achievement of higher ones. Gagné's hierarchy, however, is a much simpler theory than Piaget's. And it is not a developmental theory as such, for Gagné was not concerned with the ways that cognition develops over a child's maturation span but rather how it proceeds over the course of learning to perform a particular task.

The practical applications of learning hierarchy have been many, in both behavioral and cognitive realms. Whenever proceeding hierarchically and sequentially in doing task analyses or when instructing, a teacher is observing the hierarchical principles that Gagné championed.

Applications of the Learning Hierarchy in Remedial and Special Education

Efforts have been made to relate Gagné's learning hierarchy to remedial and special education (Gearhart, 1976; Lerner, 1981). The instructors most likely to be concerned with signal learning stage are teachers working with severely and profoundly handicapped individuals for whom orientation to learning is likely to be a major problem. Pupils at higher cognitive levels should for the most part be able to orient themselves appropriately, though teachers cannot take this for granted. Indeed, more and more pupils appear poorly motivated and poorly task oriented these days, so that the training of orientation skills should not be overlooked at any level of instruction.

Stimulus-response connections must be made in all learning. Thus a student must be able to respond orally to the numbers shown or to mark them down with a pencil. We can perhaps most clearly see breakdowns in the proper establishment of S-R units in areas of motor functioning, where many students fail to acquire stimulus-response connections effectively. Chaining problems are most likely to be demonstrated when pupils draw numbers, letters, or geometric forms, or engage in handwriting. Much of so-called perceptual-motor training involves the training of chaining.

Multiple discrimination problems, i.e., distinctions among letters, numbers, and the like, are clearly areas of concern for many learning disabled pupils. Verbal association difficulties are manifested in many encoding and decoding problems. Concept learning, i.e., similarities and differences, class membership, and principle learning and problem solving are more likely to concern remedial and special educators who work with older mildly handicapped or slow learning pupils.

Observations about Gagné's Learning Hierarchy

Gagné's conceptualization of the learning hierarchy was influential when it first appeared. Many influential psychologists and educators agreed with Klausmeier (1976), who observed that the learning hierarchy explicitly indicates "the internal conditions that are prerequisites for the successful learning of skills" (p. 190). Nevertheless not everyone has been altogether convinced as to the details of the hierarchy or its use to guide instruction in as rigid a fashion as Gagné suggested. Klausmeier advised that it should be interpreted with some flexibility. For example, he doesn't believe that pupils must specifically learn or be taught skills at each and all of the hierarchy's levels. For one, the learning of lower level skills may be implicit in the learning of higher level ones (Klausmeier, 1976). Klausmeier prefers a taxonomic approach to cognitive instruction because it allows for greater flexibility. In any case while the learning hierarchy was once hailed as a major approach to remedial and special education, it is no longer particularly influential. Indeed a new instructional theory identified as the Gagné-Briggs instructional model (1979) has been developed; it modifies the hierarchy to some considerable degree.

GAGNÉ-BRIGGS INSTRUCTIONAL MODEL

The Gagné-Briggs theory has certain features in common with Bloom's taxonomy, though Gagné claims to have arrived at his ideas independently from Bloom's model. It is also admittedly indebted to information-processing theory.

Gagné and Dick (1983) define *learning outcome* as "acquired capabilities of human learners" (p. 265). These consist of verbal information, intellectual skills, and cognitive strategies, motor skills, and attitudes.

The cognitive processes essential to these learning outcomes are ones identified by information-processing theorists. They include attention, selective perception, short- and long-term memory, rehearsal and retrieval processes. Internal (cognitive) as well as external events are essential for effective learning. In learning, the learner is assumed to be "reinforced" externally while obtaining information feedback from the environment. Thus, the Gagné-Briggs theory defines *instruction* as "a set of events external to the learner which are assigned to support the internal processes of learning" (Gagné & Dick, 1983, p. 266). Learning outcomes of instruction are conceived of as "acquired capabilities" (p. 265) in the following areas: verbal information, intellectual skills, cognitive strategies, motor skills, and attitudes.

The following approximately ordered sequence of instruction is advised by the Gagné-Briggs model as a means of achieving desired learning outcomes: gaining attention, informing the learner of the objective, stimulating the learner's recall of prerequisites to the learning of the objective, presenting the actual (stimulus) material, providing guidance to that learning, providing feedback, eliciting the performance of the task, providing feedback as to results, enhancing the retention and transfer of the task.

With younger or less able learners, the instructor is usually expected to observe the sequence of instruction systematically. Gagné, however, advises that as learners become more sophisticated, learning events, as he describes them, may increasingly be provided by the learners themselves rather than by the instructor. His new instructional model thus represents a modification from that suggested by the original learning hierarchy, which insists that all instruction proceed in a step-by-step, prescribed order.

The Gagné-Briggs theory model is not as original as the learning hierarchy. Gagné, however, claims that it is still novel from a number of standpoints: It has its roots in a learning hierarchy, it addresses all of the types of learning outcomes to which instruction is usually directed, and its rationale for instruction is a special one; i.e., it relies on the definition of instruction "as a set of events external to the learner to support the internal processes of learning" (Gagné & Dick, 1983, p. 266).

Gagné believes that the new model can be readily applied to instruction in a great number of areas. It can certainly aim itself to behavioral as well as cognitive types of instructional approaches. It has, however, not been particularly influential. And whereas Gagné's original learning hierarchy did significantly affect remedial and special education, the Gagné-Briggs model is not likely to create any great interest among remedial and special education teachers.

CONCEPT TASK ANALYSIS

Herbert Klausmeier is a distinguished educational psychologist whose more recent efforts in cognitive research and instructional psychology have been carried out in close relationships to actual class situations (Klausmeier & Allen, 1978). He has done much of his later work within a Piagetian framework (1979) and acknowledges Gagné's influences.

Klausmeier's work is not likely to be well known in remedial and special education circles since he has developed his theories and instructional programs for regular classroom purposes, often at secondary levels. At the same time it is of interest to anyone concerned with cognition and specifically with cognitive task analysis. For purpose of the latter we briefly review some of Klausmeier's ideas concerning the teaching of concepts, an instructional area with which his name has come to be strongly identified. The term *concept* as he uses it is broadly applied. Paraphrasing a statement made by Kagan in 1966, Klausmeier observes (1976), "Concepts are the building blocks not only for learning principles, problem-solving skills, and taxonomic and hierarchical relationships, but also of thinking itself." They also "comprise a substantial part of many subject matters and are the basic unit of instruction" (p. 191).

Levels of Concept Attainment

Klausmeier (1976) believes that concept teaching should respond to a child's developmental level. He has thus identified four levels of cognitive attainment (in a Piagetian vein) that should broadly guide the teaching concepts:

1. Concrete level. Achievement of a concept at this level involves attending to an object, discriminating it from other objects, and being able to recognize it as the same object at a later time.

2. Identity level. The child generalizes the object as the   same thing at the identity level of learning when the child experiences that object from a different spatio-temporal perspective or through a different sense modality. The child also acquires the name of the object and associates it with the object at both the concrete and identity levels.
3. Beginning classificatory level. The child becomes able to classify objects at this level. The lowest attainment at this level is when the child recognizes two different things as equivalents. At a more advanced, but still beginning, classificatory level the child is able to identify examples and nonexamples of the concept but cannot clearly state the reasons for categorizing the objects.
4. Mature classificatory level and formal level. A pupil at a mature classificatory level has already achieved the target concept at the previous beginning classificatory level. The student is thus ready to deal with concept learning at a beginning formal level and from there can move on to deal with concepts at a more mature level, i.e., that of advanced mathematical and scientific instruction.

Steps in Conducting a Concept Analysis

Klausmeier (1976) has recommended the following steps in concept analysis at more advanced levels of instruction:

1. The taxonomy or hierarchy to which the concepts belong should be outlined. (Klausmeier is partial to taxonomies.)
2. The concept should be defined in terms of its attributes.
3. All of the defining and some of the variables attributes of the concept should be specified.
4. Illustrative examples and nonexamples of the concept should be determined or developed.
5. Illustrative principles incorporating the concept should be identified.
6. Illustrative problem-solving exercises involving the use of the concept should be formulated.
7. A list of key vocabulary words associated with the concepts and its defining attributes should be developed.

The Teaching of Concepts

An instructor seeking to teach concepts effectively must determine the nature of the pupil's mental operations (i.e., concrete, formal, etc.). This is done on the basis of a review and synthesis of research concerning the learning of the concept and through direct behavioral analysis. Both help the instructor understand how a particular child at a particular developmental level may best learn a particular concept. Different developmental levels involve different mental operations and require different types of conceptual training.

Task Analyses for the Teaching of Concepts

Klausmeier (1976) states that three kinds of analysis should guide the preparation of instructional materials and teaching activities for the teaching of concepts. An instructional analysis is to be used so as to reach the desired terminal objectives for any ''target population of students'' (p. 192). The proper development of instructional materials requires that there be

1. A content analysis. An analysis of the concept to be taught, that is, the various facts, concepts, principles and theories that the student must acquire; these are to be embodied in the terminal objectives of the instructional program.
2. A behavioral analysis. An analysis of the cognitive behaviors and operations and skills the pupils must perform to demonstrate the learning of a particular concept at the level it is being taught. These are to be incorporated in the desired terminal objectives.
3. Instructional analysis. This is done to determine the actual instructional procedures to be used for a particular "target population of students" (1976, p. 192). The type of analysis is essential since concepts taught at different age and competency levels must be taught in different ways and achieve different terminal objectives. The concepts to be taught must be organized properly, i.e., in the form of hierarchies or taxonomies. Klausmeier usually prefers taxonomies since they can be applied more flexibly than hierarchies.

Concept Analysis and Remedial and Special Education

Klausmeier (1976) advises that with concept analysis the subject matter levels to be taught should be selected with an understanding of the topic's "structure of knowledge" (p. 192). The educator carrying out a concept analysis within a particular subject should know how the particular concept being taught fits into an appropriate taxonomy or hierarchy for that subject, how that concept is defined by experts in the particular discipline associated with the subject, and how the concept can be useful in solving various problems within the subject being taught. Remedial and special educators may be better able to apply his ideas than regular classroom teachers because their instructional methods are based on explicit instructional theories that can be applied in taxonomic or hierarchical ways, they usually know how their concepts are defined by experts, and they are more familiar with the processes and applications of task analysis than are regular education teachers.

Thus, while Klausmeier's work has been intended for normal pupils, his concepts and methods may be helpful with remedial and handicapped populations. Many seem suited to gifted pupils. Above all, Klausmeier's work is helpful to remedial and special education teachers in that he provides models for systematically establishing cognitive and behavioral objectives through task analysis. It is from this standpoint that we particularly recommend him to our readers.

NEO-PIAGETIAN TASK ANALYSIS

The term *neo-Piagetian* applies to cognitive theories research and interventions that, receiving their inspiration and some of their concepts from Piagetian theory, nevertheless go off in new directions. Klausmeier's work may be considered to be neo-Piagetian in many aspects. Another theory of instruction, clearly neo-Piagetian, that has implications for cognitive task analysis has been proposed by Case (1978a, 1978b). It is founded in Piaget's stage theory but also draws from information-processing, cognitive strategy, and metacognitive theory (Gagné & Dick, 1983).

Case proposes that intellectual development proceeds in stages. At each stage the individual's capabilities depend on the successive development of increasingly complex executive strategies. The latter's development is subject to two types of influences. The first is that of experience and instruction. The second is the gradual increase in the power of immediate short-term working memory, which is identified as *M-power*. Increases in M-power result from the automatization of the learner's basic cognitive operations. As might be expected from a stage theory, the executive cognitive strategies assembled in working memory at each stage are assembled from components developed in earlier stages. This is possible, however, only if the earlier stages have been adequately automatized.

Instructionally Case's theory provides the following guides to instructional design. In the first stage of design the instructor is to identify the goal of the task to be performed and map out the series of cognitive operations through which the pupils may achieve the goals by examining the work and introspections about that work, oral or written, of expert learners (protocol analysis).

In the second stage of instructional design the pupil's current levels of functioning are to be determined by observing how the student approaches the learning task and the nature of the student's cognitive operations, i.e., what strategies are being employed and their manner of use.

The instructor then develops an instructional program. The pupil's own cognitive strategies are first discovered and analyzed. They are then contrasted with the best "expert" cognitive strategies available, and the pupil shows how they are more effective than the pupil's own. After this the learner is provided opportunities to practice and rehearse the expert strategies. Throughout training, efforts are made to minimize cognitive complexity of the tasks being taught (which is what a good cognitive task analysis does) so as to minimize demands on the learner's limited M-power.

More specifically task analyses performed with the Case   instructional scheme observe the following guides:

- The executive strategies relevant to the particular discipline or subject matter areas within which the child is to be instructed must be specified. This first requires a determination of the goals to be achieved within the specific instructional task the child must learn to perform. It then requires a specification of the processes that skilled or expert performers use to arrive at these goals normally.

- The pupil's current level of executive functioning must be determined. This is done by studying the pupil, the way the pupil learns tasks, i.e., the processes used, and the steps in attemping to reach goals.

- The gap between the pupil's current level of performance, specifically the pupil's current use of executive strategies, and that of expert performance is to be bridged. There are three ways, instructionally: (1) presenting the pupil with tasks that demonstrate that current strategies for dealing with them are inadequate compared to other, expert strategies and helping the pupil to learn the latter; (2) teaching the pupil who is cognitively incapable of learning or using expert strategies to use simpler executive strategies that while not as good as the expert ones   will still do the job; and (3) providing the pupil with qualitatively similar tasks that can be mastered using the strategies that are already at the pupil's disposal. The intent of these three conditions is to minimize the complexity of mental operation required of the pupil.

Case's theory demonstrates Piagetian ancestry in a number of ways. Among them is its insistence that a child's level of functioning can't be addressed in instruction terms of specific strengths and weaknesses and must rather be viewed as having a distinct organizational structure of its own.

Case's approach is interesting from several standpoints. First, it appears to be a frank admission that applying classical Piagetian ideas directly to conventional academic tasks is not practical. It does not, for example, attempt to develop a pupil's general cognitive competencies but rather attempts to adapt the pupil to instruction and instruction to the pupil for specific tasks. Providing opportunities to learn strategies, it is true, is in keeping with Piaget's theory. So is the pupil's comparison of the pupil's own strategies to the more effective ones of experts. Having the pupil accept and use someone else's strategies is not, however, in keeping with classical Piagetian doctrine, according to which children must construct their own realities.

Case's theory instruction is a limited one from the standpoint of cognitive task analysis since it concerns itself exclusively with the learning of cognitive strategies. Contrast his approach to that of Gagné or Klausmeier, who have developed far more elaborate approaches to assist in cognitive task analysis. On the other hand it does suggest a useful way of approaching instruction and remediation with pupils who are cognitively capable of responding to the interactive requirements of his program.

ELABORATION THEORY OF INSTRUCTION

Reigeluth and his colleagues (Reigeluth, 1979; Reigeluth & Rodgers, 1978) have developed what they call an *elaboration theory of instruction*. It too utilizes cognitive task analytic principles.

Reigeluth's theory metaphorically conceives good instruction in using a cognitive zoom lens. Viewing an instructional scene through this lens, an instructor begins instruction with a wide angle, i.e., broad conceptual framework. The instructor then zooms down to work on specific details of instruction and zooms up to integrate the specific information gained from the detailed view within the broad framework, wherein it is related to and integrated with the context of learned information and general concepts.

The actual instructional sequence recommended by this elaboration approach is one in which all concepts, operations, etc., to be taught are first determined through task analysis; decisions are made as to the order and sequencing of the operations; appropriately sequenced lessons supporting the instructional content are developed to teach the pupil, and the pupil studies concepts both specifically and in a number of broad "synthetic" ways and practices them through a variety of applications.

Reigeluth's approach borrows many of its elements from a variety of sources including information-processing task analysis (Merrill, 1976) and Gagné's hierarchy. Its novelty is in the zooming notion. This zooming is supposed to enable the student to acquire an increasingly extended and elaborated understanding of subject matter. It has been compared to Bruner's (1966) spiral curriculum and Ausubel's (1968) notion of progressive differentiation. Bruner (1966) conceived of the same conceptual strands appearing throughout the course of instruction in a particular subject area but becoming more progressively developed and complex at higher levels of the instructional spiral. Ausubel (1969) conceived of instruction beginning with a broad general unifying concept and then moving progressively to more precise conceptual differentiations within specific instructional areas.

We are not likely to find Reigeluth's theories applied in special education. They have indeed been developed with advanced studies in mind. Nevertheless it may be helpful to remind us that we can become overanalytic in our instructional methods.

IPP COGNITIVE TASK ANALYSES

A number of the earlier cognitive task analysis approaches we have discussed employ information-processing concepts. The ones to be discussed now embody the latter in particularly vivid terms.

The information-processing paradigm (IPP) is particularly suited to cognitive task analysis. It perhaps shows its true power (and value) best in cognitive instruction when used to task analyze a pupil's cognition under actual learning situations. When this is done, a great deal may be learned about ways to improve pupils' cognitive functioning.

Two IPP approaches to task analysis for study are particularly appropriate to the interests of remedial and special educators. They are defined by Mayer as (1) a *cognitive process approach* and (2) a *cognitive structure approach*. The first is examined in an attempt to understand the pupil's cognitive processes when solving mathematics problems. The second is studied in an effort to understand how learners cognitively organize information. Mayer (1981) serves as our guide in these discussions.

COGNITIVE PROCESS ANALYSIS

Let us say we wish to task analyze the cognitive processes that a five-year-old uses in subtraction. We begin by watching the child while actually solving an arithmetic problem. Given the problem "what is eight when you take away five," we see that the child first puts out five fingers and says five and then finally extends three more fingers and counts six, seven, eight. The child then tells you the answer is three.

Using protocol analysis, i.e., interviewing the child to determine how the child arrived at the answer, we find that the child has subtracted five from eight by adding using a counting procedure. While this is an inefficient technique, it is one that can be mastered at a relatively early age and is thus quite appropriate for a five-year-old. On the basis of a task analysis we are able to develop a teaching program that embodies our pupil's methods:

- Set up your counters. Your fingers are one type of counter you will use. Your voice is another.

- Begin counting. Stick out all the fingers for the smaller number you have been given in the problem. Say nothing (the voice counter is figuratively speaking set at zero at this point).

- Ask yourself a question about the fingers. Do the fingers you stuck out equal the larger number in the problem? If yes, you should stop and tell the teacher how many times you added to the smaller number of fingers to make them as many. If the number of fingers you have out is not as many as the larger number, you should go on to Step 4.

- Increment (add to) your counters by 1. Stick out one more finger and say out loud how many times you have come to Step 3.

Using this program, the pupils keep adding fingers to the count while recycling or looping through the program between Steps 2 and 4 until giving the right answer which terminates the program. Allowing the pupil to apply this program to an eight minus five subtraction problem, we find the child begins at Step 1 by throat clearing and sticking out five fingers; then proceeds to Step 2, silently counting fingers; and then to Step 3, comparing the number of fingers counted to the number eight.

Finding that the fingers stuck out are fewer than eight, the child goes on to Step 4 to stick out an additional finger and to state how many times this was done this by saying one. The child then returns to Step 2 to stick an additional finger out. Repeating Step 3, the child finds that eight fingers haven't been extended and goes on to Step 4 to add another finger while saying two to indicate that this is the second time through the learning sequence. Again at Step 3, the child is reminded to return to Step 2 and once more to compare the number of fingers to the larger number (eight). Finding the fingers extended to be fewer than eight, the child proceeds on through Step 4 to add another finger (the third time) and finds that the fingers are now equal to the larger number begun with (eight). The child then tells the teachers how many times (three) the finger count was incremented to make them equal eight. This is the correct answer to the problem and on stating it, the pupil terminates the counting program. Figure 11–1 shows another way of demonstrating the program. This type of counting program is a primitive one. Nevertheless it may be the right one for young children or cognitively impaired ones. Older pupils usually apply much more efficient programs. They often develop them on their own, without formal instruction.

Resnick (1976), studying the way children solve arithmetic problems, found that even when pupils give the same answers to particular problems, they often do so using quite different procedural models (programs). By carrying out a cognitive task analysis of the pupils' protocols, i.e., by analyzing their gestures, their oral and written reports, and their answers, it is possible not only to determine the nature of these programs but also to decide

---

Figure 11–1 Process Model for Simple Subtraction (Flow-Chart Format)

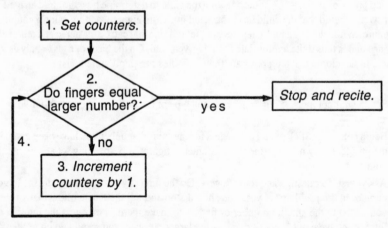

Source: Reprinted from *The Promise of Cognitive Psychology* by Richard E. Mayer with permission of W.H. Freeman and Company, © 1981.

which ones are the most efficient or effective for a particular age or type of child. (Chase suggests a similar approach from a broader instructional perspective.) Speed of solution is one way of telling which procedural programs are best for particular children. The number of errors they make is another. So are the numbers of correct and incorrect answers.

This type of cognitive task analytic approach may be particularly helpful to remedial and special educators. Brown and Burton (1978) have indeed shown that it can be applied across a broad range of arithmetic problems. Using process analysis, these researchers sought to study the different procedures pupils use to solve subtraction problems. They gave 1,325 pupils large numbers of subtraction problems and task analyzed their procedural mistakes. They uncovered four major types of problems: (1) when borrowing from a column with a zero on top, the pupil changes it to nine but doesn't subtract one from the number column to the left; (2) instead of subtracting a bottom number from a top one, the student subtracts the smaller from the larger; (3) when subtracting a bottom number from a top one that is zero, the pupil writes the bottom number as an answer; and (4) when borrowing from a column with a zero, the pupil skips the column to borrow from the next column. A particularly interesting finding was that pupils would often have difficulties in solving particular problems because they used procedures that had been successful but were inappropriate for the particular task at hand. Thus, the correct use of strategies appears as important to specific types of arithmetic instruction as it is to other types of problem solving.

Brown and Burton embodied some of their discoveries in a computer program they called BUGGY. With BUGGY a computer is programmed with all the right and wrong procedures used in particular subtraction problems. When a pupil answers a subtraction problem, the computer determines whether the answer is right or not and also whether the pupil employed the best procedures possible. Beyond that the computer can determine where the pupil's procedural problems lie and provide remedial assistance.

Other Types of Process Analysis

Other approaches to process analysis in arithmetic have also been suggested by Landa (1976) and Scandura (1977) among others; they suggest that problems first be analyzed so as to determine the best procedures, i.e., rules and algorithms for solving them, and that these procedures be taught to pupils before actually giving them problems to solve. By doing so, it may be possible to reduce pupils' errors and failure rates. A danger of this approach, one that Chase recognized, is that the best general approach may not be best for a particular child. It may, for example, be necessary to teach a particular child an inferior procedure because it is the only one that the child can use at all.

Process analysis seems to lend itself well to remedial and special education. Indeed cognitive process task analysis, directed to specific areas of study, is one of the most promising of cognitive applications to remedial and special education.

COGNITIVE STRUCTURE ANALYSIS

Much cognitive research has been devoted to the isolation of the structural components of cognition. What we call *cognitive task analysis* is a limited type of structural analysis. It is used to analyze the make-up of particular types of information in order to understand how that information is usually managed by the learners.

Cognitive structure task analysis is specifically used to analyze a person's verbal knowledge about something into its parts and to understand the latter's relationships. Structure models, often presented in the forms of tree diagrams, are used to assist in the analysis. Particular samples of verbal knowledge can be presented in tree diagrams in the form of individual units (in the form of rectangles, oval boxes, etc.) and their relationships shown (by lines drawn among these units). In using such a tree diagram (see Figure 11–2), verbal information can be readily analyzed from a hierarchical standpoint. Thus, in analyzing a sentence, the sentence is on top of the tree, clauses and phrases on the second line of branches, subjects, prepositions, noun phrases on a third branch, etc.

Certain rules govern the structural task analysis of verbal information. Thorndyke in his study of the cognitive memory structures involved in the recall of a narrative carried out an analysis according to the following rules:

- A story can be broken down into a number of distinct components: a setting, a theme, a plot, and the resolution of the story.
- The story's components can be further task analyzed along the following lines: A setting usually consists of characters, location, and time; the theme resolves into events plus a goal (a state). The plot consists of a series of episodes, each of which can be studied in terms of a subgoal, the attempts made to reach the subgoal, and the outcome of these attempts. The resolution of the story consists of an event or a state (the achievement of a particular goal).

All of these actually constitute rules for understanding narrative. Rumelhart (1975), Thorndyke (1977), and Mayer (1981) suggest that pupils continually apply such structures when they speak, write, or attempt to comprehend language information, even though they are usually unaware of doing so. And whenever pupils read, they too organize cognitively what they are reading according to structures.

Thorndyke (1977) carried out a structural task analysis called "Cognitive Structures in Comprehension and Memory of Narrative Discourse" to study the learning of a story "The Old Farmer and the Donkey." Thorndyke specifically wanted to determine how the story's structure affected its comprehension and retention. In order to do this, he had to analyze the story in particular ways. He first broke the story down into various propositions, each representing one simple event or state (Exhibit 11–1). His next step was to structure the story according to the propositions that best represented the narrative. He thus first used parsing rules to divide the story into four parts: (1) setting, (2) theme, (3) plot, and (4) resolution. He then broke the story down into the components that make up these parts (see Figure 11–3).

Analyzing the setting of the story (which may be broken down into its characters, location, and time), he found that its characters are the farmer and the donkey but that nothing in the story can be assigned a particular location or time. Dealing with the theme, which consists of the major goal of the story, Thorndyke found that it was stated entirely in Proposition 3; the farmer wanted to get the donkey into the shed. He then moved to deal with the plot, which has a number of distinguishable episodes, each with specific subgoals, attempts, and outcomes. In the first episode the subgoal was to pull the donkey; this was attempted in Proposition 4 and failed in Proposition 5. In the next episode the new subgoal was to frighten the donkey; this is stated in Propositions 10 and 15. This is achieved in Proposition 34, i.e., getting the donkey into the shed. However, in order to achieve this

Figure 11–2 Tree Structure Used with Sentences

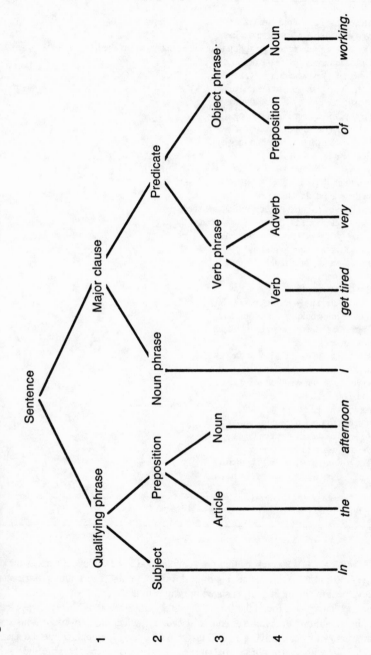

Exhibit 11-1 List of Events and States for "The Old Farmer and the Donkey"

---

1. There was once an old farmer
2. who owned a very stubborn donkey.
3. One evening the farmer was trying to put the donkey into its shed.
4. First, the farmer pulled the donkey,
5. but the donkey wouldn't move.
6. Then the farmer pushed the donkey,
7. but still the donkey wouldn't move.
8. Finally, the farmer asked his dog
9. to bark loudly at the donkey
10. and thereby frighten him into the shed.
11. But the dog refused.
12. So then, the farmer asked his cat
13. to scratch the dog
14. so the dog would bark loudly
15. and thereby frighten the donkey into the shed.
16. But the cat replied, "I would gladly scratch the dog
17. if only you would get me some milk."
18. So the farmer went to his cow
19. and asked for some milk
20. to give to the cat.
21. But the cow replied,
22. "I would gladly give you some milk
23. if only you would give me some hay."
24. Thus, the farmer went to the haystack
25. and got some hay.
26. As soon as he gave the hay to the cow,
27. the cow gave the farmer some milk.
28. Then the farmer went to the cat
29. and gave the milk to the cat.
30. As soon as the cat got the milk,
31. it began to scratch the dog.
32. As soon as the cat scratched the dog,
33. the dog began to bark loudly.
34. The barking so frightened the donkey
35. that it jumped immediately into its shed.

Source: Reprinted from "Cognitive Structures in Comprehension and Memory of Narrative Discourse" by Perry W. Thorndyke in *Cognitive Psychology,* vol. 9, with permission of Academic Press, Inc., © 1977.

---

particular subgoal (34), a number of earlier subgoals had to be achieved, such as the dog barking (Proposition 33), the cat getting milk (Proposition 30). The solution of the story, the achievement of the main goal, is stated in Proposition 35.

To sum up, Thorndyke found the story "The Old Farmer and the Donkey" was clearly divisible into a number of definite cognitive structures, which include propositions about two characters, a theme resolving around the goal of getting the donkey into the shed, a complicated plot with a variety of subgoals that resulted in an outcome of scaring the donkey and bringing about a resolution, i.e., in which the donkey was returned to the shed.

As seen in Figure 11–3 a structural tree model presents his structural analysis of "The Old Farmer and the Donkey" quite well, but how useful is it? His predictions were confirmed.

Thorndyke tested his information tree model in several ways to see whether it could be helpful in predicting the story's recall. He specifically predicted that subjects (college students) recalling the story would best remember the propositions highest on the tree and would remember those on lower "branches" less well. His predictions were confirmed. Subjects recalling the story could remember all of the Level 1 information but less and less information at lower levels. In other words, it seemed as if the students had tentatively constructed a knowledge tree as they read the story and had gradually worked their way down the tree's tip to its bottom as they organized the story in their minds and memories. In a second test of his model, Thorndyke had another group of students read the story's propositions in a random order. Finding that they recalled equal amounts of information from each of the levels, he concluded that they could not construct a knowledge tree from randomized propositions and thus were forced to recall the information in less organized ways.

In a third test of his model Thorndyke had other groups of students read and recall versions of the story that either didn't state the central theme or did so only at the story's end. He found that these students, despite the fact that they read the story in the same order as did the subjects who read it in the original version, found it difficult to recall the story. Apparently it is difficult to construct an information tree when one of its basic structures (the theme) is missing or improperly placed.

What promise does cognitive structure analysis have for remedial and special education? It enables us to break down types of verbal information in ways that clarify the organization and the relationships of their components. It can thus help instructors and students to identify the information to be learned and how it is to be learned in advance of a lesson and to manage this information better for more efficient recall and use.

The approach has potentially diagnostic implications. It can be used to distinguish the ways poor students or handicapped learners construct their knowledge trees and manage them as compared to normal pupils. It may be possible to use such knowledge to organize instruction better along individualized lines. Mayer (1981) has some useful suggestions along these lines.

COGNITIVE TASK ANALYSIS IN REMEDIAL READING

Sound traditional teaching can benefit from cognitive task analysis and from a careful analysis of the subjects being taught and of the steps and sequences that a pupil should observe to achieve the goals of instruction. In reading, the teaching of encoding and decoding skills (both cognitive processes) can readily be task analyzed for purposes of creating clearly stated objectives. This is one reason perhaps why it is possible to teach children decoding skills with a great deal of success these days and why remediation of these skills is one of the most successful educational achievements of the modern age.

Teaching reading comprehension skills, however, has been far more difficult, perhaps in part because it is more difficult to delineate appropriately the important cognitive structures and processes involved in reading. Efforts along these lines have nevertheless been made.

Otto and Smith's (1980) remedial approaches to teaching comprehension attempt to deal with the more literal aspects of reading comprehension that they believe are basic to all aspects of comprehension, as well as being a major concern in remedial education. They define *comprehension* as consisting of skill clusters that involve getting meaning from

Figure 11–3 Structural Tree Model for "The Old Farmer and the Donkey"

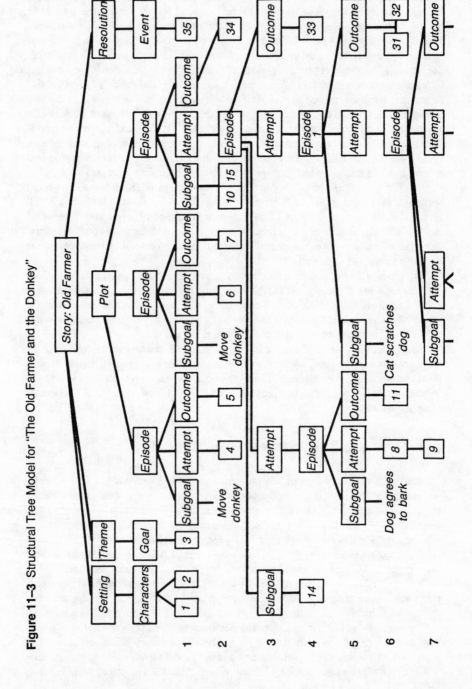

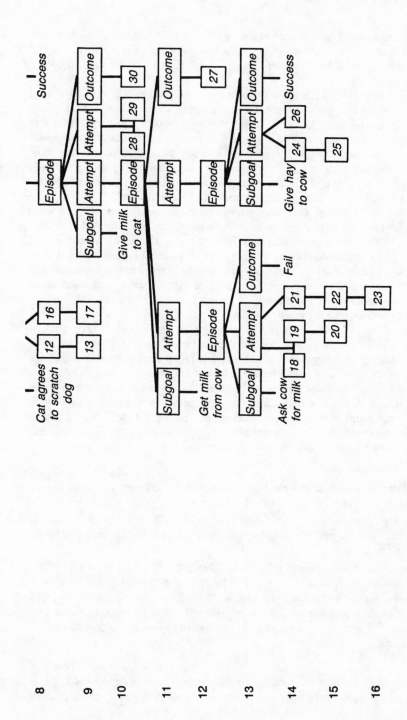

Source: Reprinted from "Cognitive structures in comprehension and memory of narrative discourse" by Perry W. Thorndyke in *Cognitive Psychology*, vol. 9, with permission of Academic Press, Inc., © 1977.

words, getting meaning from sentences, getting meaning from selections, and identifying sequence. They believe that each of the skills in each of the clusters can be assigned objectives that describe the "behavior a student should be able to exhibit in relation to a skill" (p. 257).

Otto and Smith (1980) define *comprehension* at its most basic level as an understanding of written symbols. At the observable level, comprehension deals with symbols, i.e., printed words or other visual display (S), to which the pupil responds, i.e., by oral and written statements, by checking answers on a test page, or by making gestures, or by otherwise physically performing a task (R). Mediating between the S and the R are "concepts, symbols, capacities—that help . . . [the pupil] . . . understand the symbols" (p. 254). Comprehension is a cognitive product that results from the "complex interactions of many specific skills with factors both *inside* and *outside* the head of the reader" (p. 254).

Otto and Smith (1980) advise that the cognitive aspects of reading comprehension are to be task analyzed so as to enable them to be expressed clearly in the form of behavioral responses. Verbal statements constitute legitimate behaviors. Thus a pupil's statement that expresses the comprehension of simple words represents a definition (comprehension) of those words. So does a statement of synonyms for them. Behaviors that express reading comprehension include the substitution of appropriate alternate words in sentences or the paraphrasing of statements. In such ways a student can demonstrate comprehension by expressing "a given meaning in a different way" (p. 261).

One part of Otto and Smith's (1980) task analytic approach to the teaching of comprehension skills involves the teaching of "relationships and conclusion skills/objectives." The goals of instruction are that pupils will be able to identify and interpret factual relationships in written materials and on that basis be able to form conclusions. The teacher's role in this instruction is to help the pupil identify and synthesize the statements in a reading passage that appear to be leading to a particular outcome or type of conclusions, help the pupil to focus on "statements of relationships" that support a particular conclusion, and then to decide whether the conclusion is supported by the information presented in the statement. The following objectives exemplify this type of information:

- Teaching of outcomes. The pupil synthesizes two or more events from the reading passages in order to predict   logical events.
- Drawing conclusions based on single relationships. The pupil verbally indicates whether a conclusion is correct on the basis of a single relationship that is stated in the reading passage.
- Conclusions based on direct relationships. The pupil verbally indicates whether a conclusion is correct based on directly stated relationships in the reading passage.
- Conclusions based on indirect relationships. The pupil verbally states whether particular conclusions are correctly based on the relationships that are indirectly stated in the passage (i.e., relationships that must be synthesized by the pupil from more than one statement).

Otto and Smith's approach is certainly familiar. In fact, much of remedial education is based on   cognitive task analyses of one sort or another even though it may not be identified as such.

COGNITIVE TASK ANALYSIS OF TEST ITEMS

Traditional and intelligence aptitude researchers usually attempt to determine how test items correlate with various criteria, e.g., school performance and success on the job, or analyze in terms of specific factors. In contrast, newer cognitive approaches have attempted to analyze intelligence in terms of its components.

Along these lines Carroll (1976a, 1976b) and Simon (1976) both have suggested that test items be analyzed as cognitive tasks, and a number of cognitive researchers have proceeded along these lines. Sternberg (1977), however, is the scholar whose work has perhaps most clearly been identified with what is called a "componential analysis of intelligence."

Such analysis uses psychological laboratory methods to investigate how pupils perform particular aptitude and intelligence test items. Sternberg has sought to understand the number of different cognitive components involved in solving particular test items, the number of times these components are employed in solving the items, their sequencing, and the manner of their execution. Using cognitive models to explain and predict pupils' test performances, Sternberg has found that when they were given the task of solving verbal analogies, the cognitive component of encoding stimulus terms used about half of the pupils' cognitive processing time, while only 40 percent of their processing time was devoted to the cognitive component involved in comparing the attributes of the terms. In contrast, pupils solving geometric analogies spent most of their processing time in comparing attributes. Comparing children to adults in solving analogies, he found that the former rely more on forming associations between the words in an analogy test (one type of cognitive component) while the latter spend more time in the analysis of relationships among words (another cognitive component) (Resnick, 1981). Such work is certainly interesting. Whether it will have practical implications remains to be demonstrated.

CONCLUSION

Almost all good instruction requires that the instructor proceed on the basis of clearly articulated objectives. While this statement might have been an issue of debate for previous generations of teachers, it is now almost universally accepted.

The approaches presented in this chapter as representative of cognitive task analysis are but a few of many. Many other instructional approaches though known by different names could also justify their inclusion on the basis of being cognitive and using task analytic procedures.

Good instructional objectives require four factors: (1) determination of what is to be taught, (2) analysis of what is to be taught so as to form objectives, (3) determination of the behaviors or performances that indicate achievement of the objectives, and (4) criteria by which to judge achievement of the terminal objectives. Behavioral objectives have become popular because they lend themselves easily to (2) and (3). Cognitive objectives do well on the other hand with (1) but have trouble with (2) and (3). It seems to us that both behavioral and cognitive objectives have trouble with (4). In practice, if we relate cognitive objectives to behavioral ones for instructional purposes, to take advantage of the best aspects of both types of objectives, we may be better able to accomplish all four.

Cognitive task analysis is a form of reductionism (Chapter 2). Like all forms of reductionism it has the advantage of clarifying the topics studied and of helping us to understand

and control their variables with greater precision. At the same time the cautions raised about reductionism in other areas apply to cognitive task analysis. There are thus dangers in cognitive task analysis of possible oversimplifications of cognitive issues and of possible violence to the complexity of larger cognitive units. We can reduce such dangers by judiciously applying both reductionist and nonreductionist points of view in cognitive instruction. There are times, for example, when we wish to teach our pupils systematically every point of a cognitive process or structure continuum. There are other times when we choose to teach them in more complex, dynamic, interactionist, or holistic ways. Remedial and special education teachers should approach instruction so as to maintain a proper dynamic between specific and global teaching and learning. If they do so, cognitive task analysis is sure to have an honored place but not the whole place in instruction and remediation.

Chapter 12

Cognition and Its Relation to Remedial and Special Education: Some Observations and Conclusions

The term *instructional psychology* was first used to identify a particular area of research in the 1969 *Annual Review of Psychology*. This field of instructional psychology has been characterized as "consisting of research on the acquisition of knowledge and cognitive skill and how this competence is developed through the design of conditions for learning" (Klahr, 1976, ix). It is a field that studies the integration of cognition and instruction and attempts to determine how one affects the other.

Instructional psychology in many of its aspects is identifiable with the broader field of educational psychology. It is specifically concerned with instruction, which educational psychologists at one time tended to neglect because it wasn't scientifically respectable (Klahr, 1976).

Instructional psychology in its earlier years, despite its early cognitive orientation, tended to some behavioristic overtones. This is less true during recent years. Resnick (1981) and Gagné and Briggs (1979) have identified instructional psychology as being more or less an applied branch of cognitive science. As Resnick (1981) states, instructional psychology "is now largely cognitive; it is concerned with internal mental processes and how they are enhanced through instruction" (p. 662).

Remedial and special educators who are interested in cognition are largely interested in it from the standpoint of instruction. So remedial and special educators, insofar as they are involved with cognitive processes, can regard themselves as practitioners of cognitive instructional psychology. If this statement is a legitimate one, and it is, we should evaluate remedial and special education efforts—at least insofar as they involve cognitive processes—in the broader context of instructional psychology. To do this is a sobering experience.

Instructional psychologists are legitimately enthusiastic about their field. They are also frank about its shortcomings. They agree that they have learned and are learning much about instruction by applying the methods of cognitive science to it. Many of them admit that they have not yet been able to translate effectively their understanding of cognition into methods that greatly help either to improve children's cognitive functioning or make significant improvements in academic instruction. Along these lines Resnick (1981) has observed that "even a diligent search of instructional implications of [cognitive instruction psychology] . . . yields only . . . relatively general suggestions. . . . If one were to base one's

261

prescriptions entirely on [cognitive instruction approaches] . . . [involving] . . . direct instructional interventions the suggestions would have to be more limited" (p. 692).

As Resnick (1981) puts it, instructional psychology is "largely a descriptive science, intent on analyzing performance but not upon making strong suggestions for improving it" (p. 692). A review of instructional psychology two years later suggests that no significant events have changed her opinion (Gagné & Dick, 1983).

DESCRIPTIVE AND PRESCRIPTIVE INSTRUCTIONAL SCIENCE

The distinction that Resnick made between descriptive and prescriptive instructional science, initially made by Glaser (Glaser & Resnick, 1972), appears to be an important one for remedial and special educators. Descriptive science seeks to understand the nature of the phenomena being studied to determine the relationships among them and to predict events. Prescriptive science on the other hand is interested in taking the laws and theorems established by descriptive science and in prescribing interventions on their basis. Physics and biology are descriptive sciences. Engineering and medicine are prescriptive ones. There are descriptive and prescriptive aspects to instructional psychology. The descriptive side is fairly well established. The prescriptive side, as Resnick said, is still weak.

Glaser and Resnick (1972) have listed five components that a prescriptive theory of instructional psychology needs:

1. description of the state of knowledge to be achieved by the learner, that is, a description of the instruction
2. description of the initial cognitive state in which the learner begins
3. description of the actions that are to be taken to change the initial state of learning
4. assessment of specific instructional effects
5. evaluation of generalized learning outcomes

Cognitive instructional psychology does not quite meet the requirements of prescriptive science as outlined above. Resnick (1981) observes that it has focused its attention most strongly on Components 1 and 2, and it now has the necessary tools to achieve Components 3 and 4; i.e., we can assess the task performances that are the "indicators of the understanding and knowledge that are the deeper goals of education" (p. 693). In respect to the fifth component, however, that of specifying actions to change cognitive states, Resnick believes that "cognitive instructional psychology has been almost completely silent" (p. 693).

The latter statement by Resnick may appear shocking. Are we to assume that Resnick was not aware of remedial or special education when she made this statement? Her statement rather lays bare the fact that although many educators, remedial and special educators certainly among them, believe in cognitive intervention, we have little substantial knowledge about how to do it, nor much scientific proof that it works. Despite the plethora of articles extolling the effectiveness of this or that type of cognitive intervention, there is not a strong scientific basis to support the efficiency of particular techniques of cognitive intervention.

Several questions pose themselves at this juncture. The first one is why certain cognitive interventions appear to work for some pupils, if what we wrote is true. The answer to this question is that the very act of intervention, regardless of the nature of the intervention, often has beneficial results. This has been shown again and again. When teachers try to train their pupils cognitively, they become more actively involved with their pupils and often spend time instructing them. Their pupils, seeing some new hope of success, often put forth a greater effort to learn. Intervention of any kind, cognitive or behavioral, can have strongly energizing and beneficial effects on instruction.

The second question that we might ask is whether we should continue to attempt cognitive interventions when there is really little scientific justification for their use. The answer to this is a guarded yes. Every field of human endeavor proceeds on the basis of the knowledge available to it. Physicians practiced medicine when most of what they did was scientifically invalid. Astronomers originally practiced their craft based on gross misinterpretations of planetary events. We must continue to try cognitive interventions if our interest in education proceeds beyond the training of simple skills and the inculcation of simple habits. Our efforts may eventually be productive.

Beyond this, a cognitive perspective in education is valuable even if cognitive interventions don't work. Cognitive research, theory, and models help us to understand our pupils from particular perspectives, not just what those pupils do but what they are, which means we can individualize more effectively for them.

PROXIMAL AND DISTAL EDUCATION

In addition to helping us to understand our pupils' cognitive orientations, cognitive studies provide purpose to education. Egon Brunswick (1956), a distinguished psychologist who pioneered in ecological psychology, has provided a helpful perspective from which to contrast behavioral and cognitive points of view. He wrote about proximal and distal stimuli and behaviors, somehow focused through a personal "lens." Proximal stimuli and behaviors are simple and molecular in nature. Distal stimuli and behaviors in contrast engage us in complex molar ways. To distal stimuli we respond with perceptions and thought rather than simple sensations. In distal types of behavior we are purposeful and seek to accomplish meaningful goals rather than to emit series of discrete motor movements.

Both cognitive and behavioral research take proximal and distal points of view at different times. Nevertheless behavioral education more often appears to be proximal education, cognitive education more often distal education. Thus in behavioral education the curriculum typically emphasizes the reaching of specific instructional objectives while in cognitive education instructional objectives are employed with the understanding that they are important not just of themselves but are representative of broad domains of knowledge or ability.

COMPATIBILITY OF COGNITIVE AND BEHAVIORAL PARADIGMS

Cognitive education and behavioral education are not incompatible. Each can assist the other. Along these lines Greeno (1976) has suggested that cognitive objectives for instruction enrich rather than replace behavioral objectives. Similarly Resnick (1981) states that it is "possible to treat [behavioral] task performances as indicators of the understanding and knowledge that are deeper goals of education" (p. 693).

Indeed many phenomena can be studied from different standpoints. Music can be scientifically studied from the standpoint of frequency and amplitude measures. It can also be studied objectively in terms of harmony and counterpoint. It can further be studied from the standpoint of the listener's acoustic responses and behaviors or at another level in terms of the listener's experiences and personal-emotive reactions. For that matter music can be studied in terms of the materials that constitute the instruments used to create it. Each level of study is valid for different purposes. Each level helps to explain the other levels and may partly be explained by them. But each level has its own unique characteristics that deserve study in their own right. We cannot reduce or explain an individual's exhilaration at a great piece of music simply on the basis of the resins in the violinists' instruments, the amplitudes and frequencies that help to create it, or in terms of the listener's stimulus-response associations. The esthetic experience must be studied and appreciated in its own right.

So it is with cognition and behavior. They are also most certainly related, interdependent, and essential to each other. Yet each may be usefully studied and applied separately from the other both in regular classrooms and with cognitively impaired individuals. Just as a physician or engineer chooses from different technologies to solve particular problems, so can and should we choose ours from both behavioral and cognitive domains, to fit best the needs of our educational clients.

Having stated the case in favor of cognition—which we believe—we conclude this book with some final notes. A few are cautionary. Do not believe everything you hear and read about cognition. Remember always that when dealing with cognition you are dealing with constructs and that constructs are artificial—arbitrary, hypothetical creations—not real in any physical sense. Most of them will be superseded in due time by other constructs. Do not believe, either, all the wonderful claims you read about new types of cognitive interventions. But neither should you be afraid of trying cognitive concepts because there isn't definitive proof they work. You may find that they work for you.

Bibliography

Abikoff, H. (1979). Cognitive training interventions in children: Review of a new approach. *Journal of Learning Disabilities, 12*, 123–135.

Adorno, T.W., Frenkel-Brunswik, E., Levinson, D.J., & Stanford, R.N. (1950). *The authoritarian personality.* New York: Harper & Row.

Alesandrini, K.L., Langstaff, J.J., & Wittrock, M.C. (1984). Visual-verbal strategies and analytic-holistic strategies. *Journal of Educational Research, 77* (3), 151–157.

Anastasi, A. (1976). *Psychological testing* (4th ed.). New York: Macmillan.

Anastasi, A. (1982). Coaching, test sophistication and developed abilities. *American Psychologist, 36*, 1086–1102.

Anastasi, A. (1983). Evaluating trait concepts. *American Psychologist, 38*, 175–184.

Anderson, B.F. (1975). *Cognitive psychology.* New York: Academic Press.

Anderson, J.R. (1976). *Language, memory and thought.* Hillsdale, NJ: Erlbaum.

Anderson, J.R. (1980). *Cognitive psychology and its implications.* San Francisco: W.H. Freeman and Co.

Anderson, J.R., & Bower, G.H. (1973). *Human associative memory.* Washington, DC: V.H. Winston & Sons.

Anderson, J.R., & Bower, G.H. (1974). A propositional theory of recognition memory. *Memory and Cognition, 2*, 406–41.

Arter, J.A., & Jenkins, J.R. (1979). Differential diagnostic-prescriptive teaching: A critical appraisal. *Review of Educational Research, 49*, 517–555.

Atkinson, R.C., & Shiffrin, R.M. (1968). Human memory. A proposed system and its control processes. In H.W. Spence & J.T. Spence (Eds.), *The psychology of learning and motivation* (Vol. 2). New York: Academic Press.

Ausburn, L.J., & Ausburn, F.B. (1978). Cognitive styles: Some information and implications for instructional design. *Educational Communication and Technology Journal, 26*, 337–354.

Ausubel, D.P. (1968). *Educational psychology: A cognitive view.* New York: Holt, Rinehart & Winston.

Ausubel, D.P. (1969). The use of advanced organizers in the learning and retention of meaningful material. *Journal of Educational Psychology, 51*, 267–272.

Ayres, A.J. (1972a). *Sensory integration and learning disorders.* Los Angeles: Western Psychological Services.

Ayres, A.J. (1972b). *Southern California Sensory Integration Tests.* Los Angeles: Western Psychological Services.

Ayres, A.J. (1975). The sensorimotor foundations of academic ability. In W.M. Cruickshank & D.P. Hallahan (Eds.), *Perceptual and learning disabilities in children. Vol. 2. Research and theory.* Syracuse, NY: Syracuse University Press.

Baddeley, A.D. (1978). The trouble with levels: A reexamination of Craik & Lockhart's framework for memory research. *Psychological Review, 85*, 139–152.

Baker, H.J., & Leland, B. (1935). *Detroit Tests of Learning Aptitude.* Indianapolis: Bobbs-Merrill.

Baker, L. (1982). An evaluation of metacognitive deficits in learning disabilities. *Topics in Learning and Learning Disabilities, 2*, 27–35.

Bannatyne, A. (1971). *Language, reading and learning disabilities: Psychology, neuropsychology, diagnosis and remediation*. Springfield, IL: Charles C Thomas.

Barbeau, A., Growden, J.H., & Wurtman, R.J. (Eds.). (1979). *Nutrition and the brain. Choline and lecithin in brain disorders* (Vol. 5). NY: Rowen Press.

Baron, J. (1978). Intelligence and general strategies. In G. Underwood (Ed.), *Strategies of information processing* (pp. 403–450). London: Academic Press.

Barsch, R.H. (1965). *A movigenic curriculum* (Bulletin No. 25). Madison, WI: Department of Public Instruction. Bureau for the Handicapped.

Barsch, R.H. (1967a). *Achieving perceptual-motor efficiency* (Vol. 1). Seattle: Special Child Publications.

Barsch, R.H. (1967b). *Enriching perception and cognition* (Vol. 2). Seattle: Special Child Publications.

Barsch, R.H. (1967c). *Perceptual motor curriculum* (Vol. 2). Seattle: Special Child Publications.

Bartlett, F.C. (1932). *Remembering an experimental and social study*. Cambridge: Cambridge University Press.

Bateman, B. (1964). Learning disabilities—Yesterday, today and tomorrow. *Exceptional Children, 31,* 167–177.

Baumeister, A.S., & Brooks, P. (1981). Cognitive deficits in mental retardation. In J.M. Kauffman & D.P. Hallahan (Eds.), *Handbook of special education* (pp. 87–107). Englewood Cliffs, NJ: Prentice-Hall.

Beck, A.T. (1976). *Cognitive therapy and the emotional disorders*. New York: International University Press.

Belmont, J.M., & Butterfield, E.C. (1971). Learning strategies as determinants of memory deficiencies. *Cognitive Psychology, 2,* 411–420.

Bender, L. (1938). *The Bender Visual-Motor Gestalt Test for Children*. New York: American Orthopsychiatric Association.

Bengston, J.K. (1979). Cognitive style: The individual difference variable that doesn't make a difference. *Viewpoints in Teaching and Learning, 55,* 91–97.

Bennett, C.I. (1979). Individual differences and how teachers perceive them. *Social Studies, 70,* 56–61.

Benton, A. (1963). *Revised visual retention test*. New York: Psychological Corp.

Binet, A., & Simon, T. (1908). Le développement de l'intelligence chez les enfants. *L'Année Psychologique, 11,* 193–244.

Birch, H.G., & Belmont, L. (1963). Auditory-visual integration in normal and retarded readers. *American Journal of Orthopsychiatry, 34,* 89.

Birch, H.G., & Belmont, L. (1965). Auditory visual integration, intelligence and reading abilities in school children. *Perceptual and Motor Skills, 20,* 295–305.

Birch, H.G., & Telford, A. (1963). Intersensory development in children. *Monograph of the Society for Research in Child Development, 28,* No. 89.

Blackman, S., & Goldstein, R.M. (1982). Cognitive styles and learning disabilities. *Journal of Learning Disabilities, 15,* 106–113.

Blau, T.H. (1977). Torque and schizophrenic vulnerability. *American Psychologist, 32,* 497–1005.

Block, N.J., & Dworkin, G. (1967a). IQ heritability and inequality. In N.J. Block & G. Dworkin (Eds.), *The IQ controversy: Critical readings*. New York: Pantheon.

Block, N.J., & Dworkin, G. (Eds.). (1967b). *The IQ controversy*. New York: Pantheon.

Bloom, B.S. (1976). *Human characteristics and school learning*. New York: McGraw-Hill.

Bloom, B.S., & Brader, L. (1950). *Problem solving processes of college students*. Chicago: University of Chicago Press.

Bloom, B.S., Englehart, M.B., Furst, E.J., Hill, W.H., & Krathwohl, D.R. (1956). *Taxonomy of educational objectives. The classification of educational goals. Handbook I: Cognitive domain*. New York: Longman Green.

Bogen, J.E. (1977). Some educational implications of hemispheric specialization. In M.C. Wittrock (Ed.), *The human brain*. Englewood Cliffs, NJ: Prentice-Hall.

Bolles, R.C. (1975). Learning and cognition. In W.K. Estes (Ed.), *Handbook of learning and cognitive processes*. Hillsdale, NJ: Erlbaum.

Bond, L., & Glaser, R. (1979). Review of aptitudes and instruction methods; ATI, but mostly A&T with not much of I. *Applied Psychological Measurement, 3,* 137–140.

Boring, E.G. (1923, June 6). Intelligence as the tests test it. *New Republic*, pp. 35–37.

Boring, E.G. (1950). *A history of experimental psychology* (rev. ed). New York: Appleton-Century-Crofts.

Borkowski, J.G., & Cavanaugh, J.C. (1979). Maintenance and generalization of skills and strategies by the retarded. In W.R. Ellis (Ed.), *Handbook of mental deficiency* (2nd ed.). Hillsdale, NJ: Erlbaum.

Borkowski, J.G., & Konarski, E.A. (1981). Educational implications of efforts to change intelligence. *Journal of Special Education, 15,* 289–306.

Borkowski, J.G., & Wanschura, P.B. (1974). Mediational processes in the retarded. In W.R. Ellis (Ed.), *International review of research in mental retardation* (Vol. 1). New York: Academic Press.

Bourne, L.E., Dominowski, R.L., & Loftus, E. (1979). *Cognitive processes.* Englewood Cliffs, NJ: Prentice-Hall.

Bovet, M.C. (1984). Learning research within Piagetian lines. *Learning Disability Quarterly, 7* (2), 1–9.

Bower, G.H. (1975). Cognitive psychology: An introduction. In W.K. Estes (Ed.), *Handbook of learning and cognitive processes. Introduction to concepts and issues* (Vol. 1, pp. 25–80). Hillsdale, NJ: Erlbaum.

Box, C., & Filip, D. (1981). Comprehension monitoring skills in learning disabled and average students. *Topics in Learning and Learning Disabilities, 2,* 79–85.

Braverman, D.M. (1967). Dimensions of cognitive style. *Journal of Personality, 28,* 167–185.

Bricker, W.A., Macke, P.R., Levin, J.A., & Campbell, P.H. (1981). The modifiability of intelligent behavior. *Journal of Special Education, 15,* 1.

Broadbent, D.E. (1958). *Perception and communication.* London: Pergamon Press.

Broadbent, D.E. (1971). *Decision and stress.* New York: Academic Press.

Brody, E.B., & Brody, N. (1976). *Intelligence: Nature, determinants and consequences.* New York: Academic Press.

Brown, A.C. (1978). Knowing when, where and how to remember: A problem of metacognition. In R. Glaser (Ed.), *Advances in instructional psychology.* Hillsdale, NJ: Erlbaum.

Brown, A.C., & Palincsar, A.S. (1982). Inducing strategic learning from texts by means of informed, self control training. *Topics in Learning and Learning Disabilities, 2,* 1–17.

Brown, B. (Ed.). (1978). *Found: Long-term gains from early interventions.* Boulder, CO: Westview Press.

Brown, J.S., & Burton, R.R. (1978). Diagnostic models for procedural bugs in basic mathematical skills. *Cognitive Science, 2,* 115–192.

Bruner, J.S. (1961). *The process of education.* Cambridge: Harvard University Press.

Bruner, J.S. (1966). *Toward a theory of instruction.* Cambridge: Harvard University Press.

Bruner, J.S. (1972). Nature and uses of immaturity. *American Psychologist, 27,* 1–22.

Bruner, J.S., Goodnow, J.J., & Austin, G.A. (1956). *A study of thinking.* New York: John Wiley & Sons.

Bruninks, R.H. (1971). *Bruninks-Oseretsky Test of Motor Proficiency.* Chicago: American Guidance Association.

Brunswick, E. (1956). *Perception and representative design of experiments.* Berkeley: University of California Press.

Budoff, M., Meskin, J., & Harrison, R.H. (1971). Educational test of the learning potential hypothesis. *American Journal of Mental Deficiency, 76,* 159–169.

Buros Mental Measurements Yearbook Sixth Edition. Seashore Measures of Musical Talent Revised Edition, 1965, 353.

Burt, C. (1949). The structure of the mind: A review of the results of factor analyses. *British Journal of Educational Psychology, 25,* 100–111, 176–199.

Burt, C. (1955). The evidence for the concept of intelligence. *British Journal of Educational Psychology, 25,* 15 –17.

Bush, W.J., & Giles, M.T. (1969). *Aids to psycholinguistic teaching.* Columbus, OH: Charles E. Merrill Publishing.

Butterfield, E.C., & Belmont, J.M. (1975). Assessing and improving the executive functions of mentally retarded people. In I. Bialer & M. Sternlicht (Eds.), *Psychological issues in mentally retarded people.* Chicago: Aldine.

Carroll, J.B. (1976a). *Individual difference relations in psychometric and experimental cognitive task* (ONR Tech. Rgs. 2). University of North Carolina, Chapel Hill: Thurstone Psychometric Laboratory.

Carroll, J.B. (1976b). Psychometric tests as cognitive tasks. In L.B. Resnick (Ed.), *The nature of intelligence.* Hillsdale, NJ: Erlbaum.

Case, R. (1978a). A developmentally based theory and technology of instruction. *Review of Educational Research, 48,* 439–463.

Case, R. (1978b). Piaget and beyond: Toward a developmentally based theory and technology of instruction. In R. Glaser (Ed.), *Research and development and school change* (pp. 167–228). Hillsdale, NJ: Erlbaum.

Cattell, R.B. (1971). *Abilities: Their structure, growth and action.* Boston: Houghton Mifflin.

Cattell, R.B. (1979). Are culture free tests possible and necessary? *Journal of Research and Development in Education, 12,* 3–13.

Cattell, R.B., & Horn, J.L. (1981). On the scientific basis of ability testing. *American Psychologist, 36,* 1012–1020.

Cavanaugh, J.C., & Borkowski, J.G. (1980). Searching for meta-memory corrections. A developmental study. *Developmental Psychology, 4,* 41–53.

Chalfant, J.C., & Scheffelin, M.A. (1969). *Central processing dysfunctions in children. A review of research* (NINDS Monographs No. 9). Bethesda, MD: U.S. Department of Health, Education and Welfare.

Chall, J.S., & Mirsky, A.F. (Eds.). (1978). *Education and the brain: The seventy-seventh yearbook of the National Society for the Study of Education: Part II.* Chicago: University of Chicago Press.

Charlesworth, W.R. (1976). Human intelligence as adaptation: An ethological approach. In Lauren B. Resnick (Ed.), *The nature of intelligence.* Hillsdale, NJ: Erlbaum.

Chein, I. (1945). On the nature of intelligence. *Journal of General Psychology, 32,* 111–126.

Chomsky, N. (1957). *Syntactic structures.* The Hague: Montour.

Chomsky, N. (1968). *Language and mind.* New York: Harcourt Brace Jovanovich.

Cofer, C.N. (1976). An historical perspective. In C.N. Cofer (Ed.), *The structure of memory.* San Francisco: W.H. Freeman & Co.

Cohen, P.R., & Feigenbaum, E.A. (Eds.). (1982). *The handbook of artificial intelligence* (Vol. 3). Stanford, CA: Kaufman.

Colarusso, R., & Hammill, D.D. (1972). *The Motor Free Test of Visual Perception.* San Rafael, CA: Academic Therapy Publication.

Collins, A., & Loftus, E.F. (1975). A spreading activation theory of semantic processing. *Psychological Review, 82,* 407–428.

Collins, A., & Quillian, M.R. (1969). Retrieval time from semantic memory. *Journal of Verbal Learning and Verbal Behavior,* 240–247.

Conger, J.J. (1959). The meaningful measurement of intelligence. *Rocky Mountain Medical Journal.*

Cooley, W.W. (1976). Who needs general intelligence. In L.B. Resnick (Ed.), *The nature of intelligence* (pp. 57–61). Hillsdale, NJ: Erlbaum.

Coop, R., & Sigel, I. (1971). Cognitive style: Implications for learning and instruction. *Psychology in the Schools, 8,* 152–161.

Covington, M.V., & Osrelich, C.R. (1979). Effort: The double edged word in school achievement. *Journal of Educational Psychology, 71,* 169–182.

Craik, F.I.M. (1979a). Levels of processing: Overview and closing comments. In L.S. Cermak & F.I.M. Craik (Eds.), *Levels of processing in human meaning.* Hillsdale, NJ: Erlbaum.

Craik, F.I.M. (1979b). Human memory. *Annual Review of Psychology, 30,* 63–102.

Craik, F.I.M., & Lockhart, R.S. (1968). Levels of processing: A framework for memory research. *Journal of Verbal Learning and Verbal Behavior, 7,* 16–19.

Cratty, B.J. (1967). *Developmental sequences of perceptual motor tasks.* Freeport, NY: Educational Activities.

Cratty, B.J. (1969a). *Movement, perception and thought.* Palo Alto, CA: Peek.

Cratty, B.J. (1969b). *Perceptual-motor behavioral and educational processes.* Springfield, IL: Charles C Thomas.

Cratty, B.J. (1971). *Active learning: Games to enhance academic abilities.* Englewood Cliffs, NJ: Prentice-Hall.

Cratty, B.J., & Martin, M.M. (1969). *Perceptual-motor efficiency in children. The measurement and improvement of movement attributes.* Lea & Felige.

Cronbach, L.J., & Snow, R.E. (1977). *Aptitudes and instructional methods.* New York: Irvington.

Cruickshank, W.M. (1961). A teaching method for brain injured and hyperactive children. *Special Education and Rehabilitations (Monograph, Series No. 6).* Syracuse, NY: Syracuse University Press.

Cruickshank, W.M., & Silver, A. (1981). *Bridges to tomorrow* (Vols. 1–2). Syracuse, NY: Syracuse University Press.

Delacato, C.H. (1966a). *Neurological organization and reading.* Springfield, IL: Charles C Thomas.

Delacato, C.H. (1966b). *The diagnosis and treatment of speech and reading problems.* Springfield, IL: Charles C Thomas.

Day, M.C., & Parker, R. (Eds.). (1977). *The preschool in action: Exploring early childhood programming.* Boston: Allyn & Bacon.

Denney, D.R. (1972). Modeling effects upon conceptual style and cognitive tempo. *Child Development, 43,* 105–119.

Denney, D.R. (1974). Relationship of three cognitive style dimensions to elementary reading abilities. *Educational Psychology, 66,* 702–709.

Denney, D.R., Denney, N.W., & Ziobrowski, M.J. (1973). Alterations in the information processing strategies of young children following observation of adult models. *Developmental Psychology, 8,* 202–208.

Detterman, D.K., & Sternberg, R.J. (1982). *How and how much can intelligence be increased?* Norwood, NJ: Ablex Pub.

Dollard, J., & Miller, N.E. (1950). *Personality and psychotherapy: An analysis in terms of learning, thinking and culture.* New York: McGraw-Hill.

Doman, R., Spitz, E., Zuchman, E., Delacato, C.H., & Doman, G. (1967). Children with severe brain injuries: Neurological organization in terms of mobility. *Journal of American Medical Association, 174,* 119–124.

Douglas, V.J. (1972). Stop, look and listen: The problem of sustained attention and in public control in hyperactive and normal children. *Canadian Journal of Behavior Science, 4,* 259–282.

Douglas, V.J., Parry, P., Marton, P., & Garson, C. (1976). Assessment of a cognitive training program for hyperactive children. *Journal of Abnormal Child Psychology, 4,* 389–410.

Duane, D.D. (1981). Towards the demystification of the clinical electroencephalogram. In W.A. Cruickshank and A. Silver (Eds.), *Bridge to Tomorrow* (Vol. 2). Syracuse, NY: Syracuse University Press.

Dunker, K. (1945). On problem solving. *Psychological Monograph, 58* (No. 270).

Dunn, R. (1983). Learning styles and its relation to exceptionality at both ends of the spectrum. *Exceptional Children, 40,* 496–506.

Dunn, R., & Dunn, K. (1975). Learning styles, teaching styles. *NASSP Bulletin, 59,* 37–49a.

Dunn, R., & Dunn, K. (1977). How to diagnose learning styles. *Instructor, 87,* 123–4, 126, 128, 130, 132, 134, 136, 140, 142, 144.

Dunn, R., & Dunn, K. (1979). Learning styles teaching styles: Should they . . . can they . . . be matched. *Educational Leadership, 36,* 238–244.

Dunn, R., Dunn, K., & Price, G. (1977). Diagnosing learning styles: A prescription for avoiding malpractice suits. *Phi Delta Kappan, 58,* 418–420.

Dunst, C.J. (1978a, October). *The organization of sensorimotor intelligence among organically impaired children.* Unpublished study, George Peabody College for Teachers.

Dunst, C.J. (1978b, October). *Sensorimotor development among Down's syndrome infants.* Unpublished study, George Peabody College for Teachers.

Dunst, C.J., & Brassell, W.R. (1977, December). *The structural features of sensorimotor development among developmentally delayed infants and toddlers.* Unpublished study, Western Carolina Infant's Program, Morgantown, NC.

Durrell, D.D. (1955). *Analysis of reading difficulty: Manual of directions.* New York: Harcourt, Brace and World.

Durrell, D.D. (1967). Learning factors in beginning reading. In W.G. Cutts (Ed.), *Teaching young children to read* (Bulletin No. 19). Washington, DC: U.S. Department of Health, Education and Welfare.

Ebel, R.L. (1979). Intelligence: A skeptical view. *Journal of Research and Development in Education, 2,* 14–21.

Eisner, E.W., & Vallance, E. (1974). *Conflicting conceptions of curricula.* Berkeley, CA: McCutchan Publishing Corp.

Elkind, D. (1976). *Child Development and education: A Piagetian perspective.* New York: Oxford University Press.

Elkind, D. (1979). Piaget and developmental psychology. In F.B. Murray (Ed.), *The impact of Piagetian theory.* Baltimore: University Park Press.

Elliot, A., & Donaldson, M. (1978a). Interchange. Elliot and Donaldson reply to Sinclair. In S. Modgil & C. Modgil (Eds.), *Jean Piaget: Consensus and controversy* (p. 178). New York: Praeger Publishing.

Elliot, A., & Donaldson, M. (1978b). Piaget on language. In S. Modgil & C. Modgil (Eds.), *Jean Piaget: Consensus and controversy* (pp. 157–166). New York: Praeger Publishing.

Ennis, R. (1982). Children's ability to handle Piaget's propositional logic: A conceptual critique. In S. Modgil & C. Modgil (Eds.), *Jean Piaget: Consensus and controversy* (pp. 101–130). New York: Praeger.

Erickson, K.A., & Simon, H.A. (1981). Sources of evidence on cognition: A historical overview. In T.V. Merluzzi, C.R. Glass, & M. Genest (Eds.), *Cognitive assessment*. New York: Guilford Press.

Evarts, E.V. (1979). Brain mechanisms of movement. *Scientific American, 241,* 164–179.

Eysenck, H.J. (1952). The effects of psychotherapy: An evaluation. *Journal of Consulting Psychology, 16,* 329–334.

Eysenck, H.J. (1959). Learning theory and behavioral therapy. *Journal of Mental Science, 61,* 75, 105.

Eysenck, H.J. (1973). *The inequality of man.* London: Temple Smith.

Fantini, M.D. (1980). A contemporary approach to individualization. *Theory and Practice, 19,* 28–31.

Farnhan-Diggory, S. (1978). *Learning disabilities.* Cambridge: Harvard University Press, 63.

Fass, L.A. (1981). *Children with learning problems.* Boston: Houghton Mifflin.

Feingold, B.F. (1976). Hyperkinesis and learning disabilities linked to the ingestion of artificial broad colors and flavors. *Journal of Learning Disabilities, 9,* 551–559.

Fernald, G. (1943). *Remedial techniques in basic school subjects.* New York: McGraw-Hill.

Feuerstein, R., Rand, Y., & Hoffman, M.B. (1979). *The dynamic assessment of retarded performers.* Baltimore: University Park Press.

Feuerstein, R., Rand, Y., Hoffman, M.B., & Miller, R. (1980). *Instrumental Enrichment.* Baltimore: University Park Press.

Feuerstein, R., Miller, R., Hoffman, M.B., Rand, Y., Mintzler, M.A., & Jersen, M.R. (1981). Cognitive modifiability in adolescence cognitive structure and the effects of intervention. *Journal of Special Education, 15,* 167–287.

Filskov, S.B., Grimm, B.H., & Lewis, J.A. (1980). Brain-behavior relationships. In S. Filskov & T.J. Boll (Eds.), *Handbook of neuropsychology.* New York: John Wiley & Sons.

Finch, A.J., Wilkinson, M.D., Nelson, W.M., & Montgomery, L.E. (1975). Modification of an impulsive cognitive tempo in emotionally disturbed boys. *Journal of Abnormal Child Psychology, 3,* 49–52.

Fincham, F. (1982). Piaget's theory and the learning disabled: A critical analysis. In S. Modgil & C. Modgil (Eds.), *Jean Piaget: Consensus and controversy* (pp. 360–390). New York: Praeger.

Fincher, J. (1981). *The brain.* Washington, DC: U.S. News Books.

Fischer, C.T. (1969). Intelligence defined as effectiveness of approach. *Journal of Consulting and Clinical Psychology, 33,* 668–674.

Fisher, M.A., & Zeaman, D. (1973). An attention-retention theory of retardate discrimination learning. In N.R. Ellis (Ed.), *International review of research in mental retardation* (Vol. 6). New York: Academic Press.

Flavell, J.H. (1970). Developmental studies of mediated memory. In H.W. Reese & L.P. Lipsitt (Eds.), *Advances in child development and behavior.*

Flavell, J.H. (1976). Metacognitive aspects of problem solving. In L.B. Resnick (Ed.), *The nature of intelligence.* Hillsdale, NJ: Erlbaum.

Flavell, J.H. (1977). *Cognitive development.* Englewood Cliffs, NJ: Prentice-Hall.

Flavell, J.H. (1979). Metacognition and metacognitive monitoring: A new area of cognitive developmental inquiry. *American Psychologist, 34,* 906–911.

Flavell, J.H. (1982). In W.A. Collins (Ed.), The concept of development. *The Minnesota symposia on child psychology* (Vol. 15). Hillsdale, NJ: Erlbaum.

Flavell, J.H., Beach, D.R., & Chimsky, J.M. (1966). Spontaneous verbal rehearsal in a memory task as a function of age. *Child Development, 37,* 283–299.

Flavell, J.H., & Wellman, T.M. (1977). Metamemory. In R.V. Kail & J.H. Hagan (Eds.), *Perspectives on the development of memory and cognition.* Hillsdale, NJ: Erlbaum.

Fleishman, E.A., & Herpel, W. (1956). Factorial analyses of complex psychomotor performance and related skills. *Journal of Applied Psychology, 40,* 96–104.

Flexser, A.J., & Tulving, E. (1978). Retrieval independence in recognition and recall. *Psychological Review, 85,* 153–171.

Fodor, J.A. (1975). *The language of thought.* New York: Crowell.

Fogelman, C.J. (Ed.). (1974). *AAMD adaptive behavior scale manual.* Washington, DC: American Association on Mental Deficiency.

Frailberg, S., & Frailberg, L. (1979). *Insights from the blind: Comparative studies of blind and sighted infants*. New York: NAL.

Frank, G. (1976). Measures of intelligence and conceptual thinking. In I.B. Weinver (Ed.), *Clinical methods in psychology*. New York: John Wiley & Sons.

Freeman, F.N. (1925). What is intelligence? *School Review, 33,* 253–263.

Freeman, R. (1967). Controversy over "patterning" as a treatment for brain damage in children. *Journal of the American Medical Association, 202,* 385–388.

French, J.W. (1951). The description of aptitude and achievement tests in terms of rotated factors. *Psychometric Monographs, 5.*

French, J.W., Tucker, L.R., Newman, S.H., & Bobbitt, J.M. (1952). A factor analysis of aptitude and achievement entrance tests and course grades at the United States Coast Guard Academy. *Journal of Educational Psychology, 43,* 65–80.

Frostig, M. (1967). Testing as a basis for educational therapy. *Journal of Special Education, 2,* 15–34.

Frostig, M. (1968). Education for children with learning disabilities. In H. Myklebust (Ed.), *Progress in learning disabilities*. New York: Grune & Stratton.

Frostig, M. (1969). *Move-grow-learn*. Chicago: Follett.

Frostig, M. (1974). Futures in perceptual training. In M. Krasnoff (Ed.), *Learning disabilities*. Ann Arbor, MI: Institute for the Study of Mental Retardation and Related Disabilities.

Frostig, M., & Horne, D. (1967). *The Frostig program for the development of visual perception*. Chicago: Follett.

Frostig, M., Maslow, P., Lefever, W., & Whittlesey, J.R. (1964). *Marianne Frostig Developmental Test of Visual Perception*. Palo Alto, CA: Consulting Psychologists Press.

Fulkerson, S.C. (1965). Some implications of the new cognitive theory for projective tests. *Journal of Consulting Psychology, 29,* 191–197.

Furth, H., & Wachs, H. (1977). *Thinking goes to school: Piaget's theory in practice*. New York: Oxford University Press.

Gage, N.L., & Berliner, D.C. (1979). *Educational psychology* (2nd ed). Boston: Houghton Mifflin.

Gagné, R.M. (1965). *The conditions of learning*. New York: Holt, Rinehart & Winston.

Gagné, R.M., & Briggs, L.J. (1979). *Principles of instructional design*. New York: Holt, Rinehart & Winston.

Gagné, R.M., & Dick, W. (1983). Instructional psychology. In M.R. Rosenzweig & L.W. Porter (Eds.), *Annual Review of Psychology, 34,* 261–295.

Gallagher, J.J. (1979). The interdisciplinary sharing of knowledge. *Journal of Special Education, 13* (1), 41–43.

Galton, F. (1870). *Hereditary genius: An inquiry into its laws and consequences*. New York: D. Appleton.

Garber, H., & Heber, R. (1973). *The Milwaukee Project: Early intervention as a technique to prevent mental retardation*. (National leadership institute teacher education/early childhood technical paper). Storrs: University of Connecticut.

Garber, H., & Heber, R. (1978, July). *The efficacy of early intervention with family rehabilitation*. Paper presented at the Conference on Prevention of Retarded Development in Psycho-Socially Disadvantaged Children, Madison, WI.

Garcia, J. (1981). The logic and limits of mental aptitude testing. *American Psychologist, 35,* 1172–1180.

Gardner, H. (1983). *Frames of mind, the theory of multiple intelligences*. New York: Basic Books.

Gardner, R.W. (1953). Cognitive styles in categorizing behavior. *Journal of Personality, 22,* 214–233.

Gardner, R.W., Holzman, P.S., Klein, G.S., Linton, H., & Spence, D.S. (1959). Cognitive control: A study of individual consistencies in cognitive behavior. *Psychological Issues, 1* (4).

Gardner, R.W., Jackson, D.N., & Messick, S.J. (1960). *Personality organization in cognitive controls and intellectual abilities*. *Psychological Issues, 2* (8), 1–149.

Gardner, R.W., & Moriarity, R.A. (1968). Dimensions of cognitive control at preadolescence. In R. Gardner (Ed.), *Personality development at preadolescence*. Seattle: University of Washington Press.

Gardner, R.W., & Schoen, D. (1962). Differentiation and abstraction in concept formation. *Psychological Monographs, 76* (No. 560).

Garrett, H.E. (1946). A developmental theory of intelligence. *American Psychologist, 1,* 372–378.

Gates-Mikillop Reading Diagnostic Tests. (1962). Joplin, Mo.: College Press.

Gavelik, J.R., & Raphael, T.E. (1982). Instructing metacognitive awareness of question-answer relationships. *Topics in Learning and Learning Disabilities,* (2) 69–77.

Gazzaniga, M., & Ledoux, J. (1978). *The integrative mind.* New York: Plenum.

Gearhart, B.R. (1973). *Learning disabilities educational strategies.* St. Louis: C.V. Mosby Co.

Gearhart, B.R. (1976). *Teaching the learning disabled.* St. Louis: C.V. Mosby Co.

Geogoric, A.F. (1979). Learning/teaching styles: Potent forces behind them. *Educational Leadership, 36,* 234–236.

Gerschwind, N. (1980). Neurological knowledge and complex behaviors. *Cognitive Science, 4,* 185–193.

Gesell, A., & Amatruda, C. (1974). Developmental diagnosis: Normal and abnormal child development. In H. Knoblock & B. Pasaminck (Eds.), *Gesell & Amatruda's developmental diagnosis.* New York: Harper & Row.

Getman, G.N. (1965). The visuomotor complex in the acquisition of learning skills. In J. Hellmuth (Ed.), *Learning Disorders* (Vol. 1). Seattle: Special Child Publications.

Getman, G.N., & Hendrickson, H.H. (1966). The needs of teachers for specialized information on the development of visual-motor skills in relation to academic performance. In W.M. Cruickshank (Ed.), *The teacher of brain injured children* (pp. 153–168). Syracuse, NY: Syracuse University Press.

Gillingham, A., & Stillman, B. (1966). *Remedial training for children with specific difficulty in reading, spelling, and penmanship* (7th ed.). Cambridge, MA: Educators Publishing Services.

Ginsburg, H., & Opper, S. (1979). *Piaget's theory of intellect development. An introduction* (2nd ed). Englewood Cliffs, NJ: Prentice-Hall.

Glaser, R. (Ed.). (1978). *Advances in instructional psychology* (Vol. 1). Hillsdale, NJ: Erlbaum.

Glaser, R., & Bond, L. (Eds.). (1981). Testing: Concepts, policy, practice and research. *American Psychologist 36* (10).

Glaser, R., & Resnick, L.B. (1972). Instructional psychology. In P.H. Mussen & M.R. Rosenzweig (Eds.), *Annual Review of Psychology,* (23) 207–271.

Goldfarb, W., et al. (1978). Psychotic children grown up: A prospective follow-up study in adolescence and childhood. *Issues in Child Mental Health,* 108–183.

Goldman, R., Fristoe, M.A., & Woodcock R. (1976). *Goldman-Fristoe-Woodcock Test of Auditory Discrimination.* Circle Pines, MN: American Guidance Service.

Goldstein, E.B. (1980). *Sensation and perception.* Belmont, CA: Wadsworth.

Goldstein, K. (1939). *The organism.* New York: American Book.

Goldstein, K., & Scheerer, M. (1941). Abstract and concrete behavior. *Psychological Monographs, 53* (239).

Goldstein, K.M., & Blackman, S. (1977). The assessment of cognitive styles. In P. McReynolds (Ed.), *Advances in psychological assessment* (Vol. 4). San Francisco: Jossey-Bass.

Goldstein, K.M., & Blackman, S. (1978). *Cognitive styles: Five approaches to theory and research.* New York: John Wiley & Sons.

Gomez, A.J. (1978). *Basic informational concepts in neuroanatomy and neurophysiology.* In A.J. Gomez & B.B. Podhajski (Eds.), *Common neurological and language disorders* (pp. 120–145).

Goodard, H.H. (1911). *The Binet-Simon Measuring Scale for Intelligence* (rev. ed.). Vineland, NJ: Training School.

Graham, F., & Kendall (1960). *Memory-for-design test.* Missorda, MT: Psychological Test Specialists.

Greeno, J.G. (1976). Indefinite goals in well structured problems. *Psychological Review,* (83), 479, 491.

Greeno, J.G. (1978). Nature of problem solving abilities. In W.K. Estes (Ed.), *Handbook of learning and cognitive processes* (vol. 5, pp. 239–270). Hillsdale, NJ: Erlbaum.

Greeno, J.G. Preliminary steps toward a model of learning primary arithmetic. In K.C. Ferson & W.E. Geeslin (Eds.), *Explorations in the modeling of the learning of mathematics.* [Monograph from Georgia Center, Learning-teaching math]. Columbus, OH: ERIC/SMEAC Sci. Math, Inf. Anal. Center.

Greeno, J.G. (1980a). Psychology of learning, 1960–1980. Used participant's observations. *American Psychology, 35,* 713–718.

Greeno, J.G. (1980b). Some examples of cognitive task analysis with instructive implications. In R.E. Snow, P.A. Federico, & W.E. Montague (Eds.), *Aptitudes, learning and instruction* (vol. 7). Hillsdale, NJ: Erlbaum.

Guilford, J.P. (1959). The three faces of intellect. *American Psychologist, 14,* 464–479.

Guilford, J.P. (1967). *The nature of human intelligence.* New York: McGraw-Hill.

Guilford, J.P. (1979). Intelligence isn't what it used to be: What to do about it. *Journal of Research and Development in Education, 12,* 33–46.

Guilford, J.P. (1981). Higher-order structure of intellect abilities. *Multivariate Behavioral Research, 16,* 411–435.

Gilford, J.P., & Hoepfner, R. (1971). *The analysis of intelligence.* New York: McGraw-Hill.

Gutkin, T.B., & Reynolds, C.R. (1981). Factorial similarity of the WISC-R for white and black children from the standardization sample. *Journal of Educational Psychology, 73,* 227–231.

Hagen, J.W., Barclay, C.R., & Newman, R.S. (1982). Metacognition, self knowledge, and learning disabilities: Some thoughts on knowing and doing. *Topics in Learning and Learning Disabilities, 2,* 17–19.

Hall, R.J. (1980). Cognitive behavior modification and information-processing skills of exceptional children. *Exceptional Education Quarterly, 1,* 9–15.

Hallahan, D.P., & Cruickshank, W. (1973). *Psychoeducational foundations of learning disabilities.* Englewood Cliffs, NJ: Prentice-Hall.

Hallahan, D.P., Lloyd, J., Rosenweicz, M., Kaufman, J., & Gravers, A. (1979). Self monitoring of attention as a treatment for a learning disabled boy's off-task behavior. *Learning Disability Quarterly, 2,* 24–32.

Hamlyn, D.W. (1971). Epistemology and conceptual development. In T. Mischel (Ed.), *Cognitive development and epistemology.* New York: Academic Press.

Hammill, D.D. (1972). Training visual perceptual processes. *Journal of Learning Disabilities, 5,* 552–559.

Hammill, D.D., & Bartell, N.D. (1982). *Teaching children with learning behavior problems.* Boston: Allyn & Bacon.

Hayes, J.R. (1978). *Cognitive psychology: Thinking and creating.* Homewood, IL: Dorsey.

Heckelman, R.G. (1968). The neurological impress methods of remedial reading instruction. *Academic Therapy, 4,* 277–282.

Hermon, V.A.C. (1921). Intelligence and its measurement: A symposium. *Journal of Educational Psychology, 12,* 195–198.

Hildreth, G. (1955). *Teaching spelling: A guide to principles and practices.* New York: Holt.

Hilliard, A.G. III. (1979). Standardization and cultural bias as impediments to the scientific study and validation of "intelligence." *Journal of Research and Development in Education, 12,* 47–58.

Hinton, G.E., & Anderson, J.A. (1981). *Parallel models of associative memory.* Hillsdale, NJ: Erlbaum.

Hirst, W., Spelke, E., Reaves, C., Caharack, G. (1980). Dividing attention without alteration or automaticity. *Journal of Experimental Psychology, 109* (1), 98–117.

Hiscock, M. (1983). Do learning disabled children lack functional hemispheric laterization? *Topics in Learning and Learning Disabilities, 3,* 14–28.

Hiscock, M., & Kinsbourne, M. (1980a). *Individual differences in verbal lateralization: Are they relevant to learning disability?* Syracuse, NY: Syracuse University Press.

Hiscock, M., & Kinsbourne, M. (1980b). Individual differences in cerebral lateralization. In W.M. Cruickshank & A. Silver (Eds.), *Approaches to learning* (Vol. 1). Syracuse, NY: Syracuse University Press.

Hobbs, S.A., Moguin, L.E., & Troyler, N. (1980). Parameters of investigations of cognitive behavior therapy with children. *Catalog of Selected Documents in Psychology, 10,* 62–63.

Hodges, W., & Cooper, M. (1981). Head-Start and Follow-Through. Influences on intellectual development. *Journal of Special Education, 15,* 221–238.

Holland, R.P. (1982). Learner characteristic and learner performance: Implications for instructional placement decision. *Journal of Special Education, 16,* 7–10.

Holman, J., & Bear, D.M. (1978). Facilitating generalization of on-task behavior through self monitoring of academic tasks. *Journal of Autism and Developmental Disorders, 7,* 429–446.

Holt, E.B. (1914). *The Freudian wish and its place in ethics.* New York: Macmillan.

Horn, J.L. (1968). Organization of abilities and the development of intelligence. *Psychological Review, 75,* 242–259a.

Horn, J.L. (1978a). Human ability system. In P.B. Baltes (Ed.), *Life-span development and behavior* (Vol. 1). New York: Academic Press.

Horn, J.L. (1978b). Some correctable defects in research on intelligence. *Intelligence, 3,* 307–322.

Horn, J.L. (1978c). The rise and fall of human abilities. *Journal of Research and Development in Education, 12,* 59–78.

Horn, J.L. (1979). Trends in the measurement of intelligence. *Intelligence, 3,* 229–240.

Horn, J.L., Donaldson, G., & Engstrom, R. (1981). Apprehension, memory and fluid intelligence decline in adulthood. *Research on aging, 3,* 33–84.

Houston, J.P. (1976). *Fundamentals of learning*. New York: Academic Press.

Houts, P.L. (Ed) (1973). *The myth of measurability*. New York: A. & W. Publishers.

Howe, M. (1980). *The psychology of human learning*. New York: Harper & Row.

Hubel, D.H. (1979). The brain. *Scientific American, 241* (45), 453.

Hubel, D.H., & Wiesel, T.N. (1959). Receptive fields, binocular interaction and functional architecture in the cat's visual cortex. *Journal of Physiology, 160*, 106–154.

Hull, C.L. (1943). *Principles of behavior*. New York: Appleton-Century-Crofts.

Hull, C.L. (1952). *A behavior system*. New Haven: Yale University Press.

Hulmes, C. (1981). *Reading retardation and multisensory teaching*. London: Routledge & Kegan Paul.

Humphreys, L.G. (1979). The construct of general intelligence. *Intelligence, 3*, 105–120.

Humphreys, L.G. (1981). The primary mental ability. In M.P. Friedman, J.P.N. O'Connor (Eds.), *Intelligence and learning*. New York: Plenum.

Hunt, D.E. (1971). Matching models in education. *The coordination of teaching methods with student characteristics*. Toronto: Ontario Institute for Studies in Education.

Hunt, D.E. (1974). Learning styles and teaching strategies. *Behavioral and Social Science Teacher, 2*, 22–24.

Hunt, D.E. (1975a). The B-P-E paradigm for theory, research, and practice. *Canadian Psychological Review, 16*, 185–197.

Hunt, D.E. (1975b). Person-environment interaction: A challenge found wanting before it was tried. *Review of Educational Research, 45*, 209–230.

Hunt, D.E. (1976). Varieties of cognitive power. In L.B. Resnick (Ed.), *The nature of intelligence*. Hillsdale, NJ: Erlbaum.

Hunt, D.E. (1977). *A paradigm for developing and analyzing differential treatment in drug and alcohol counseling program*. Palm Springs, CA: ETC Publications.

Hunt, D.E. (1977–78). Conceptual level theory and research as guides to educational practice. *Interchange, 8*, 78–90.

Hunt, D.E. (1978). Mechanics of verbal ability. *Psychological Review, 85*, 109–130.

Hunt, D.E. (1979). A conceptual level matching model for coordinating learner characteristics with educational approaches. *Interchange, 1*, 68–82.

Hunt, D.E., Butler, L.F., Noy, J.E., & Rosser, M.E. (1978). *Assessing conceptual level by the paragraph completion method*. Toronto: Ontario Institute for Studies in Education.

Hunt, E.N., Frost, N., & Lenneberg, C. (1973). Individual differences in cognition: A new approach to intelligence. In M.G. Bower (Ed.), *The psychology of learning and motivation* (Vol. 7). New York: Academic Press.

Hunt, E.N., Lenneberg, C., & Lewis, J. (1975). What does it mean to be high verbal? *Cognitive Psychology, 7*, 194–227.

Hunt, J. McV. (1961). *Intelligence and experience*. New York: Ronald Press.

Hynd, G.N., & Obrzut, J.E. (Eds.). (1981). *Neuropsychological assessment of the school age child*. New York: Grune & Stratton.

Inhelder, B. (1982). Outlook. In S. Modgil & C. Modgil (Eds.), *Jean Piaget: Consensus and controversy* (pp. 411–418). New York: Praeger Publishing.

Jacobs, P.S., & Vandeventer, M. (1971). The learning and transfer of double classification skills: A replication and extension. *Journal of Experimental Psychology, 11*, 140–157.

Jensen, A.R. (1969). How can we boost IQ and scholastic achievement? *Harvard Educational Review, 38*, 1–123.

Jensen, A.R. (1973). *Educability and group differences*. New York: Harper & Row.

Jensen, A.R. (1979). The nature of intelligence and its relation to learning. *Journal of Research and Development in Education, 12*, 79–95.

Jensen, A.R. (1981). *Straight talk about mental tests*. New York: Free Press.

Jensen, A.R. (1982). Level I/Level II: Factors or categories. *Journal of Educational Psychology, 74* (6), 868–873.

Johns, E.R., & Schwartz, E.L. (1978). The neurophysiology of information processing and cognition. In M.R. Rosenzweig & L.W. Porter (Eds.), *Annual review of psychology, 29*, 1–30.

Johnson, C. (1981). *The diagnosis of learning disabilities*. Boulder, CO: Pruett Publishing.

Johnson, D.J., & Myklebust, H.R. (1969). *Learning disabilities: Educational principles and practices*. New York: Grune & Stratton.

Johnson, E.G. (1980). A battery of tasks to examine Luria's theory of the development of verbal control of motor behavior. *Genetic Psychology Monographs, 102,* 269.

Johnson, P., & Myklebust, H.R. (1967). *Learning disabilities: Educational principles and practices.* New York: Grune & Stratton.

Johnson, S.W., & Morasky, R.L. (1980). *Learning disabilities* (2nd ed.). Boston: Allyn & Bacon.

Kagan, J. (1965). Reflection-impulsivity and reading ability in primary grade children. *Child Development, 36,* 609–628.

Kagan, J., & Kogan, N. (1970). Individual variation in cognitive processes. In P.H. Mussen (Ed.), *Carmichael's manual of child psychology* (Vol. 1). New York: John Wiley & Sons.

Kagan, J., & Messler, S.B. (1975). A reply to "Some misgivings about the Matching Familiar Figures Test as a measure of reflection-impulsivity." *Developmental Psychology, 11,* 244–248.

Kagan, J., Moss, H.A., & Sigel, J.F. (1963). Psychological significance of styles of conceptualization. In J.C. Wright & J. Kagan (Eds.), Basic cognitive processes in children. *Monographs of the Society for Research in Child Development, 28* (Serial No. 86).

Kagan, J., Rosman, B.L., Day, D., Albert J., & Phillips, W. (1964). Information processing in the child: Significance of analytic and reflective attitudes. *Psychological Monographs, 78* (No. 578).

Kagan, S., & Zahn, G.L. (1975). Field dependence and the school achievement gap between Anglo-American and Mexican-American children. *Journal of Educational Psychology, 67,* 643–650.

Kagan, S., Zahn, G.L., & Gealy, J. Competition and school achievements among Anglo-American and Mexican-American children. *Journal of Educational Psychology, 69,* 432–441.

Kalish, H. (1981). *From behavioral science to behavior modification.* New York: McGraw-Hill.

Kamii, C., & DeVries, R. (1978). *Physical knowledge in preschool education: Implications of Piaget's theory.* Englewood Cliffs, NJ: Prentice-Hall.

Kamin, L.J. (1974). *The science and politics of IQ.* New York: John Wiley & Sons.

Kandel, E.R. (1979). Small systems of newborns. *Scientific American, 241,* 56–87.

Karnes, M. (1972). *Goal program development game.* Springfield, MA: Milton Bradley.

Karplus, R. (1974). *Science curriculum improvement study: Teachers handbook.* Berkeley, CA: Lawrence Hall of Science.

Kaufman, A.S. (1979). *Intelligent testing with the WISC-R.* New York: John Wiley & Sons.

Kaufman, A.S., & Kaufman, N.L. (1983). *The Kaufman Assessment Battery for Children.* Chicago: American Guidance Association.

Kaufman, J.M. (Ed.). (1981). Attention disorders: Implications for the classroom. *Exceptional Education Quarterly, 2.*

Kausler, D.H. (1974). *Psychology of verbal learning and memory.* New York: Academic Press.

Kavale, K.A. (1984). Potential advantages of the meta-analysis technique for research in special education. *Journal of Special Education, 18* (1), 61–72.

Kavale, K.A., & Forness, S.R. (1984). A meta-analysis of the validity of Wechsler Scale profiles and recategorizations: Patterns or parodies? *Learning Disability Quarterly, 7* (2), 136–156.

Kelley, T.L. (1928). *Crossroads in the mind of man: A study of differentiable mental abilities.* Stanford University Press.

Kendall, C.R., Borkowski, J.G., & Cavanaugh, J.C. (1980). Metamemory and the transfer of an interrogative strategy by E.M.R. children. *Intelligence, 4,* 255–270.

Kendler, H.H., & D'Amato, M.F. (1955). A comparison of reversal shifts and non-reverse shifts in human concept formation behavior. *Journal of Exceptional Child Psychology, 13,* 195–209.

Kendler, H.H., & Kendler, T.S. (1975). From discrimination learning to cognitive development: A neobehaviorist odyssey. In W.K. Estes (Ed.), *Handbook of learning and cognitive processes.* Hillsdale, NJ: Erlbaum.

Kendler, H.H., & Spence, J.T. (1971). Tenets of neobehaviorism. In H.H. Kendler & J.T. Spence (Eds.), *Essays in neobehaviorism: A memorial value to Kenneth W. Spence* (pp. 11–40). New York: Appleton-Century-Crofts.

Kendler, H.H., & Vineberg, R. (1954). The acquisition of compound concepts as a function of previous training. *Journal of Experimental Psychology, 48,* 242–258.

Kendler, T.S. (1970). An ontogeny of mediation deficiency. *Child Development, 41,* 1–27.

Kendler, T.S., & Kendler, H.H. (1949). Reversal and nonreversal shifts in kindergarten children. *Journal of Experimental Psychology, 58,* 56–60.

Kennedy, B.A., & Miller, D.J. (1976). Persistent use of verbal rehearsal as a function of information about its value. *Child Development, 47,* 566–569.

Keogh, B., & Glover, A.T. (1980). The generalizability and durability of cognitive training effects. *Exceptional Education Quarterly, 1,* 75–82.

Kephart, N.C. (1971). *The slow learner in the classroom* (2nd ed.). Columbus, OH: Charles E. Merrill.

Kimura, D. (1961). Cerebral dominance and the perception of verbal stimuli. *Canadian Journal of Psychology, 15,* 166–171.

Kimura, D. (1963). Speech lateralization in young children as determined by an auditory test. *Journal of Comparative and Physiological Psychology, 56,* 799–890.

Kimura, D. (1967). Functional asymmetry of the brain in dichotic listening. *Cortex, 3,* 163–178.

Kinsbourne, M. (1980). Lateral input may shift activation balance in the integrated brain. *American Psychologist, 38,* 228–229.

Kinsbourne, M. (1983). Do learning disabled children lack functional hemispheric lateralization? *Topics in Learning and Learning Disabilities, 3,* 14–28.

Kintsch, W. (1977). *Memory and cognition* (2nd ed.). New York: John Wiley & Sons.

Kirby, J.A., & Briggs, J.B. (1980). *Cognition, development and instruction.* New York: Grune & Stratton.

Kirk, S.A. (1940). *Teaching reading to slow learning children.* Boston: Houghton Mifflin.

Kirk, S.A. (1968). *The diagnosis and remediation of psycholinguistic learning disabilities.* Urbana: University of Illinois Press.

Kirk, S.A., & Kirk, W.D. (1971). *Psycholinguistic learning disabilities. Diagnosis and remediation.* Urbana: University of Illinois Press.

Kirk, S.A., McCarthy, J.J., & Kirk, W.D. (1971). *Illinois Test of Psycholinguistic Abilities* (rev. ed.). Urbana: University of Illinois Press.

Klahr, D. (Ed.). (1976). *Cognition and instruction.* Hillsdale, NJ: Erlbaum.

Klausmeier, H. (1976). Instructional design and the teaching concepts. In J.R. Levin & V.L. Allen (Eds.), *Cognitive learning in children.* New York: Academic Press.

Klausmeier, H. (1979). *Cognitive learning and development: Information processing and Piagetian perspectives.* Cambridge, MA: Ballinger.

Klausmeier, H., & Allen, P.S. (1978). *Cognitive development of children and youth: A longitudinal study.* New York: Academic Press.

Knashen, S.D. (1977). *The left hemisphere of the human brain.* Englewood, NJ: Prentice-Hall.

Kneedler, R.D. (1980). The use of cognitive training to change social behavior. *Exceptional Education Quarterly, 1,* 65–73.

Knickerbocker, B. (1980). *A holistic approach to the treatment of learning disorders.* Thorofare, NJ: Slack.

Kogan, N. (1973). Creativity and cognitive style. In P.B. Baltes and K.W. Schaie (Eds.), *Life-span development psychology: Personality and socialization.* New York: Academic Press.

Kogan, N. (1976). *Cognitive styles in infancy and early childhood.* Hillsdale, NJ: Erlbaum.

Kogan, N. (1980a). A cognitive style approach to metaphoric thinking. In R.E. Snow, P.A. Federico, & W.E. Montague (Eds.), *Aptitude, learning and instruction: Cognitive process analyses.* Hillsdale, NJ: Erlbaum.

Kogan, N. (1980b). Cognitive styles and reading performance. *Bulletin of the Orton Society, 39,* 63–77.

Kogan, N., Connor, K., Gross, A., & Fava, D. (1980). *Understanding visual metaphor.*

Krupski, A. (1980). Attention processes: Research theory, and implications for special education. In B.K. Keogh (Ed.), *Advances in special education* (Vol. 1). Greenwich, CT: JAI Press.

Kuhn, D. (1978). The application of Piaget's theory of cognitive development to education. *Harvard Educational Review, 3* (49), 340–360.

Lachman, R., Lachman, J.L., & Butterfield, E.C. (1979). *Cognitive psychology and information processing.* Hillsdale, NJ: Erlbaum.

Landa, L.M. (1976). *Instructional regulation and control.* Englewood Cliffs: Educational Technology.

Lavatelli, C. (1970). *Piaget's theory applied to an early childhood curriculum.* Boston: American Science and Engineering.

Lawson, A., & Wollman, W. (1975). Encouraging the transition from concrete to a formal cognitive functioning—an experiment. *Advancing education through science-oriented programs* (Report ID-15). Berkeley: Lawrence Hall of Science, University of California.

Ledwidge, B. (1978). Cognitive behavior modification: A step in the wrong direction. *Psychological Bulletin, 85* (2), 353–375.

Lenneberg, E.H. (1967). *Biological foundation of language*. New York: John Wiley & Sons.

Lenneberg, E.H. (1974). Language and brain: Developmental aspects, neuroscience research. *Pragna Bulletin, 12*, 513–656.

Lerner, J. (1981). *Learning disabilities* (3rd ed.). Boston: Houghton Mifflin.

Lesgold, A.M., Pelligreno, J.W., Fokkema, S.D., & Glaser, R. (1978). *Cognitive psychology and instruction*. New York: Plenum Press.

Levin, J.R., & Allen, V.L. (1976). *Cognitive learning in children theories and strategies*. New York: Academic Press.

Lewontin, R.C., Steven, R.P., & Kamin, L.J. (1984). *Not in our genes: Biology, ideology, and human nature*. New York: Pantheon Books.

Lindsly, P.H., & Norman, D.A. (1972). *Human information processing*. New York: Academic Press.

Lloyd, J. (1980). Academic instruction and cognitive behavior modification: The need for attack strategy training. *Exceptional Education Quarterly, 1*, 53–67.

Loftus, E.F. (1973). Leading questions and the eye-witness report. *Cognitive Psychology, 97*, 70–74.

Loftus, E.F., & Loftus, G.R. (1980). On the permanence of stored information in the human brain. *American Psychologist, 35*, 409–420.

Loftus, G.R., & Loftus, E.F. (1976). *Human memory: The processing of information*. Hillsdale, NJ: Erlbaum.

Loper, A. (1980). Metacognitive development. *Exceptional Education Quarterly, 1*, 1–15.

Loper, A. (1982). Metacognitive training to correct academic deficiency. *Topics in Learning and Learning Disabilities, 2*, 61–68.

Lovitt, T. (1972). Applied behavior analysis and learning disabilities. Part II. Specific research recommendation and suggestions for practitioners. *Journal of Learning Disabilities, 8*, 504–518.

Luria, A.R. (1961). *The role of speech in the regulation of normal and abnormal behavior*. Oxford: Pergamon Press.

Luria, A.R. (1966). *Higher cortical functions in man*. New York: Basic Books.

Luria, A.R. (J.V. Vertsch, Ed.). (1982). *Language and cognition*. Washington, DC: Winston & Sons.

Maccoby, E., & Zellner, M. (1970). *Experiments in primary education*. New York: Harcourt Brace Jovanovich.

McGuignon, F.J. (1978). *Cognitive psychophysiology: Principles of covert behavior*. Englewood Cliffs, NJ: Prentice-Hall.

McMullen, R.E., & Giles, T.R. (1981). *Cognitive-behavior therapy*. New York: Grune & Stratton.

McNemar, Q. (1964). Lost: Our intelligence. Why? *American Psychologist, 18*, 871–882.

Mahlios, M.C. (1978). *Implications of cognitive style for teachers and learners*. Tempe: Arizona State University. (ERIC Document Reproduction Services No. 152 704)

Mahoney, M.J. (1974). *Cognition and behavior modification*. Cambridge, MA: Bollinger.

Mandler, G. (1955). *Mind and emotion*. New York: John Wiley & Sons.

Mandler, G., & Boeck, W.J. (1974). Retrieval processes in recognition. *Memory and Cognition, 2*, 613–615.

Mann, L. (1979). *On the trail of process*. New York: Grune & Stratton.

Mann, P.H., & Suiter, R. (1974). *A handbook in diagnostic teaching: A learning disabilities approach*. Boston: Allyn & Bacon.

Markman, E.M. (1979). Realizing that you don't understand: Elementary school children's awareness of inconsistencies. *Child Development, 50*, 643–655.

Markus, H. (1977). Self-schemata and processing information about the self. *Journal of Personality and Social Psychology, 35*, 63–78.

Markus, H. (1980). The self-thought and memory. In D.M. Wegner & R.R. Vallocher (Eds.), *The self in social psychology*. Oxford: Oxford University Press.

Masserman, J.H. (1940). Is the hypothalamus a center of emotion? *Psychomatic Medicine, 3*, 3–25.

Masserman, J.H. (1943). *Behavior and neurosis*. Chicago: University of Chicago Press.

Masson, M.E.J. (1982). A framework of cognitive and metacognitive determinant of reading skill. *Topics in Learning and Learning Disabilities, 2,* 37–43.

Matarazzo, J.D. (1972). *Wechsler's measurement and appraisal of adult intelligence* (5th ed.). Baltimore: Williams & Wilkins.

Mayer, R.E. (1981). *The promise of cognitive psychology.* San Francisco: W.H. Freeman & Co.

Meeker, M.N. (1965). A procedure for relating Stanford-Binet behavior sampling to Guilford's structure of the intellect. *Journal of School Psychology, 3,* 26–36.

Meeker, M.N. (1975). A paradigm for special education diagnostics: The cognitive areas. In K.F. Kramer & R. Rosonke (Eds.), *State of the art: Diagnosis and treatment* (pp. 35–77). Lexington, KY: Coordinating Office of Regional Resource Centers.

Meeker, M.N., & Meeker, R.S. (1973). Strategies for assessing intellectual patterns of black, anglo, and Mexican-American boys—or other children—and implications for education. *Journal of School Psychology, 11,* 341–360.

Meichenbaum, D. (1977). *Cognitive-behavior modification.* New York: Plenum Press.

Meichenbaum, D. (1979). Teaching children self-control. In B.B. Lakey & A.E. Kazden (Eds.), *Advances in clinical child psychology* (Vol. 2). New York: Plenum.

Meichenbaum, D. (1980). Cognitive behavior modification with exceptional children: A promise yet unfulfilled. *Exceptional Educational Quarterly, 1,* 83–88.

Meichenbaum, D., & Goodman, T. (1977). Training impulsive children to talk to themselves. *Journal of Abnormal Psychology, 77,* 115–126.

Mercer, J.R. (1973). *Labeling the mentally retarded.* Berkeley: University of California Press.

Mercer, J.R. (1978–79). Test "validity," "bias," and "fairness": An analysis from the perspective of the sociology of knowledge. *Interchange, 9,* 1–16.

Mercer, J.R., & Lewis, J.F. (1979). *System of multicultural pluralistic assessment.* New York: Psychological Corp.

Merluzzi, T.V., Rudy, T.E., & Glass, C.R. (1981). The information processing paradigm: Implications for clinical science. In T.V. Merluzzi, C.R. Glass, & G. Myles, (Eds.). *Cognitive Assessment.* New York: Guilford Press.

Merrill, P.F. (1976). Task analysis—An information processing approach. *NSPI, J., 15,* 7–11.

Messick, S.B. (1976). Reflection-impulsivity: A review. *Psychological Bulletin, 83,* 1026–1052.

Metfessel, N.S., Michael, W.B., & Kirsner, D.A. (1969). Instrumentation of Bloom's and Krathwol's taxonomies for the writing of behavioral objectives. *Psychology in the School, 16,* 227–231.

Meyer, D.E. (1970). On the representation and retrieval of stored semantic information. *Cognitive Psychology, 1,* 242–300.

Miles, F.N., & Evarts, E.V. (1979). Concepts of motor organization. *Annual Review of Psychology, 30,* 327–362.

Miller, G.A. (1956). The magic number seven, plus or minus two: Some limits on our capacity or processing information. *Psychological Review, 63,* 81–97.

Miller, G.A., Galanter, E., & Pribam, K.H. (1960). *Plans and the structure of behavior.* New York: Holt, Rinehart & Winston.

Miller, T.L. (Ed.). (1981). The training of intelligence: Implications for special educators. *Journal of Special Education, 15* (2).

Minskoff, E.H., Wiseman, D.E., & Minskoff, J.A. (1972). *The MWM program for developing language abilities.* Ridgefield, NJ: Educational Performance Associates.

Moates, D.R., & Schumacher, G.M. (1979). *An introduction to cognitive psychology.* Belmont, CA: Wadsworth Publishing Co.

Modgil, S., & Modgil, C. (1976). *Piagetian research compilation and commentary.* Windsor: NFER Publishing Co.

Modgil, S., & Modgil, C. (Eds.). (1982). *Jean Piaget: Consensus and controversy.* New York: Praeger Publishing.

Moray, N. (1978). The strategic control of information processing. In G. Underwood (Ed.), *Strategies of information processing* (pp. 301–328). London: Academic Press.

Moses, N. (1981). Using Piagetian principles to guide instruction of the learning disabled. *Topics in Learning and Learning Disabilities, 1,* 11–20.

Murray, F. (1978). *The impact of Piagetian theory.* Baltimore: University Park Press.

Myklebust, H.R. (1973). *Developmental and disorders of written language* (Vol. 2). New York: Grune & Stratton.

Nebes, R.D. (1977). Man's so-called minor hemisphere. In M.C. Wittrock (Ed.), *The human brain.* Englewood, NJ: Prentice-Hall.

Neisser, U. (1967). *Cognitive psychology*. New York: Appleton-Century-Crofts.

Neisser, U. (1976a). *Cognition and reality*. San Francisco: W.H. Freeman & Co.

Neisser, U. (1976b). General and artificial intelligence. In Lauren B. Resnick (Ed.), *The nature of intelligence* (pp. 135–144). Hillsdale, NJ: Erlbaum.

Newcomer, P.L., & Hammill, D.D. (1976). *Psycholinguistics in the schools*. Columbus, OH: Charles E. Merrill.

Newell, A. (1979). One final word. In D.T. Tuma & F. Reid (Eds.), *Problem solving and education: Issues in teaching and research*. Hillsdale, NJ: Erlbaum.

Newell, A., & Simon, H.A. (1972). *Human problem solving*. Englewood Cliffs, NJ: Prentice-Hall.

Norman, D.A. (1980). Twelve issues for cognitive science. *Cognitive Science, 4*, 1–31.

Oakland, T., Deluna, C., & Morgan, C. (1977). Annotated bibliography of language dominance measures. In T. Oakland (Ed.), *Psychological and educational assessment of minority children*. New York: Brunner-Mazel.

Obrzut, J., Hynd, G.W., & Obrzut, A. (1980). Development of cerebral dominance in learning disabled children. In W. Cruickshank (Ed.), *Approaches to learning* (Vol. 1). Syracuse, NY: Syracuse University Press.

Olds, J., & Olds, M.E. (1965). Promises, rewards and the brain. In T.M. Newcomb (Ed.), *New directions in psychology* (Vol. 2, pp. 327–410). New York: Holt.

Orton, S.T. (1928). Specific reading disability-strephosymbolia. *Journal of the American Medical Association, 90*, 1095–1099.

Orton, S.T. (1973). *Reading, writing, and speech problems in children*. New York: Brunner-Mazel.

Osgood, C.E. (1957). A behavioristic analysis of perception and language as cognitive phenomena. *Contemporary approaches to cognition: A symposium held at the University of Colorado*. Cambridge: Harvard University Press.

Otto, W., & Smith, R.J. (1980). *Corrective and remedial teaching* (3rd ed.). Boston: Houghton Mifflin.

Oxford universal dictionary (3rd ed.).

Paivio, A. (1975). Imagery and verbal processes. In A. Kennedy & A. Wiekes (Eds.), *Studies in long term memory*. London: Wiley.

Paivio, A. (1979). *Imagery and verbal processes*. New York: Holt, Rinehart & Winston.

Paraskenopoulas, J.N., & Kirk, S.A. (1965). *The development and psychometric characteristics of the revised Illinois Test of Psycholinguistic Abilities*. Urbana: University of Illinois Press.

Parrill-Burnstein, M. (1981). *Problem solving and learning disabilities*. New York: Grune & Stratton.

Parsons, J.E. (1981). Expectancies, values, and academic choice. In J.T. Spence (Ed.), *Assessing achievement*. San Francisco: W.H. Freeman & Co.

Pavlov, I.P. (1927). *Conditioned reflexes*. Oxford: Oxford University Press.

Pegley, R., & Adler, C. (1977). Compensating educations in Israel: Conceptions, attitudes and trends. *American Psychologist, 32*, 945–958.

Peterson, J. (1922). Intelligence and learning. *Psychological Review, 29*, 366–389.

Peterson, J. (1925). *Early conceptions and tests of intelligence*. Yonkers, NY: World Book.

Pew, R. (1974). The experimental psychological series. *Journal of Verbal Learning and Learning Behavior, 7*.

Phillips, D. (1982). Perspectives on Piaget as philosopher: The tough, tender-minded syndrome. In S. Modgil & C. Modgil (Eds.), *Jean Piaget: Consensus and controversy* (pp. 13–30). New York: Praeger Publishing.

Phillips, J.L. (1981). *Piaget's theory: A primer*. San Francisco: W.H. Freeman & Co.

Piaget, J. (1950). *The psychology of intelligence* (T. Percy & D.E. Berlyne, Trans.). London: Routledge and Kegan Paul Ltd.

Piaget, J. (1952). *Genetic epistemology*. New York: Columbia University Press.

Piaget, J. (1972). *The principles of genetic epistemology* (W. Mays, Trans.). London: Routledge and Kegan Paul Ltd.

Piaget, J. (1973). "Preface," in A. Binet, *Les Ideés modernes sur les enfants*. Paris: Flammarion.

Pieron, H. (1926). The problem of intelligence. *Pedigogic Seminar, 33*, 50–60.

Pintner, R. (1923). *Intelligence testing: Methods and results*. New York: Holt.

Polya, G. (1957). *How to solve it*. Garden City, NY: Doubleday.

Polya, G. (1968). *Mathematical discovery*. New York: John Wiley & Sons.

Popper, K.R., & Eccles, J.C. (1977). *The self and the brain*. New York: Springer-Verlag.

Posner, J.S., Boies, W., Eichelman, W., & Taylor, R. (1969). Retention of visual and name codes of single letters. *Journal of Experimental Psychology Monographs, 79* (1, Pt. 21).

Premack, D. (1982). Animal cognition. In M.R. Rosenzweig & L.W. Porter (Eds.), *Annual review of psychology*, 351–362.

Pressley, M. (1977). Imagery and children's learning: Putting the picture in developmental perspective. *Review of Educational Research, 47*, 585–622.

Pribam, K.H. (1977). Human consciousness and the functions of the brain. *Somatics, 7*, 5–7.

Pribam, K.H. (1978). Consciousness: A scientific approach. *Indian Psychology, 21*, 95–118.

Price, G., Dunn, R., & Dunn, K. (1977, April). *Summary of research on learning style based on the learning style inventory.* Paper presented at the annual meeting of the American Educational Research Association, New York. (ERIC Document Reproduction Service No. 137, 329)

Quillian, M.R. (1968). Semantic memory. In M. Minsky (Ed.), *Semantic information processing.* Cambridge: MIT Press.

Rabinowitz, J.C., Mandler, G., & Patterson, K.E. (1977). Determinants of recognition and recall: Accessibility and generation. *Journal of Experimental Psychology: General, 106*, 302–329.

Random House dictionary (1966 ed.). New York: Random House.

Raven, J.C. (1938). *Progressive matrices: A perceptual test of intelligence.* London: Lewis.

Readence, J.F., & Bean, T.W. (1978). Modification of impulsive cognitive styles: A survey of the literature. *Psychological Reports, 43*, 327–337.

Reed, H.B. (1979). Biological defects and special education: An issue in personnel preparation. *Journal of Special Education, 13* (1), 9–33.

Reese, H.W. (1962). Verbal mediation as a function of an age level. *Psychological Bulletin, 59*, 502–509.

Reese, H.W. (1968). *The perception of stimulus relations. Discrimination learning and transportation.* New York: Academic Press.

Reese, H.W. (1970). Acquired distinctiveness and equivalence of cues in young children. *Journal of Experimental Child Psychology, 10*, 263–278.

Reese, H.W. (1976). *Basic learning processes in childhood.* New York: Holt, Rinehart & Winston.

Reese, H.W., Parnes, S.J., Treffinger, D.J., & Kaltsounis, G. (1937). Effects of a creative studies program on structure of intellect factors. *Journal of Educational Psychology, 39*, 287–292.

Reese, H.W., Parnes, S.J., Treffinger, D.J., & Kaltsounis, G. (1976). Effects of a creative studies program on structure of intellect factors. *Journal of Educational Psychology, 68*, 401–410.

Reid, D.K. (1978). Genevan theory and the education of exceptional children. In J.M. Gallagher & J.A. Easley (Eds.), *Knowledge and development: Piaget and education* (Vol. 2). New York: Plenum.

Reid, D.K. (1979). Toward an application of developmental epistemology to special education. *Proceedings of the Eighth Interdisciplinary International Conference on Piagetian Theory and the Helping Professions.* Baltimore: University Park Press.

Reid, D.K., & Hresko, W.P. (1981). *A cognitive approach to learning disabilities.* New York: McGraw-Hill.

Reigeluth, C.M. (1979). In search of a better way to organize instruction. The elaboration theory of instructional development, *2*, 8–15.

Reigeluth, C.M., & Rodgers, C.A. (1978). The elaboration theory of instruction: Prescriptions for task analysis and design. *NSPIJ, 19*, 16–26.

Reinert, H. (1976). One picture is worth a thousand words? Not necessarily! *Modern Language Journal, 60* (4), 162–168.

Renzulli, J.S. (1973). *New directions in creativity.* New York: Harper & Row.

Resnick, L.B. (1976). Task analysis in instructional design. Some cases from mathematics. In D. Klasko (Ed.), *Cognition and instruction.* Hillsdale, NJ: Erlbaum.

Resnick, L.B. (1981). Instructional psychology. In M.R. Rosenzweig & L.W. Porter (Eds.), *Annual Review of Psychology, 32*, 659–704.

Reschly, D.J. (1981). Psychological testing in educational classification and placement. *American Psychologist, 36*, 1094–1102.

Reynolds, C., & Miller, T. (Eds.). (1984). The K-ABC. *Journal of Special Education.*

Rice, B. (1979, September). Brave new world of intelligence testing. *Psychology Today*, pp. 27–41.

Rimland, B. (1964). *Infantile autism.* New York: Appleton-Century-Crofts.

Rimm, D.C., & Masters, J.C. (1974). *Behavior therapy techniques and empirical findings.* New York: Academic Press.

Roach, C., & Kephart, W. (1966). *The Purdue Perceptual-Motor Survey*. Columbus, OH: Charles E. Merrill.

Robinson, N.M., & Robinson, H.B. (1976). *The mentally retarded child*. New York: McGraw-Hill.

Ross, D.M., & Ross, S.A. (1978). *Pacemaker curriculum*. Belmont, CA: Fearon.

Royes, S. (1977). Characteristics of the cognitive development of profoundly retarded children. *Child Development*, *48*, 837–843.

Rosenzweig, M.R. (1981). Neural bases of intelligence and training. *Journal of Special Education, 15*, 105–123.

Rumelhart, D.E. (1975). Notes on a schema for stories. In D.G. Bobram & A.M. Collins (Eds.), *Representation and understanding studies in cognitive science*. New York: Academic Press.

Runion, H.I., & McNett-McGowan. (1981). An illustrated review of normal brain anatomy and physiology. In W.M. Cruickshank & A.A. Silver (Eds.), *Bridges to tomorrow* (Vol. 2). Syracuse, NY: Syracuse University Press.

Ryan, E.B., Ledger, G.W., Short, E.J., & Weed, K.A. (1982). Promoting the use of active comprehension strategies by poor readers. *Topics in Learning and Learning Disabilities, 2*, 53–60.

Sabatino, D.A. (1973). Auditory perception: Development, assessment, and intervention. In L. Mann & D.A. Sabatino (Eds.), *First Review of Special Education*. Philadelphia: JSE Press.

Sabatino, D.A. (1974). The construction and assessment of an experimental test of auditory perception. *Journal of Learning Disabilities, 6*, 115–121.

Sabatino, D.A., & Dorfman, N. (1974). Matching learner aptitudes to the commercial reading programs. *Exceptional Children, 41*, 85–90.

Sabatino, D.A., & Miller, P.F. (1978). *Describing learner characteristics of handicapped children and youth*. New York: Grune & Stratton.

Sabatino, D.A., Miller, P.F., & Schmidt, C. (1981). Can intelligence be modified through cognitive training? *Journal of Special Education, 2*, 125–144.

Sagotsky, G., Patterson, C., & Lepper, M. (1978). Training children in self control: A field experiment in self monitoring and goal setting in the classroom. *Journal of Experimental Child Psychology, 25*, 242–253.

Salvia, J., & Ysseldyke, J.E. (1981). *Assessment in special and remedial education*. Boston: Houghton Mifflin.

Samuels, S.J. (1979). The method of repeated readings. *Reading Teacher, 32*, 403–408.

Santostefano, S., & Paley, E. (1964). Development of cognitive controls in children. *Child Development, 35*, 939–949.

Santostefano, S., Rutledge, L., & Randall, D. (1965). Cognitive styles and reading disability. *Psychology in the Schools, 2*, 57–62.

Sattler, J.M. (1982). *Assessment of children's intelligence and special abilities* (2nd ed.). Boston: Allyn & Bacon.

Satz, P. (1976). Cerebral dominance and reading disability: An old problem revisited. In R.M. Knight, D.J. Bakker, & P. Satz (Eds.), *Specific reading disability: Advances in theory and method*. Baltimore: University Park Press.

Scandura, J.M. (1977). A structural approach to instructional problems. *American Psychologist, 32*, 33–53.

Scandura, J.M. (1980). Theoretical foundations of instruction. A systems alternative to cognitive psychology. *Journal of Structure Learning, 6*, 347–393.

Scarr, S. (1981). Testing for children: Assessment and the many determinants of intellectual competence. *American Psychologist, 36*, 1159–1166.

Schmidt, R.A. (1982). *Motor control and learning: A behavioral emphasis*. Champaign, IL: Human Kinetics.

Schultz, D.P. (1969). *A history of modern psychology*. New York and London: Academic Press.

Science Research Associates. (1962). *Primary mental abilities test*. Chicago: Science Research Associates.

Scott, W.A., & Osgood, D.W. (1979). *Cognitive structure: Theory and measurement of individual differences*. Washington, DC: V.H. Winston & Sons.

Shannon, C.E., & Weaver, W. (1949). *The mathematical theory of communication*. Urbana: University of Illinois Press.

Sherrington, C.S. (1906). *The integrative action of the nervous system*. New Haven: Yale University Press.

Shiffrin, R.N., & Atkinson, R.C. (1969). Storage and retrieval processes in long term memory. *Psychological Review, 76*, 179–193.

Siegel, L., & Hodkin, B. (1982a). Interchange. Siegel and Hodkin reply to Voneche and Bovet. In S. Modgil & C. Modgil (Eds.), *Jean Piaget: Consensus and controversy* (p. 95). New York: Praeger Publishing.

Siegel, L., & Hodkin, B. (1982b). The garden path to the understanding of cognitive development: Has Piaget led us into the poison ivy? In S. Modgil & C. Modgil (Eds.), *Jean Piaget: Consensus and controversy* (pp. 57–82). New York: Praeger Publishing.

Silver, A.A., & Hagin, R.A. (1976). *Search*. New York: Walker.

Simon, H.A. (1976). Identifying basic abilities underlying intelligent performance of complex tasks. In L. Resnick (Ed.), *The nature of intelligence*. Hillsdale, NJ: Erlbaum.

Simon, H.A. (1978). Information processing theory of human problem solving. In W.K. Estes (Ed.), *Handbook of learning and cognitive processes* (Vol 5). *Human information processing*. Hillsdale, NJ: Erlbaum.

Sinclair, H. (1976). Quoted in T.C. O'Brien (Ed.), *Implications of Piagetian research in education*. Interview with Elizabeth M. Hitchfield. St. Louis, MO: *Teachers Center*.

Sinclair, H. (1982). Interchange. Sinclair replies to Elliot and Donaldson. In S. Modgil & C. Modgil (Eds.), *Jean Piaget: Consensus and controversy* (p. 178). New York: Praeger Publishing.

Singer, D.G., & Revenson, T.A. (1978). *A Piaget primer: How a child thinks*. New York: New American Library.

Skinner, B.F. (1957). *Verbal behavior*. New York: Appleton-Century-Crofts.

Skinner, B.F. (1977). *About behaviorism*. New York: Knopf.

Skinner, B.F. (1978a). *Reflections on behaviorism and society*. Englewood Cliffs, NJ: Prentice-Hall.

Skinner, B.F. (1978b). Why I am not a cognitive psychologist. *Behaviorism, 5* (2), 1–10.

Smith, D.C. (Ed.). (1981). Attention disorder: Implications for the classroom. *Exceptional Educational Quarterly, 2, 3*.

Smith, E.E., Shoben, E.J., & Rips, L.J. (1974). Structure and process in semantic memory: A featural model for semantic decisions. *Psychological Review, 81,* 214–241.

Smith, G.J.E., & Klein, G.S. (1953). Cognitive controls in serial behavior patterns. *Journal of Personality, 22,* 188–213.

Snyder, J.J., & White, M.J. (1979). The use of cognitive self instruction in the treatment of behaviorally disturbed adolescents. *Behavior Therapy, 19,* 227–235.

Spear, W.E., & Miller, R.R. (1981). *Information processing in animals: Memory mechanisms*. Hillsdale, NJ: Erlbaum.

Spearman, C. (1904). "General intelligence," objectively determined and measured. *American Journal of Psychology, 15,* 201–293.

Spearman, C. (1914). The theory of two factors. *Psychological Review, 21,* 101–115.

Spearman, C. (1927). *The abilities of man: Their nature and measurement*. New York: Macmillan.

Spence, K.W. (1950). Cognitive vs. stimulus-response theories of learning. *Psychological Review, 57,* 159–172.

Sperry, R.W. (1974). Later specialization in the surgically separated hemispheres. In F.Q. Schmidt & F. Worden (Eds.), *The neurosciences: Third study program* (pp. 71–74). Cambridge: MIT Press.

Sperry, R.W., Gazzaniga, M.S., & Bogen, J.E. (1969). Interhemispheric disconnection. *Handbook of Clinical Neurology,* 273–290.

Stankov, L., Horn, J.L., & Ray, T. (1980). On the relationship between GF/Cc theory and Jensen's level I/II theory. *Journal of Educational Psychology, 72,* 796–809.

States, A.W., & Burns, G.L. (1981). Intelligence and child development: What intelligence is and how it is learned and functions. *Genetic Psychology Monographs, 104,* 237–301.

Stauffer, R. (1969). *Directing reading maturity as a cognitive process*. New York: Harper & Row.

Stern, W. (1974). The psychological method of testing intelligence. *Educational Psychology Monographs* (No. 13).

Sternberg, R.J. (1977). *Intelligence, information processing, and analogical reasoning: The componential analysis of human reasoning*. Hillsdale, NJ: Erlbaum.

Sternberg, R.J. (1979). The nature of mental abilities. *American Psychologist, 34,* 214–230.

Sternberg, R.J. (1981a). Cognitive behavioral approaches to the training of intelligence in the retarded. *Journal of Special Education, 15,* 165–184.

Sternberg, R.J. (1981b). Nothing fails like success: The search for an intelligent paradigm for studying intelligence. *Journal of Educational Psychology, 73,* 142–155.

Sternberg, R.J., & Wagner, R.K. (1981). Automatization failure in learning disabilities. *Topics in Learning and Learning Disabilities, 1,* 1–22.

Sternberg, R.J., & Wagner, R.K. (1984). Alternative conceptions of intelligence and their implications for education. *Review of Educational Research, 54* (1), 179–223.

Sternberg, S. (1969). Memory-scanning: Mental processes revealed by reaction time experiments. *American Scientist, 57,* 421–445.

Stevens, C.F. (1979). The neuron. *Scientific American, 241,* 66–87.

Stoddard, G.D. (1941). On the meaning of intelligence. *Psychological Review, 48,* 250–260.

Strong, S.R., & Claiborn, C.D. (1982). *Change through intervention: Social psychological processes of counseling and psychotherapy.* New York: John Wiley & Sons.

Stroop, J.R. (1935). Studies of intelligence in serial verbal reactions. *Journal of Experimental Psychology, 18,* 643–662.

Tenopyr, M. (1981). The realities of employment testing. *American Psychologist, 36,* 1120–1127.

Terman, L.M. (1916). *The measurement of intelligence.* Boston: Houghton Mifflin.

Terman, L.M. (1917). *The Stanford revision and extension of the Binet-Simon Scale for measuring intelligence.* Baltimore: Warwick & York.

Teuber, H.L. (1914). Why two brains? In Francis O. Schmitt & F.G. Worden (Eds.), *The neurosciences third study program* (pp. 71–74). Cambridge: MIT Press.

Teyler, T. (1977). An introduction to the neurosciences. In M.C. Wittrock (Ed.), *The human brain.* Englewood Cliffs, NJ: Prentice-Hall.

Thomson, G.H. (1948). The factorial analyses of human ability. Darby, PA: Arden Lib.

Thorndike, E.L. (1926). *The measurement of intelligence.* New York: Columbia Teachers College.

Thorndike, E.L. (1931). *Human learning.* New York: Appleton-Century Crofts.

Thorndike, E.L., Terman, L.M., Freeman, F.N., Calver, S.S., Pistner, R., Rummel, B., Pressey, S.L., Hermon, A.C., Peterson, J., Thurstone, L.L., Woodrow, H., Dearboon, W.F., & Haggerty, M.E. (1921). Intelligence and its measurement: A symposium. *Journal of Educational Psychology, 12,* 123–147, 195–216.

Thorndyke, P.W. (1977). Cognitive structures in comprehension and memory of narrative discourse. *Cognitive Psychology, 9,* 77–110.

Thornell, J.G. (1976). Research on cognitive styles: Implications for teaching and learning. *Educational Leadership, 33,* 503–504.

Thurstone, L.L. (1924). *The nature of intelligence.* New York: Harcourt Brace.

Thurstone, L.L. (1936a). The factorial isolation of primary abilities. *Psychometrika, 1,* 175–182.

Thurstone, L.L. (1936b). A new conception of intelligence. *Educational Record, 17,* 441–450.

Thurstone, L.L. (1938). *Primary mental abilities.* Chicago: University of Chicago Press.

Thurstone, L.L. (1940). Current issues in factor analysis. *Psychological Bulletin, 37,* 189–236.

Thurstone, L.L. (1944). A factional study of perception. *Psychometric Monographs* (No. 4). Chicago: University of Chicago Press.

Thurstone, L.L. (1948). Psychological implications of factor analysis. *American Psychologist, 3,* 402–408.

Thurstone, L.L., & Thurstone, G. (1941). Factorial studies of intelligence. *Psychometric Monographs* (No. 2).

Torgeson, J.K. (1979). What shall we do with psychological processes? *Journal of Learning Disabilities, 12,* 514–521.

Torgeson, J.K. (1981). The relationship between memory and attention in learning disabilities. *Exceptional Education Quarterly,* 58–59.

Torgeson, J.K. (1982). The learning disabled child as an inactive learner: Educational implications. *Topics in Learning and Learning Disabilities, 2,* 455–521.

Traver, S.G., & Ellsworth, P.S. (1981). Written and oral language for verbal children. In J.M. Kaufman & D.P. Hallahan, *Handbook of Special Education.* Englewood Cliffs, NJ: 1981.

Travers, R. (1977). *Essentials of learning.* New York: Macmillan.

Tryson, W.W., & Jacobs, R.S. (1980). *Effects of basic learning skill training on Peabody Picture Vocabulary Test scores of severely disruptive, low functioning children.* Paper presented at meeting of the Eastern Psychological Association, Hartford, CT.

Tulving, E. (1972). Episodic and semantic memory. In E. Tulving & C.W. Donaldson (Eds.), *Organization of memory.* New York: Academic Press.

Tulving, E., & Madigan, S.A. (1970). Memory and verbal learning. *Annual Review of Psychology, 21,* 437–484.

Turvey, M.T. (1974). Perspectives in vision: Conception on perception. In D.D. Duane & M.B. Rawson (Eds.), *Reading, perception and language* (pp. 131–194). Baltimore: York Press.

Ullmann, L.P., & Krasner, L. (1968). *Case studies in behavior modification*. Boston: Houghton Mifflin.

Underwood, G. (Ed.). (1978a). *Strategies of information processing*. London: Academic Press.

Underwood, G. (1978b). Concepts in information processing theory. In G. Underwood (Ed.), *Strategies of information processing* (pp. 1–22). London: Academic Press.

U.S. President's Committee on Mental Retardation. *Mental Retardation: Century of decision* (DHEW Publication No. COHD 76-21013) (1976).

Uzigris, I., & Hunt, J. McV. (1975). *Assessment in infancy ordinal scales of psychological development*. Urbana: University of Illinois Press.

Vallett, R.E. (1964). A clinical profile for the Stanford-Binet. *Journal of School Psychology,* 49–54.

Vallett, R.E. (1966a). *A psychoeducational profile of basic learning abilities*. Palo Alto, CA: Consulting Psychologists Press.

Vallett, R.E. (1966b). *Vallett developmental survey of basic learning disabilities*. Palo Alto, CA: Consulting Psychologists Press.

Vallett, R.E. (1967). *The remediation of learning disabilities*. Palo Alto, CA: Fearon.

Vallett, R.E. (1968). *A psychoeducational inventory of basic learning abilities*. Palo Alto, CA: Fearon.

Vellutino, F.R. (1974). How the perceptual hypotheses led us astray. *Journal of Learning Disabilities, 7,* 103–110.

Vernon, P.A. (1981). Level I & Level II: A review. *Educational Psychologist*.

Vernon, P.A. (1983). Recent findings on the nature of *g. Journal of Special Education, 17* (4).

Vernon, P.E. (1961). *The structure of human abilities* (rev. ed.). London: Methuen.

Vernon, P.E. (1969). *Intelligence and cultural environment*. London: Methuen.

Vigotsky, L.S. (1962). *Thought and language*. (E. Hanfman & G. Vakar, Eds. and Transl.) Cambridge: MIT Press. (Original work published in 1923).

Voneche & Bovet. (1982). Interchange. Voneche and Bovet reply to Siegel and Hodkin. In S. Modgil & C. Modgil (Eds.), *Jean Piaget: Consensus and controversy* (p. 96). New York: Praeger Publishing.

Wadsworth, B.J. (1978). *Piaget for the classroom teacher*. New York: Longman.

Wadsworth, B.J. (1979). *Piaget's theory of cognitive development*. New York: Longman.

Wallas, G. (1926). *The art of thought*. New York: Harcourt.

Watson, J.B. (1913). Psychology as behaviorists view it. *Psychological Review, 20,* 158–177.

Webster's third new international dictionary (1971 ed.) Springfield, MA: C.G. Merriam.

Watson, J.B. (1925). *Behaviorism*. New York: W.W. Norton.

Wechsler, D. (1944). *The measurement of adult intelligence (3rd ed.)*. Baltimore: Williams & Wilkins.

Wechsler, D. (1955). *Manual for the Wechsler adult intelligence scale*. New York: Psychological Corp.

Weckelgren, W.A. (1977). *Learning and memory*. Englewood Cliffs, NJ: Prentice-Hall.

Weikart, D. (1971). *The cognitively oriented curricula*. Urbana, IL: ERIC-NAEYC.

Weiner, B. (1979). A theory of motivation for some classroom experience. *Journal of Educational Psychology, 71,* 3–25.

Weiner, B.A., Russell, D., & Lerman, D. (1979). The cognition emotion process in achievement related contexts. *Journal of Personality and Social Psychology, 37,* 1211–1220.

Weisz, J.R., & Zigler, E. (1979). Cognitive development in retarded and non-retarded persons: Piagetian tests of the similar sequence hypothesis. *Psychological Bulletin, 86* (4), 831–851.

Wepman, J. (1958). *Auditory discrimination tests*. Chicago: Language Research Associates.

Wertheimer, M. (1959). *Productive thinking*. New York: Harper.

Wickelgren, W.A. (1977). *Learning and memory*. Englewood Cliffs, NJ: Prentice-Hall.

Winschel, J.F., & Lawrence, E.A. (1975). Short-term memory: Curricular implications for the mentally retarded. *Journal of Special Education, 9,* 395–408.

Wittrock, M.C. (Ed.). (1977). *The human brain*. Englewood Cliffs, NJ: Prentice-Hall.

Wolpe, J. (1978). Cognition and causation in human behavior and its therapy. *American Psychologist*.

Woodrow, H. (1921). Intelligence and its measurement: A symposium. *Journal of Educational Psychology, 12,* 207–210.

Wozniak, R.H. (1972). Verbal regulation of motor behavior—Soviet research and non Soviet replications. *Human Development, 15,* 13.

Wurtman, R.J., & Wurtman, J.J. (Eds.). (1979a). *Nutrition and the brain. Vol. 3. Disorders of eating and nutrients in treatment of brain disorder.* New York: Raven Press.

Wurtman, R.J., & Wurtman, J.J. (Eds). (1979b). *Nutrition and the brain. Vol. 4: Toxic effects of food constituents on the brain.* New York: Raven Press.

Young, R.M. (1978). Strategies and the structure of a cognitive skill. In G. Underwood (Ed.), *Strategies of information processing* (pp. 357–401). London: Academic Press.

Ysseldyke, J., & Algozzine, B. (1982). *Critical issues in special and remedial education.* Boston: Houghton Mifflin.

Zeaman, D., & House, B.J. (1963). An attention theory of retardate discrimination learning. In N.R. Ellis (Ed.), *Handbook of mental deficiency.* New York: McGraw-Hill.

Zenhausern, R. (1983). Lateralized presentation and hemispheric integration. *American Psychologist, 38,* 227–228.

Zigler, E., & Balla, D. (1971). Luria's verbal deficiency theory of mental retardation and performance on sameness, symmetry and opposition tasks: A critique. *American Journal of Mental Deficiency, 74,* 400.

Index